P9-CEZ-300

Patient-Centered Interviewing
An Evidence-Based Method

SECOND EDITION

Robert C. Smith, M.D., SC.M.

Professor of Medicine and Psychiatry
Michigan State University
College of Human Medicine
East Lansing, Michigan

LIPPINCOTT WILLIAMS & WILKINS
A **Wolters Kluwer** Company
Philadelphia • Baltimore • New York • London
Buenos Aires • Hong Kong • Sydney • Tokyo

Acquisitions Editor: Richard Winters
Developmental Editor: Joanne Bersin
Production Editor: Christiana Sahl
Manufacturing Manager: Colin Warnock
Cover Designer: Mark Lerner
Compositor: Maryland Composition
Printer: R.R. Donnelley/Crawfordsville

© 2002 by LIPPINCOTT WILLIAMS & WILKINS
530 Walnut Street
Philadelphia, PA 19106 USA
LWW.com

All rights reserved. This book is protected by copyright. No part of this book may be reproduced in any form or by any means, including photocopying, or utilized by any information storage and retrieval system without written permission from the copyright owner, except for brief quotations embodied in critical articles and reviews. Materials appearing in this book prepared by individuals as part of their official duties as U.S. government employees are not covered by the above-mentioned copyright.
Printed in the USA

Library of Congress Cataloging-in-Publication Data

Smith, Robert C. (Robert Charles), 1937-
    Patient centered interviewing / Robert C. Smith—2nd ed.
      p. ; cm.
    Rev. ed. of: The patient's story. 1st ed. c1996.
    Includes bibliographical references and index.
    ISBN13 978-0-7817-3279-6
    ISBN10 0-7817-3279-4
    1. Medical history taking. 2. Physician and patient. I. Smith, Robert C. (Robert Charles), 1937- Patient's story. II. Title.
    [DNLM: 1. Medical History Taking—methods. 2. Physician-Patient Relations. WB 290 S658p 2002]
    RC65 .S65 2002
    616.07'51—dc21
                                                                  2001033877

Care has been taken to confirm the accuracy of the information presented and to describe generally accepted practices. However, the author and publisher are not responsible for errors or omissions or for any consequences from application of the information in this book and make no warranty, expressed or implied, with respect to the currency, completeness, or accuracy of the contents of the publication. Application of this information in a particular situation remains the professional responsibility of the practitioner.

The author and publisher have exerted every effort to ensure that drug selection and dosage set forth in this text are in accordance with current recommendations and practice at the time of publication. However, in view of ongoing research, changes in government regulations, and the constant flow of information relating to drug therapy and drug reactions, the reader is urged to check the package insert for each drug for any change in indications and dosage and for added warnings and precautions. This is particularly important when the recommended agent is a new or infrequently employed drug.

Some drugs and medical devices presented in this publication have Food and Drug Administration (FDA) clearance for limited use in restricted research settings. It is the responsibility of the health care provider to ascertain the FDA status of each drug or device planned for use in their clinical practice.

10 9 8 7 6 5 4

*In memory of **George L. Engel**,*
my friend, teacher, and inspiration,
who always had enough time.

As in the first edition, this book is also dedicated to the following:

In memory of my first
and most enduring medical influence,
*my father, **Elmer M. Smith**.*

To my first teacher of humanity
and so many other important things,
*my mother, **Mary Louise Smith**.*

To my guide, friend, and the love of my life,
*my wife, **Susan Sleeper-Smith**.*

Contents

Appendices

Foreword

Introduction

"The Interview is the most powerful, encompassing and versatile instrument available to the physician."

George L. Engel (1)

For thousands of years and across virtually all cultures, the response of people who experience "dis-ease" has been to seek counsel and care from physicians and healers. In contemporary Western culture, the concept of care has been defined primarily in terms of pathophysiology with an attendant focus on outcomes of treatment (either symptoms resolve or they do not). Less attention has been paid to the experience of care as an unfolding communication process in which a panoply of emotions, expectations, and reactions come into play. Ask any group of physicians, "What is the most frequently performed medical procedure?" and you are likely to hear responses such as the physical exam, urinalysis, and blood testing. In fact, the most common procedure is the medical interview, which is performed 140,000 to 160,000 times by the average American physician during a practice lifetime (2).

Because it is so frequently employed and so often unacknowledged, the reader may ask what is actually known about the interview, its impact on both the process and the outcomes of care, and the extent to which it can be taught, learned, and put into practice. A growing body of evidence supports Dr. Engel's claim and demonstrates that the interview exerts powerful and measurable influences on both biomedical and psychosocial outcomes of care. The good news is that virtually all of the most important interviewing skills can be learned and then improved upon. Evidence from a variety of studies points to the fact that interviewing is *not* an innate, immutable skill but rather one that develops over time, takes practice, and requires proper nurturing. Qualities like empathy, active listening, and open-ended questioning may seem artificial and even unnatural given personal experiences with these phenomena in everyday conversations. Learning the skills of professional communication and therapeutic interviewing will require you, as the reader, to place what you already know into a different framework. If you have ever tried to learn to play a musical instrument, you know that some fundamentals need to be mastered in order to perform optimally. These include *content* (being able to produce the notes to a piece of music), *timing* (placing the notes into a metric or time structure), and *style* (how the notes and timing are made unique by a particular performer). The medical interview consists of the same basic skills; you must learn the following: what questions to ask, how these questions relate to one another in time, and how to develop an interviewing style that suits your particular level of comfort and expertise.

Patient-Centered Interviewing will guide you step-by-step through this process. Its author, Robert Smith, M.D., has devoted most of his professional career to teaching and scholarship about the medical interview, a field that has grown rapidly in the past two decades. For example, the Index Medicus now lists over 20,000 articles on the physician–patient relationship and communication. Few physician educators have been as comprehensive and as careful as Dr. Smith in establishing the validity of their methods of training. As a result, this volume contains information and instruction that is wise, practical, and scientifically valid.

Mastering complex interviewing skills that require emotional intelligence, maturity, personal involvement, and judgement is inherently risky—it can leave learners feeling exposed, vulnerable, and anxious. Therefore, understanding the background context in which *Patient-Centered Interviewing* was written and the fact that hundreds and thousands of physicians have come before you and have struggled to master the medical interview without the benefit of guidance, a validated framework, or support is important.

Medical education has made great strides over the past 20 years. Today we are using new techniques from fields far-removed from medicine, such as aviation and nuclear power. For example, as awareness of the generic importance of patient safety has grown, several scholars such as Leape (3) and Helmreich and Schaefer (4) have compared how other professions educate their practitioners on dealing with errors. The results are striking. In medical practice, mistakes, including those that arise from poor interviewing practice, have traditionally been treated as occasions for blame, shame, and guilt. Under these conditions, individuals who commit errors, wary of being blamed, are reticent about discussing what happened. This pattern is established through formal and informal education, faculty modeling, and peer pressure. In aviation, mistakes are a different story. Recognizing that everyone in the industry has something to gain by understanding what went wrong in the cockpit, crew members are encouraged early in training to view errors as occasions for learning. Coupled with an anonymous national reporting system and error analysis that is available industry-wide, this view of the positive potential for learning from errors has led to a significant improvement in safety. Learning in this context is collaborative, collective, and blame-free. Using a similar approach, *Patient-Centered Interviewing* represents the cutting edge of change in medical education.

The Interview in History

No one knows when the first interview was conducted, who its participants were, or what its focus was. According to the *Oxford English Dictionary* (5), the earliest recorded definition of the interview in 1498 refers to "a meeting of persons face-to-face, especially one sought or arranged for the purpose of formal conference on some point." Early interviews involved persons of high status who likely had prior knowledge about one another even if they had never met face-to-face. A case consultation between two well-known medical specialists from different medical centers who know of one another by reputation but who have never met captures a sense of this early definition.

A more modern definition of the interview is "to talk with or question so as to elicit statements or facts for publication." In its modern guise the interview is treated more as a *technique* used by one person in order to obtain information from another. In addition, the role of the interviewer has evolved into one of gathering and reporting information rather than one of conferring about it.

Medical encounters differ from other types of interviews in a number of ways. First, the interaction is highly personal and confidential, so much so that access to the content and records of physician–patient conversations is protected by law. Another important difference between medical interviews and other types is the use of information for solving problems. Press and personal interviews typically focus on information gathering that is used exclusively for others' interests, not for collaborative problem solving. Although the following may seem like common sense, one should note that a therapeutic interview differs from a survey or news interview by virtue of the fact that the *interviewee* in a clinician–patient encounter seeks, or is required to obtain, the services of an interviewer whom they hope and expect can solve a practical problem of disequilibrium or disease. In other types of interviews, the *interviewer* seeks his or her respondent. A little reflection on this point should make clear the differences in emphasis and obligation that characterize the medical interview.

The Patient's Story Is a Key to the Medical Interview

Wiesel reminds us of this in a wonderful story (6).

> *"When the great Rabbi Israel Baal Shem-Tov saw misfortune threatening the Jews, it was his custom to go into a certain part of the forest to meditate. There he would light a fire, say a special prayer, and the miracle would be accomplished and the misfortune averted.*
>
> *Later when his disciple, the celebrated Magid of Mezritch, had occasion, for the same reason, to intercede with heaven, he would go to the same place in the forest and say, 'Master of the Universe, listen! I do not know how to light the fire, but I am still able to say the prayer.' And again the miracle would be accomplished.*
>
> *Still later, Rabbi Moshe-Leib of Sasov, in order to save his people once more, would go into the forest and say, 'I do not know the prayer, but I know the place and this must be sufficient.' It was sufficient and the miracle was accomplished.*
>
> *Then it fell to Rabbi Israel of Rizhyn to overcome misfortune. Sitting in his armchair, his head in his hands, he spoke to God, 'I am unable to light the fire and I do not know the prayer; I cannot even find the place in the forest. All I can do is to tell the story and this must be sufficient.' And it was sufficient. God made man (and woman) because he loves stories."*

Physicians and healers have always sought to understand suffering by listening to their patients' stories and then acting on the basis of what they learn. Historically, this was often done with surprising sophistication and knowledge of the role and impact of the physician–patient relationship. In his book entitled *The Laws,* Plato, who was both a philosopher and a physician, observed that a physician to slaves never gave an account of his findings to his patients nor asked for any. Instead, the physician "gives an empirical injunction in the brusque fashion of a dictator." By contrast, physicians who cared for free men and women did so by going into things thoroughly and by using the relationship to persuade the sufferer into compliance. Plato understood the power of relationships to effect change, as well as the fact that these relationships were a right or privilege of some groups in society but not others. This distinction rings eerily true today in terms of the debate about national health insurance and because of an overall increase in demands on physicians' time, which is a limiting factor in developing relationships.

Although the Greek physicians and others were aware of the physician–patient relationship, the interview itself did not become a topic of scholarly interest until the early to mid-twentieth century. Stoeckle and Billings (7) identify the work of Deutsch and Murphy (8), two psychiatrists who began to train residents by making sound recordings of their interviews with patients as a basis for feedback and improvement, as the starting point for research and scholarship in this area. Since that time, clinician–patient communication research has grown dramatically in scope, sophistication, and scientific rigor.

I will briefly review what we know about the interview and its relationship to processes and outcomes of care in a moment, but first, observing how the profession's view of the interview has changed since scholarship in the area began is instructive. In his book, *Talking With Patients* (9), Eric Cassell, an internist and ethicist, writes, "In the 1930s my grandmother saw a specialist about a melanoma on her face. During the course of the visit when she asked him a question, he slapped her face, saying, 'I'll ask the questions here.' Can you imagine such an event occurring today? Melanomas may not have changed very much in the last 50 years, but the profession of medicine has."

Three features of Dr. Cassell's observation are worth noting. The first has to do with the *structure* of the medical interview and the speaking roles each person plays; second is the *dynamics* of the interview, or who does what to whom; and third is the effect of structure and dynamics in creating or improving *outcomes* of care.

Structure

In casual conversation, questions abound. We ask a stranger, "Can you tell me what time it is?" Someone asks us, "How far is it to the Carter Street Mall?" Questions also abound in professional discourse; however, a different set of rules applies as to who gets to ask and who is expected to answer. The courtroom provides the clearest example of the differences. As an attorney addressing a witness, I have the right to ask questions, such as "Where were you on the night of August 23?" The witness does not have the same right. He or she may not ask me, "Where were *you* on the night of August 23?" This difference in rights is not trivial; in fact, it carries the force of law. If the witness does ask such a question, she or he can, and almost surely will, be found in contempt of court.

The medical encounter, while not as highly constrained as a legal proceeding, does have a structure that is similar. Generally speaking, the structure of the medical encounter consists of physicians asking and patients answering questions. Evidence in research literature shows that patients prefer to convey information using formats other than questions (10) and that patients who ask too many questions are viewed by their physicians as "difficult" or "challenging." What is it about questions or, more precisely, chains of questions that accounts for their skewed distribution in physician–patient dialogues? From an interactional perspective, questions represent the first action in a two-part sequence. In essence, a question places an obligation on its recipient to provide an answer. If one person (a physician) chronically initiates the sequence and obliges another (a patient) to answer, the effect creates a system of deference in which the patient is repeatedly expected to respond to rather than to initiate action. Research confirms this observation. A study by West (11) and another by Frankel (10) showed that 91% and 99%, respectively, of what physicians do during primary care encounters is to ask questions, while patients answer questions a similar amount of the time.

In constrained speech activity systems, questions and question-asking can take on great significance in terms of completeness and accuracy of information. At one end of the spectrum is the view that questions are "dangerous" because of where they may lead. As a result, they may be completely discouraged. Frank McCourt captures this view of questions brilliantly in his memoir *Angela's Ashes* (12). "Brendan Quigley raises his hand . . . and asks, 'What's sanctifying grace?' The master rolls his eyes to heaven . . . 'Never mind what's sanctifying grace, Quigley. That's none of your business. You're here to learn catechism and do what you're told. You're not here to be asking questions. There are too many people wandering the world asking questions, and that's what has us in the state we're in; and if I find any boy in this class asking questions, I won't be responsible for what happens.'"

At the other end of the spectrum, psychologists like Carl Rogers (13,14) have developed techniques of questioning that are open-ended, inclusive, and collaborative. An open-ended response to a patient who is tearfully describing the loss of his spouse (e.g., "I don't know how I'll carry on.") might simply be to repeat the statement in the form of a question, such as, "You don't know how you'll carry on?" The research literature in this area is clear. Patients who are asked open-ended questions perceive their physicians as more caring and concerned than those who ask narrowly focused, close-ended questions. The difference between these two approaches has actually been measured, and visits with higher levels of patient participation have been found to be associated with higher satisfaction levels and better outcomes, both biomedical and psychosocial (15).

Dynamics

"The patient–physician relationship is the center of medicine (16)." Relationships are central to medical practice, and the dynamic interplay of talk, touch, and feelings between patient and physician creates, sustains, and terminates those relationships.

At the core of any therapeutic relationship is the feeling that an individual can safely expose his or her vulnerability and that he or she is genuinely cared for. These qualities are not merely a matter of having a good "bedside" manner or of "being nice." They have actually been associated with outcomes of care. For example, Milmoe and Rosenthal (17) showed that the tone of voice used by the clinician in making referrals for alcohol treatment predicted success and failure. Clinicians whose tone of voice was warm, friendly, and accepting were much more likely to have patients who followed through on the referral than were those whose tone of voice was neutral or negative.

The core skill of relationship-building is empathy, which is an accurate recognition and acceptance of another's emotional state. Two recent studies, one by Branch and Malik (18) and the other by Suchman et al. (19), point to the importance of this skill in creating successful therapeutic relationships, as well as the extent to which the skill is used in practice.

Branch and Malik were interested in knowing what behaviors characterized physicians who were nominated by their peers as having "outstanding" communication skills. Reviewing audiotapes of visits from their sample, the investigators found that "outstanding" communicators almost always used what they called "windows of opportunity." At some point in each of their visits, these physicians provided an open-ended opportunity for patients to speak about their feelings, fears, and other concerns. This behavior was not present in reports about interviews with trainees and other less-skilled physicians.

Suchman et al. went one step further by defining moments in the encounter where empathy might logically occur. These were moments of frank emotion (e.g., "I was really scared I was going to die.") or hints about emotional states (e.g., "The doctor said it was touch-and-go."). In both cases the investigators found that the most frequent physician response was to shift the topic abruptly and focus on facts rather than feelings. An example from their paper illustrates as follows:

> **PT:** I'm thinking of retiring next year. I'll be 65.
> **DOC:** Do you have Medicare?

In this example, the patient's statement about retiring is an indirect cue or hint that retiring may in some way be problematic. Rather than focus on the issue or concern, the physician pursues a factual line of questioning by saying, "Do you have Medicare?" Suchman et al. suggests that such responses leave patients feeling less well understood and less cared for than does an exploration of the emotions and concerns that underlie the hint. Although theirs was not designed as a population-based study, it is worth noting that empathic responses occurred in less than 5% of the identified empathic opportunities or moments. These two studies and a host of others like them identify an opportunity for training young physicians to become more aware of, and responsive to, relationship issues in the clinician–patient encounter.

Outcomes

A growing amount of scholarship uses highly sophisticated, randomized control trial (RCT) designs that link specific elements of communication with specific outcomes of care. I briefly review three studies that illustrate this. Greenfield and his colleagues (20,21) designed a series of RCTs to test the effect of patient participation on biomedical and psychosocial outcomes of care. Increased participation was based on the patient asking questions during an index visit. The intervention consisted of a 20-minute coaching session prior to the encounter, in which the coach and patient collaboratively developed a strategy to increase nonconfrontational question-asking. Based on a single coaching session, the investigators found highly significant differences between "activated" and "nonactivated" patients in three out of four disease categories—hypertension, diabetes, ulcer disease, and breast cancer. Although a trend for activated breast cancer patients to live longer was observed, the differences did not reach statistical significance. For the other three diseases, however, activation during the encounter led to improved biomedical, as well as functional, outcomes.

The second study, conducted by Stewart (22), was a systematic review of communication studies designed to answer whether scientific evidence demonstrates that communication and the relationship make a difference in terms of outcomes of care. Stewart reviewed 23 analytic and/or RCT studies and found that the majority of patient-centered communication interventions produced positive effects on outcomes of care, in contrast to those interactions in which the doctor was in total control and asked the questions. These effects included symptom reduction, increased satisfaction, improved functional status, and better adherence to medical recommendations. Stewart's use of metaanalysis is the highest scientific standard that one can apply to test intervention effects.

The final study, by Levinson (23), compared the communication behaviors of groups of physicians who had been sued for medical malpractice at least twice in the past with those who had never been sued. The researchers found significant differences in communication between the two groups. Physicians who had never been sued took, on average, 3 minutes longer than those who had (18.3 minutes vs. 15 minutes). The national average is 16.1 minutes. In addition, nonsued physicians oriented their patients to the nature and process of the visit and demonstrated more sociability than did sued physicians. This study clearly indicates that some physician communication behaviors are associated with extreme dissatisfaction and the decision to litigate.

Conclusion

In his foreword to the first edition of *Patient-Centered Interviewing* [then called *The Patient's Story* (24)], George Engel speculated that the link between the science of relationships and medical outcomes was in its infancy and would require more and better evidence to be able to draw any viable conclusions (25). In the world of medical practice, increasingly clear and sophisticated evidence shows that communication makes a measurable difference in outcome without adding significantly to the length of visits.

Whether these skills can be taught, learned, and put into practice by trainees has also been addressed recently by the author of this book and his colleagues (26). In the first RCT to test the effect of an interviewing method, the same one described in *Patient-Centered Interviewing: An Evidence-Based Method*, the researchers found significant differences in outcome between residents who had received training and those who had not. The results of this study are extremely encouraging in addressing the question of transferability of skills and learning and suggest that trainees at all levels can indeed benefit from a comprehensive approach to communication and enhancement of their relationship skills.

I invite you to experience the world of human relations that we as medical professionals are privileged to enter when caring for the bodies, hearts, and minds of our patients. We are fortunate to be living in an era in which the consensus, on both sides of the stethoscope, is that optimal medical care should involve personal awareness, participation, and partnership. We are more fortunate still to have a practical, scientifically sound resource such as *Patient-Centered Interviewing* to help make that ideal a reality.

Richard M. Frankel, PH.D.
Professor of Medicine and Community and Preventive Medicine,
University of Rochester School of Medicine and Dentistry
Rochester, New York;
Vice President for Program Evaluation,
The Fetzer Institute,
Kalamazoo, Michigan

References

1. Engel GL. How much longer must medicine's science be bounded by a seventeenth century world view? In: White KL, ed. *The task of medicine: dialogue at Wickenburg.* Menlo Park, CA: The Henry Kaiser Foundation; 1988:113–136.
2. Lipkin JM, Frankel R, Beckman H, Charon R, Fein O. Performing the interview. In: Lipkin M, Putnam M, Lazare A, eds. *The medical interview.* New York: Springer-Verlag; 1995:65–82.
3. Leape L. Error in medicine. *JAMA* 1994;272:1851–1857.
4. Helmreich RS, Schaefer H. Team performance in the operating room. In: Bogner MS, ed. *Human error in medicine.* Hillsdale, NJ: Lawrence Erlbaum; 1994:225–254.

5. Oxford English Dictionary. *Oxford English dictionary*, compact ed. Oxford: Oxford University Press, 1985.
6. Wiesel E. *The gates of the forest*. New York: Henry Holt; 1966.
7. Stoeckle JD, Billings A. A history of history-taking: the medical interview. *J Gen Intern Med* 1987; 2: 119–127.
8. Deutsch F, Murphy WF. *The clinical interview*. New York: International Universities Press, Inc.; 1954.
9. Cassell EJ. *Talking with patients*. Vol. 1. Cambridge: MIT Press; 1985.
10. Frankel RM. Talking in interviews: a dispreference for patient-initiated questions in physician–patient encounters. In: Psathas G, ed. *Interactional competence*. Washington, D.C.: University Press of America; 1990.
11. West C. Ask me no questions. An analysis of queries and replies in physician–patient dialogs. In: Fisher S, Todd A, eds. *The social organization of doctor–patient communication*. Washington, D.C.: Center for Applied Linguistics; 1984.
12. McCourt F. *Angela's ashes: a memoir*. New York: Scribners; 1996.
13. Rogers CR. *Client-centered therapy*. Boston: Houghton-Mifflin; 1951.
14. Rogers CR. *On becoming a person*. Boston: Houghton-Mifflin; 1961.
15. Kaplan SH, Gondek B, Greenfield S, Rogers W, Ware J. Patient visit characteristics related to physicians' participatory decision-making style: results from the Medical Outcome Study. *Med Care* 1995;32:1176–1187.
16. Glass RM. The patient–physician relationship. JAMA focuses on the center of medicine. *JAMA* 1996;275:147–148.
17. Milmoe S, Rosenthal R. The doctor's voice: predictor of successful referral of alcoholic patients. *J Abnorm Psychol* 1967;72:78–84.
18. Branch WT, Malik TK. Using 'windows of opportunities' in brief interviews to understand patients' concerns. *JAMA* 1993;269:1667–1668.
19. Suchman AL, Markakis K, Beckman HB, Frankel R. A model of empathic communication in the medical interview. *JAMA* 1997;277:678–682.
20. Greenfield S, Kaplan S, Ware JE Jr. Expanding patient involvement in care—effects on patient outcomes. *Ann Intern Med* 1985;102:520–528.
21. Greenfield S, Kaplan SII, Ware JE Jr, et al. Patients' participation in medical care: effects on blood sugar control and quality of life in diabetes. *J Gen Intern Med* 1988;3:448–457.
22. Stewart MA. Effective physician–patient communication and health outcomes: a review. *Can Med Assoc J* 1995;152:1423–1433.
23. Levinson W, Roter DL, Mullooly JP, et al. Physician–patient communication—the relationship with malpractice claims among primary care physicians and surgeons. *JAMA* 1997;277:553–559.
24. Smith RC. *The patient's story: integrated patient–doctor interviewing*. Boston: Little, Brown and Company; 1996.
25. Engel GL. Foreword. In: Smith RC. *The patient's story: integrated patient–doctor interviewing*. Boston: Little, Brown and Company; 1996:ix–xxi.
26. Smith RC, Lyles JS, Mettler J, et al. The effectiveness of intensive training for residents in interviewing. A randomized, controlled study. *Ann Intern Med* 1998; 128:118–126.

Preface

Interviewing is the most important and most difficult skill learners in medicine and nursing must master. As a primary care physician, I have worked for over 20 years to establish a method that includes the patient as a person, as well as his or her disease. Doing so required formulating a detailed, step-by-step description of medical interviewing from start to finish, which is the subject of this book. To further assist with learning this skill, my colleagues and I have developed a videotape to complement and parallel the book so that teachers and learners now have a detailed demonstration of the specific interviewing behaviors the book describes.[*]

I designed the book for training members of medical, nursing, nurse practitioner, physician assistant, and other health-related disciplines where communication and relational skills are central. These users and their teachers have particularly valued the following two unique aspects of the book:

1. *Patient-Centered Interviewing* synthesizes the literature into **one comprehensive and efficient method,** as educators and other scientists commonly request for complex topics (1-18). A behaviorally defined, step-by-step method provides a basic infrastructure for both communication and the provider–patient relationship.

2. The book further addresses educators' and scientists' requests (9–22) by providing **evidence for the specific method** it recommends (23–27).

[*]*The videotape will be published by Lippincott Williams & Wilkins concurrently with this book. It is also available from the Marketing Division of the Instructional Media Center at Michigan State University. Contact them in writing at P.O. Box 710, East Lansing, MI 48826; by phone at 517-353-9229; by fax at 517-432-2650; or on the Web at http://www. msuvmall.msu.edu/imc.*

Our research, which spanned 20 years, culminated with a focus on testing the specific method presented here (23–27). Appendix A contains the full text of one paper from the randomized, controlled trial that demonstrates the effectiveness of the method presented in this book.

I thus present **an evidence-based infrastructure for teaching and practicing the basic science of health care communication** in response to the needs identified by Korsch (28), Engel (11–13,29), McWhinney (9,10), Feinstein (14–18), Inui (19), and others (20–22).

The users of the book have also commented frequently on two additional features as follows:

1. The 5-step method in the book is user-friendly and is easily learned, as our research also shows (23–27). Learners and teachers using the method have been pleased with the structure provided. Learners typically are taught the basic skills in one session and the requisite interviewing steps in the next two teaching sessions; and they progress rapidly thereafter. Educators comment that the method is "more substantive" and "less diffuse" in comparison to previous methods. Learners with prior interviewing training say things like "now I see how this all goes together" and "this is much easier to learn." Both learners and teachers have been pleased with the results, especially with the level of confidence that it gives the learners.

2. Teachers using the method report that it fosters both the interviewer's and the patient's individuality and that it greatly enhances the humanistic dimension for each, which our research also shows (23,26,27). Similarly, the educational literature reports that explicit, behaviorally defined methods for complex tasks allow learners not only to be more effective and confident but also to be more themselves when faced with complex and otherwise insurmountable tasks (1–8).

As a result of a corporate merger, the second edition has a new publisher, Lippincott Williams & Wilkins. The title also is new, changing from *The Patient's Story* to *Patient-Centered Interviewing: An Evidence-Based Method*, reflecting the publication of our research data since the first edition in 1996 (23–27). I have extensively reformatted the text and have added more graphics to enhance learning and to make the book more reader-centered. Each chapter and its references have been updated, and I have added **Learning Exercises** and **Practice Exercises** at the end of each chapter.

Patient-Centered Interviewing works best when used in the order presented. Chapter 1 orients the reader to interviewing, provides necessary background material, and presents an overview of integrated patient-centered and doctor-centered interviewing, which is the unified interviewing approach presented in this book. Chapter 2 describes individual interviewing skills, which are synthesized in Chapter 3 as the patient-centered process of integrated interviewing; this chapter presents the *basic patient-centered infrastructure.* Chapter 4 outlines symptom-defining skills, which are then synthesized in Chapter 5 as the doctor-centered process of integrated interviewing; this chapter presents the *basic doctor-centered infrastructure.* Chapter 6 addresses more *advanced interviewing* issues, especially fine-tuning one's interviewing skills in widely varied circumstances. Chapter 7 addresses *advanced interviewing* concerning the doctor-patient relationship, with a focus on interviewer self-awareness, patient personality styles, and nonverbal communication. Chapter 8 describes how interviewers synthesize the information obtained from the patient and, in turn, present it to others in both verbal and written forms. Chapter 9 describes how the clinician gives the patient different types of information, from routine information to bad news to motivating patients to change behaviors. Appendices A and B, respectively, print in their entirety a research paper supporting the method described in this book and Dr. George L. Engel's foreword to the first edition. Appendix C presents examples of emotions. Appendix D gives a complete write-up of the case of Mrs. Jones that was presented throughout the text as an example of the interviewing process. Appendix E explains the mental status evaluation.

I intend the book for use in all years of student training. Chapters 1–3 (basic patient-centered interviewing) are typically presented first, and Chapters 4 and 5 (basic doctor-centered interviewing) are taught either a year later or later in the same year. Chapter 6 (advanced interviewing: adapting the interview to many different situations) and Chapter 7 (advanced interviewing: provider-patient relationships) follow; while they are sometimes introduced with earlier chapters, they are designed for later in training, often for advanced interviewing experiences during clinical training. Chapter 8 (presenting the patient's story verbally and as a write-up) and Chapter 9 (patient education) require expertise with the preceding chapters and usually are presented in clinical years, although they can be introduced sooner. Training graduate learners and learners outside medical and/or nursing professions typically does not involve Chapters 4, 5, and 8 either because learners are already familiar with this material or because interviewing for disease is not part of their discipline. Other chapters are relevant to all learners.

References

1. Maguire P. Teaching interviewing skills to medical students. *Medical Encounter* 1992;8:4–5.
2. Schunk DH. Self-efficacy and classroom learning. *Psychology in the Schools* 1985;22:208–223.
3. McKeachie WJ, Pintrich PR, Lin Y, Smith DAF, Sharma R. *Teaching and learning in the college classroom*, 2nd ed. Ann Arbor, MI: Regents of the University of Michigan; 1990.
4. Feinstein AR. Clinical judgement revisited: the distraction of quantitative models. *Ann Intern Med* 1994;120:799–805.
5. Flaherty JA. Education and evaluation of interpersonal skills. In: Rezler AG, Flaherty JA, eds. *The interpersonal dimension in medical education*. New York: Springer Publishing Co.; 1985:101–146.
6. Stewart M, Roter D. Conclusions. In: Stewart M, Roter D, eds. *Communicating with medical patients*. London: Sage Publications, Inc.; 1989:252–255.
7. Westberg J, Jason H. *Teaching creatively with video: fostering reflection, communication and other clinical skills*. New York: Springer Publishing Co.; 1994.
8. Carroll JG, Monroe J. Teaching clinical interviewing in the health professions—a review of empirical research. *Evaluation Health Professions* 1980;3:21–45.
9. McWhinney I. The need for a transformed clinical method. In: Stewart M, Roter D, eds. *Communicating with medical patients*. London: Sage Publications, Inc.; 1989:25–42.
10. McWhinney I. *An introduction to family medicine*. New York: Oxford University Press; 1981.
11. Engel GL. The need for a new medical model: a challenge for biomedicine. *Science* 1977;196:129–136.
12. Engel GL. The care of the patient: art or science? *Johns Hopkins Med J* 1977; 140:222–232.
13. Engel GL. Physician-scientists and scientific physicians. *Am J Med* 1987;82: 107–111.
14. Feinstein AR. The intellectual crisis in clinical science: medaled models and muddled mettle. *Perspect Biol Med* 1987;30:215–230.
15. Feinstein AR. An additional basic science for clinical medicine: I. The constraining fundamental paradigms. *Ann Intern Med* 1983;99:393–397.
16. Feinstein AR. An additional basic science for clinical medicine: II. The limitations of randomized trials. *Ann Intern Med* 1983;99:544–550.
17. Feinstein AR. An additional basic science for clinical medicine: III. The challenges of comparison and measurement. *Ann Intern Med* 1983;99:705–712.
18. Feinstein AR. An additional basic science for clinical medicine: IV. The development of clinimetrics. *Ann Intern Med* 1983;99:843–848.
19. Inui TS, Carter WB. Problems and prospects for health services research on provider–patient communication. *Med Care* 1985;23:521–538.
20. Hart I. Best evidence medical education (BEME). *Medical Teacher* 1999;21: 453–454.

21. Harden RM, Grant J, Buckley G, Hart IR. BEME Guide No. 1: Best evidence medical education. *Medical Teacher* 1999;21:553–562.

22. Aspegren K. BEME Guide No. 2: Teaching and learning communication skills in medicine—a review with quality grading of articles. *Medical Teacher* 1999;21: 563–570.

23. Smith RC, Lyles JS, Mettler J, et al. The effectiveness of intensive training for residents in interviewing. A randomized, controlled study. *Ann Intern Med* 1998; 128:118–126.

24. Smith RC, Marshall-Dorsey AA, Osborn GG, et al. Evidence-based guidelines for teaching patient-centered interviewing. *Patient Education and Counseling* 2000; 39:27–36.

25. Smith RC, Dorsey AM, Lyles JS, Frankel RM. Teaching self-awareness enhances learning about patient-centered interviewing. *Acad Med* 1999;74:1242–1248.

26. Smith RC, Lyles JS, Mettler JA, et al. A strategy for improving patient satisfaction by the intensive training of residents in psychosocial medicine: a controlled, randomized study. *Acad Med* 1995;70:729–732.

27. Smith RC, Mettler JA, Stoffelmayr BE, et al. Improving residents' confidence in using psychosocial skills. *J Gen Intern Med* 1995;10:315–320.

28. Korsch BM. Current issues in communication research. *Health Communications* 1989;1:5–9.

29. Engel GL. The clinical application of the biopsychosocial model. *Am J Psychiatry* 1980;137:535–544.

Instructor's Preface

Because *Patient-Centered Interviewing* presents a comprehensive, detailed approach to interviewing, a **companion teaching supplement** is available for teachers and other interested faculty. The supplement considers how educators might teach the material presented in this book. It extensively details one possible way to teach beginning students in medicine and/or nursing disciplines the patient-centered interviewing approach in ten sessions. Each is a one-hour lecture and/or demonstration, followed by a two-hour skill-oriented small group experience. The teaching supplement also describes in considerable detail how to teach self-awareness to students and others and how to integrate self-awareness training into the ten-session patient-centered interviewing course.

The 61-page supplement is available from the author at no cost at the following address:

> Robert C. Smith
> B312 Clinical Center
> East Lansing, MI 48824.

I also invite questions and feedback at the above address or via e-mail at Robert.Smith@ht.msu.edu.

Because I received feedback following the first edition that an actual demonstration of the interviewing method described in this book would be helpful, I have developed a *companion teaching videotape*. It will be published by Lippincott Williams & Wilkins concurrently with this book. It is also available from the Marketing Division at the Instructional Media Center of Michigan State University by mail at P.O. Box 710, East Lansing, MI 48826; by phone at 517-353-9229; by fax at 517-432-2650; or on the Internet at http://www.msuvmall.msu.edu/imc.

Acknowledgments

George L. Engel died recently, and I, with many, grieve his loss. But his influence will not wane, nor will fond recollections of our many interactions. The University of Rochester Program in Biopsychosocial Medicine, which he founded and led for many years, powerfully influenced me. I knew that the psychosocial dimensions of medicine were important, but I was not sure how to act upon that interest while still remaining scientific. George facilitated my move from full-time practice to Rochester for a fellowship and the start of an academic career in 1978 and had a tremendous influence on my life and work thereafter.

I have dedicated this edition to him as a small tribute to a wonderful man who made fundamental observations about the science of medicine in the biopsychosocial model and elsewhere and who was one of the great teachers of all time. George was characterized not only by his intellect and humanity but also by his willingness to spend whatever amount of time was needed to teach a new concept or skill in all its essential complexity. His unending support challenged many to stretch themselves to work out the logical next steps that built upon his seminal work. We who were privileged to learn from him were both blessed by our association with him and humbled by the magnitude of his work and the new direction we must take to advance it—to operationalize the biopsychosocial model through interviewing or, in other words, to make the model relevant, practical, and usable on a daily basis with each patient. Achieving that goal will be the ultimate tribute to one of the truly great physicians of the century.

Rich Winters, Acquisitions Editor at Lippincott Williams & Wilkins, deserves special mention. He became my new editor when the previous publisher, Little, Brown and Company, was sold to Lippincott Williams &

Wilkins. Rich took charge of several problems attending this transfer and turned a potentially chaotic situation around completely, using not only his consummate professional skills but also a calm, caring, and respectful approach that could be the model for this book. In addition, he valued and encouraged what he called my "passion" for the subject material and supported the promulgation of a new evidence-based method for interviewer training. Rich's influence continued as I put this edition together in an increasingly user-friendly way.

I also thank many course directors for their helpful feedback on how the first edition worked and for what could make it better. I am equally indebted to many other colleagues for their input about both the book and the companion videotape. Direct feedback from many students, residents, and graduate professionals also has been invaluable, as has feedback from the ultimate judges, our patients.

I am especially grateful to many friends from the American Academy on Physician and Patient, the Fetzer Institute, and Michigan State University. I have learned much from them, and I hope that I have satisfactorily reflected their rich input over many years. The organizations and institutions that they represent are unique, and they are the vanguard for ensuring that the Engel revolution and legacy thrive. They are the leaders in creating a new way for medicine. Their impact upon me both personally and professionally has been of inestimable importance.

Patient-Centered Interviewing

An Evidence-Based Method

1 Interviewing

"How are you feeling? Are you sick?" We, as human beings, know when something is wrong but how do we convey our problem to others? Then, how does the medical student diagnose it? The student learns what is wrong by interviewing the patient and by identifying his or her symptoms and personal concerns (1). Although uniquely private and subjective, symptoms and concerns are the primary data—the hard data of the science of medicine—and clinicians and students can enhance their scientific value by good interviewing.

These human data lead to most diagnoses and determine most treatments (2–6). By "human data," I mean information that the patient communicates either in words or by nonverbal, but uniquely human, ways, such as a frown. These data are found in no other domain. Height, weight, an enlarged liver, elevated cholesterol, or high blood sugar, whether observed directly or indirectly by the interviewer, are not examples of data that are uniquely human; however, a patient's report of a symptom or personal concern is. Human medicine is the only scientific field in which the subject literally tells the scientist what the problem is (1). A diseased plant or animal, a collapsing rock structure, or an aberrant molecule cannot. If the science of human medicine was similar to professions dealing with those items or beings, the doctor would simply perform a physical examination and run some tests. Therefore, I offer these challenges to both clinicians and students: keep human data foremost and do not rely primarily on the physical examination or laboratory tests. Interviewing is the key skill of the physician. The data obtained from interviews markedly enlarge the scope of medical science.

Most students enjoy interviewing. It launches their clinical careers and often provides the brightest spot in the first 2 years. Interviewing puts the student at the heart of medicine—working with a patient. Certainly, seeing a patient for the first time can provoke anxiety in the student; but living the reality of the student's dream of becoming a physician far outweighs the fear. Most students say something like "Now I'm beginning to see where all this basic science stuff is going; I'm starting to see the light at the end of the tunnel."

Students possess many of the skills necessary for interviewing, although mastering interviewing is difficult. Not only have they cleared multiple hurdles to get this far in their careers, but they also have a lifetime of experience with communication. In addition, students have many interpersonal and relational skills, which are among the most important abilities required for successful interviewing. Nor are students completely unfamiliar with the vicissitudes of life that their patients will present. Students do not come to the interview process unprepared; nevertheless, they need to develop their existing expertise further in the medical setting and to learn some new skills.

Interviewing consists of an exchange of relevant information about the patient for the interviewer's professional purposes. Why is interviewing so important (7,8)? First, it provides the vehicle for the interaction and exchange of information in nearly all circumstances. Second, the greatest portion of information about a patient comes from the interview (2). In fact, interviewing produces data needed for diagnoses more often than do the physical examination and laboratory investigation combined (3–6). Third, interviewing generates most of the data essential to treatment and prevention, and it becomes the major means by which all types of information are transmitted to the patient (9). Finally, and probably most importantly, interviewing itself determines how the doctor–patient relationship evolves (9). This relationship is important because the quality of the relationship with the patient correlates with the quality of data exchanged (10,11). One should note that clinicians perform up to 200,000 interviews during their careers (12). Sir William Osler captured the role of the interview long ago when he said, "By historical method [the interview] alone can many problems in medicine be approached profitably" (13). Therefore, interviewing is worth doing well and efficiently (2).

In summation, interviewing is the most fundamental of all medical skills. Not only does it provide most diagnostic and therapeutic information about the patient, but it also is the major determinant of the doctor–patient relationship and outcome of care. Nothing in medicine requires greater expertise and mastery than this skill, which is the core skill of medicine.

Interviewing Permits Us to Synthesize the Biopsychosocial Story

The focus of this book is an interviewing method that elicits relevant personal and symptom data about the patient. After obtaining these human data, the clinician or student can synthesize them into a description of the patient, called the biopsychosocial story.

The Biopsychosocial Model

The *biomedical model* (disease model, biotechnical model) describes patients only in terms of diseases, both psychiatric and physical, but it excludes most psychological and social aspects of the person (14,15). Although it is responsible for many of medicine's successes, the biomedical model has also caused much damage because it ignores the human dimension. When one integrates the psychosocial dimensions of the patient, it evolves into a *biopsychosocial model.*

George L. Engel proposed the biopsychosocial model in order to describe a person as an integrated mix of her or his biological, psychological, and social components (16,17). This model includes the person with the disease (e.g., the unique personal features of the patient, the doctor–patient relationship, the family, the community, and the spirit), as well as the disease itself, because it integrates the psychological and social dimensions with the biomedical aspects (9,10,16–20). This says, in a roundabout way, that the mind and body are not separable and that the modern caretaker can best understand the patient only as a whole person (10).

Yet, students often become frustrated when learning the biopsychosocial model. Students observe that the biopsychosocial model by itself "doesn't give a clue" about how to obtain the biological, psychological, and social data that the model prescribes. Engel's model identifies content without addressing the interviewing process by which one elicits the data necessary to synthesize that content.

The Interviewing Approach

Students trained in the biomedical model are taught to elicit symptoms of disease by using a *doctor-centered* interviewing process. Doctor-centered interviewing means that the student or physician takes charge of the interaction to meet her or his own need to acquire the symptoms, their details, and the other data that will help her or him identify a disease. By eliciting many bits of these nonpersonal data, the student can synthesize them into a description of the patient's disease. Personal concerns are largely ignored and are, in fact, discouraged so that the student can focus solely on making a disease diagnosis. Thus, a doctor-centered interview takes the lead away from the patient and prevents most personal information about the patient from arising, therefore limiting one's ability to develop an adequate psychosocial description (14,15,21,22).

To correct this, a new process that generates personal data—*patient-centered* interviewing (23–29) or the relationship-centered approach (29,30)—has evolved. Patient-centered interviewing encourages patients to express what is most important to them. They express their personal concerns in addition to symptoms. The interviewer can synthesize a psychosocial description of the patient by eliciting these personal data. Not only does the student or clinician avoid an isolated focus on symptoms, but she or he also allows the patient to lead and direct the conversation to important personal data, which usually includes the personal context of the patient's symptoms and disease (10). This means the patient's ideas and concerns, rather than the doctor's, are paramount. This interviewing process was developed to complement doctor-centered interviewing; I do not recommend its use in isolation.

The issue is not which method works best—clinicians need both. This text teaches readers how to integrate both the patient-centered and doctor-centered interviewing processes to elicit both personal and symptom data. The student or clinician must then interpret and synthesize these data, using his or her knowledge of medicine, with available data from the physical examination and laboratory, to produce the biopsychosocial description—the patient's story (9).

The term "patient-centered" can be used in two ways. In a general sense, every action with the patient is patient-centered because everything is done in the patient's interest. Therefore, to term one of the processes for achieving this "patient-centered interviewing" (to contrast it to "doctor-centered interviewing") is confusing. However, rather than introducing new terminology, these terms will suffice as long as the reader recalls that both ultimately are employed toward meeting the patient's foremost needs.

In summary, the biopsychosocial model completely describes the patient. This text outlines the integrated interviewing method that we as clinicians and students use to obtain the human data that we can then synthesize to make a biopsychosocial description.

Clinical Approach

The patient's needs should always take precedence (23–27,31,32), yet, as clinicians and students, we recognize that a patient can have many different needs, many of which are detailed in Table 1.1. We scrutinize the patient for obvious symptoms of an urgent disease problem that would dictate immediate doctor-directed input (e.g., unconscious condition; acute chest pain; profound shortness of breath; overtly disruptive, extremely anxious, or actively psychotic behavior) before the interview is begun and during its early parts. If these features are present, we take charge and act immediately to address

TABLE 1.1. NEEDS COMMUNICATED BY PATIENTS

A. Needs to express symptoms, concerns, fears, interests, desire for information, and other ideas (e.g., worry about cancer, sore throat, feeling down, desire to lose weight, fever, refill of medications)*—**Very Common**.

B. Special communication needs (e.g., deaf, blind, mute, cognitively impaired)[†]—**Common**.

C. Urgent, sometimes life-threatening needs requiring immediate attention**—**Uncommon**.

    1. Medical (e.g., unconscious, hematemesis, symptoms of acute myocardial infarction, recent history of syncope, severe pain, severe nausea and vomiting, marked shortness of breath, fracture).

    2. Psychosocial (e.g., suicidal, homicidal, very disruptive, overtly psychotic, severe organic brain syndrome, agitated, or very anxious).

*Addressed in Chapters 1 to 5.
[†]Addressed in Chapter 6.
**Not addressed in this book.

the problem. In these unusual and almost always very obvious circumstances, the patient needs us to take over direction of the process.

The vast majority of patients, however, have no acute, life-threatening problem; they can communicate, do not exhibit prohibitive anxiety, and desire to talk about their symptoms, interests, fears, and concerns. In these more common situations, the interviewer initially meets these needs, not by taking control, but rather by allowing the patient to lead the conversation and to discuss the symptoms or personal issues that she or he prefers. Ideas in the initial dialogue originate in the patient's mind rather than in the interviewer's; later, the doctor or student inserts her or his ideas into the exchange.

I address the common circumstance first in Chapters 2 through 5 and consider the interviewing approach to communication problems in Chapter 6; the approach to emergency medical and psychological conditions is considered elsewhere in clinical training.

The Rationale for Integrating Patient-Centered Interviewing

A strong rationale exists for integrating patient-centered interviewing with doctor-centered interviewing rather than using a doctor-centered approach in isolation, which is still an all-too-common practice. Table 1.2 summarizes the argument that follows.

The humanistic argument. Most clinicians and students recognize that a powerful humanistic rationale exists for integrating patient-centered principles and for first addressing patients' needs. We then hear and understand our patients in a way that validates them as human beings rather than as objects of study (33). As we strengthen the involvement of our patients, their sense of

TABLE 1.2. PATIENT-CENTERED INTERVIEWING IS MORE HUMANISTIC AND SCIENTIFIC THAN ISOLATED DOCTOR-CENTERED INTERVIEWING

A. More humanistic
  1. It validates the patient as a human being, not as an object of study.
  2. Self-sufficiency and responsibility, sharing power with the doctor, and patient autonomy occur.
  3. Caretakers can recognize and address their own human attributes of caring, concern, respect, and empathy.
  4. Connectedness between doctor and patient is found; both feel better.
B. More scientific
  1. Isolated doctor-centered interviewing is deficient.
    a. Doctor interrupts early.
    b. Doctor omits nearly all personal information about the patient.
    c. Doctor takes control.
    d. Doctor's agenda precludes patient's.
  2. Integrated patient-centered interviewing leads to the following:
    a. Improved satisfaction.
    b. Improved compliance, knowledge, understanding, and recall.
    c. Decreased malpractice suits and doctor-shopping.
    d. Improved health outcomes (e.g., diabetes, hypertension, perinatal care, postoperative results, cancer).
  3. Integrated patient-centered interviewing better meets general scientific principles because the following are true:
    a. Data are more reliable (less biased and more consistent).
    b. Data are more valid (more complete and more representative of the patient).
    c. The biopsychosocial model on which patient-centered interviewing is based operationalizes general system theory.

self-sufficiency, and their feeling of responsibility, they are more likely to share power with us and to feel more autonomy (34), an essential feature of positive patient outcomes (35). Thus, effective communication involves a patient who is the expert on her or his needs and a doctor who is the expert at translating these needs into diagnoses of disease and treatment (9,10,34).

Physicians and students also benefit. They can fully express human attributes, such as respect, empathy, humility, and sensitivity. Because these qualities seem to have less value in the isolated doctor-centered approach, physicians often feel guilty for expressing them; they often surreptitiously employ them and even admonish colleagues "not to tell anyone." The ideal of developing a feeling of connectedness between the doctor and patient can become reality with a patient-centered approach and, at times, allows previously unheard of dimensions of caring and spirituality to enter (36,37). Both the doctor and patient feel better (36,38,39).

The scientific argument. By far, the most common question I hear from teachers is, "How do I convince learners that patient-centered interviewing is important and that they need to learn it and take it seriously?" In this day and age of evidence-based medicine (40,41) and of evidence-based medical education (42–44), as instructors, we must acknowledge that students are sometimes dubious and that they view areas like interviewing as soft, ambiguous, and opinion-based (42–45)—with some justification (42–44,46). Therefore, we need rigorous methods that are supported by scientific evidence to justify what we do with our patients and to substantiate the use of valuable teaching time in busy curricula.

In this book, I present the **only evidence-based interviewing method** (see our randomized controlled trial in Appendix A) (47). In addition to that, I now make this argument: **the integration of patient-centered interviewing is more scientific than is isolated doctor-centered interviewing.** The converse also is true—isolated doctor-centered practices, while very common, are less scientific. Because, as students and clinicians, we integrate patient-centered with doctor-centered practices, we lose none of the impressive benefits of disease-oriented interviewing. Rather, we simply add to them in a way that further improves the services that we provide to the patient. I urge learners and practioners to have the scientific argument that follows at the tip of their tongue so that they can answer those who might question this "touchy-feely" approach.

Deficiencies of an Isolated Doctor-Centered Approach

1. Physicians do not allow patients to complete their opening statement of symptoms and concerns in 69% of visits and interrupt patients after a mean time of 18 seconds (48). Information is obtained almost entirely through doctor-centered inquiry.

2. Isolated doctor-centered interviewing elicits only 6% of the primary problems that ultimately have been determined to be psychosocial (49).

3. Incomplete databases result from omitting personal information and then using a "high control" style of isolated doctor-centered interactions (50). These and many other studies show that much patient data from isolated doctor-centered practices are determined by physicians, are skewed toward physical symptoms, and are directed away from the personal dimension and the patient's concerns (22).

Superior Results from Integrating Patient-Centered and Doctor-Centered Approaches

1. Many studies show increased *patient satisfaction* when patient-centered approaches are included in care in comparison to the use of isolated doctor-centered approaches (38,39,51,52).

2. Patient-centered approaches enhance *patient compliance* (21,39,51), and *patients' knowledge* and *recall* are greater (38,39,51).

3. Clinicians and students also frequently observe decreased *malpractice* suits (53–55) and decreased *doctor shopping* (56) when patient-centered approaches are integrated into care.

4. Improved *health outcomes* are regularly reported when we integrate patient-centered approaches in our diagnosis and treatment. For example, **patient-centered approaches produce better blood pressure and diabetic control (57), improved perinatal outcomes (58), shortened and less complicated postoperative courses (59–61), and improved cancer outcomes (62–65).** Recent reviews provide much more research material (35,66,67).

5. Patient-centered interviewing even produces much of the physical symptom data ordinarily obtained via doctor-centered inquiry (6), and in addition, it produces some physical symptom information that is not elicited at all by doctor-centered approaches but that is often of great value for diagnosing organic diseases (68).

Integrating Patient-Centered Interviewing Is More Compatible with General Scientific Principles

1. An isolated doctor-centered approach is at odds with scientific requirements because it produces biased data about the patient. This flaunts basic scientific requirements that data about the subject of any science be reliable (consistent, unbiased) (69–71). Experience shows that patient-centered interviewing is more consistent and less biased because it is far less influenced by the interviewer and his or her perceptions (9).

2. Patient-centered interviewing produces much personal data and emotional material omitted by isolated doctor-centered interviewing (72–74). This meets basic science requirements that data about the subject of any science be valid (complete, fully representative) (69–71) much better than does the isolated doctor-centered approach. An integrated approach that includes psychosocial aspects demonstrably produces more complete and, therefore, more valid data about the patient—who is, after all, the subject of the science of medicine (9,15,48–50,75,76).

3. Not only are data more reliable and valid, but patient-centered inter viewing also produces a biopsychosocial description of the patient in- stead of just a simple disease description. Biopsychosocial medicine stems from the guiding theory of modern science—general system the- ory—rather than from the old, simple cause–effect model (18–20) that produced the disease-oriented biomedical model.

An additional attribute of a patient-centered approach that the reader will be relieved to learn is that it elicits both personal and symptom data that are highly relevant for developing a biopsychosocial description of the patient quickly (9). In fact, these data efficiently point to the most important problem that the patient has at a given time (9,77). Indeed, research data show that in- cluding the patient-centered aspect does not take more time (78).

To summarize, integrating patient-centered interactions is not only more humanistic, which virtually everyone accepts, but it also is research-based and more scientific. I urge you to know the preceding argument well and to spread the word to others. If you do not have time to give the entire argument to a doubter, simply tell him or her that integrating patient-centered interviewing improves our patients' health outcomes. The opportunity to become a better physician convinces most.

Integrated Interviewing

Figure 1.1 provides an overview of the integrated interview. The patient-cen- tered process precedes the doctor-centered process. The amount of time spent in each varies with the circumstances but, generally, the doctor-centered pro- cess takes much longer. As shown in Fig. 1.1, from research, I estimate that approximately 10% of the time will be patient-centered and that 90% will be doctor-centered. I discourage interviewers from starting with the doctor-cen- tered process, except in the rare emergency situations that were noted earlier. Even if the interviewer later introduces the patient-centered process, the order suggests that the doctor's agenda is more important.

Figure 1.1 depicts a new patient interview, so all components of the his- tory are included: the chief complaint (CC), the history of present illness (HPI), other current active problems (OCAP), health issues (HI), past medical history (PMH), social history (SH), family history (FH), and review of sys- tems (ROS). In patients who have been previously evaluated, we usually need only the CC and HPI because other data are already known; sometimes, how- ever, a brief updating of the other components is necessary.

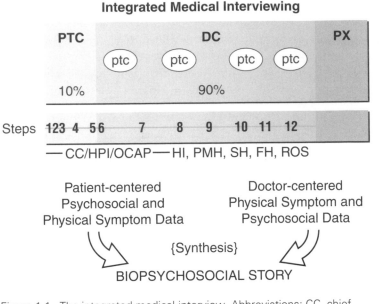

Figure 1.1. The integrated medical interview. Abbreviations: CC, chief complaint; DC, doctor-centered; FH, family history; HI, health issues; HPI, history of the present illness; OCAP, other current active problems; PMH, past medical history; PTC, patient-centered; PX, physical examination; ROS, review of systems; SH, social history.

The CC is the patient's most bothersome complaint. The HPI is usually the most helpful historical component; it is where the patient gives both the physical symptoms of the possible disease and the personal context in which they occur. When patients have more than one current medical concern, the interviewer obtains these in OCAP. In HI, the interviewer inquires about relevant ethical-social-spiritual issues, functional capacity, health-promoting behaviors, and health hazards. In the PMH, the patient gives important past information that is not germane to the HPI or OCAP. In the SH, the patient provides routine personal data that has not already been obtained as relevant; the FH does the same with routine family data. In the ROS, the student or clinician screens for any physical symptoms or other problems that have not already been discussed.

Ordinarily, the CC/HPI/OCAP takes approximately half the total time available. **The CC and initial portions of the HPI/OCAP develop using a patient-centered process, whereas the latter portions of the HPI/OCAP result from a doctor-centered process.** The HI, PMH, FH, SH, and ROS develop largely by using a doctor-centered process. The interviewer, however, should not remain entirely doctor-centered during this time but rather should periodically return to patient-centered skills. For example, if you are interviewing a patient and you ask the father's age during the FH and the patient begins to cry, saying that his father died last month, the next question is not "How old is your mother?" Rather, you should again become patient-centered (shown in Fig. 1.1 by the small PTC pockets), support the patient, and try to understand further her or his sadness before going on with additional doctor-centered questions, such as the mother's age. If the initial patient-centered process has been effective, most highly charged issues will already have arisen and these returns to patient-centeredness will be brief. Thus, the interview should begin as patient-centered and should then go back and forth between the two processes, spending most of the time as doctor-centered.

The interviewer will find that the patient-centered process produces psychosocial and, to a lesser extent, physical symptom data. Conversely, the doctor-centered process produces physical symptoms and, to a lesser extent, psychosocial data (which are of a more routine type than are psychosocial data obtained in patient-centered interviewing). Using a knowledge base in medicine, the interviewer can then synthesize these data into a description of the patient—his or her biopsychosocial story.

Integrated interviewing is the basis for most interactions—both with new and returning patients, in the ward setting or the clinic, in surgery or medicine, with tertiary or primary care, at an emergency room, or for a consultation visit. The student or clinician determines the specific amount of time that should be spent with the opening patient-centered process by the extent and urgency of an individual patient's personal issues.

With this process and content of the interview, asking about its intended functions is logical. Three distinct functions of the interview are found: data gathering, establishing a relationship with the patient, and patient education (79–81). I show the specific method subserving the first two functions in Chapters 1 through 5; I address the third function in Chapter 9. Unfortunately, some clinicians see data gathering, which is the act of obtaining relevant information about the patient, as the only function of the interview. However, relationship building, which deals with emotional issues and establishes a relationship with the caretaker, is equally important. Furthermore, the function of education provides the patient with necessary information and motivates him or her to action when it is required.

Having identified the general interviewing process, its content, and expected functions, the reader still is left with an unanswered question—"What actually goes on at the bedside or in the clinic? What do we do and how do we do it?" We are now ready to begin learning the 5 steps of patient-centered interviewing and the 7 steps of doctor-centered interviewing.

LEARNING EXERCISES

1. Define interviewing.
2. Human data are contrasted to what other types of data? What is unique about human data?
3. Define the biopsychosocial model, patient-centered interviewing, and doctor-centered interviewing. How are they related? How does the biomedical model relate to the biopsychosocial model?*
4. Give examples of some needs that can be overlooked with the use of isolated doctor-centered interviewing.
5. Under what circumstances would you not begin an interaction with a patient-centered approach?
6. Give three problems encountered with isolated doctor-centered interviewing.
7. List the benefits from integrating patient-centered and doctor-centered interviewing. How do they make interviewing more scientific and humanistic, as compared to isolated doctor-centered interviewing?*
8. Draw the full diagram of the interview and label the following: patient-centered and doctor-centered portions, CC and HPI/OCAP, HI, PMH, SH, FH, ROS.*
9. What are the functions of each interview component listed in question #8?
10. Where does important disease information first arise in the interview? Would you expect personal and psychosocial information to arise in the doctor-centered process? Why or why not?
11. How do you think the interviewer might feel in an isolated doctor-centered interview compared to an interview where he or she integrates patient-centered with doctor-centered processes? Why is this the case?

*Good test questions.

References

1. Engel GL. White coats, intimacy, and medicine as a human science. Presentation to The Program for Biopsychosocial Studies, The University of Rochester School of Medicine and Dentistry, Rochester, NY, June 3, 1994.
2. Simpson M, Buckman R, Stewart M, et al. Doctor-patient communication: the Toronto consensus statement. *Br Med J* 1991;303:1385–1387.
3. Peterson MC, Holbrook JH, Von Hales DE, et al. Contributions of the history, physical examination, and laboratory investigation in making medical diagnoses. *West J Med* 1992;156:163–165.
4. Schmitt BP, Kushner MS, Wiener SL. The diagnostic usefulness of the history of the patient with dyspnea. *J Gen Intern Med* 1986;1:386–393.

5. Hampton JR, Harrison MJG, Mitchell JRA, et al. Relative contributions of history-taking, physical examination, and laboratory investigation to diagnosis and management of medical outpatients. *Br Med J* 1975;2:486–489.
6. Linfors EW, Neelon FA. Interrogation and interview: strategies for obtaining clinical data. *J Royal Coll Gen Practit* 1981;31:426–428.
7. Lipkin M. The medical interview as core clinical skill: the problem and the opportunity. *J Gen Intern Med* 1987;2:363–365.
8. Stoeckle JD, Billings A. A history of history-taking: the medical interview. *J Gen Intern Med* 1987;2:119–127.
9. Smith RC, Hoppe RB. The patient's story: integrating the patient- and physician-centered approaches to interviewing. *Ann Intern Med* 1991;115:470–477.
10. Watzlawick P, Bavelas JB, Jackson DD. *Pragmatics of human communication: a study of interactional patterns, pathologies, and paradoxes.* New York: WW Norton, 1967.
11. Foss L, Rothenberg K. *The second medical revolution: from biomedicine to infomedicine.* Boston: Shambhala, 1987.
12. Davidoff F, Deutsch S, Egan KL, et al. *Who has seen a blood sugar? Reflections on medical education.* Philadelphia: American College of Physicians, 1996.
13. Bean RB, Bean WB, eds. *Sir William Osler. Aphorisms: from his bedside teachings and writings.* Springfield, IL: Charles C Thomas, 1961.
14. Schwartz MA, Wiggins O. Science, humanism, and the nature of medical practice: a phenomenological view. *Perspect Biol Med* 1985;28:331–361.
15. Feinstein AR. The intellectual crisis in clinical science: medaled models and muddled mettle. *Perspect Biol Med* 1987;30:215–230.
16. Engel GL. The clinical application of the biopsychosocial model. *Am J Psychiatry* 1980;137:535–544.
17. Engel GL. The need for a new medical model: a challenge for biomedicine. *Science* 1977;196:129–136.
18. von Bertalanffy L. *General system theory: foundations, development, application,* rev. ed. New York: George Braziller, 1968.
19. Weiss PA. *The science of life: the living system—a system for living.* Mount Kisco, NY: Futura, 1973.
20. Brody H. The systems view of man: implications for medicine, science, and ethics. *Perspect Biol Med* 1973;17:71–92.
21. Lazare A. Hidden conceptual models in clinical psychiatry. *N Engl J Med* 1973;288:345–351.
22. Waitzkin H. *The politics of medical encounters: how patients and doctors deal with social problems.* New Haven: Yale University Press, 1991.
23. Levenstein JH, McCracken EC, McWhinney IR, et al. The patient-centered clinical method. 1. A model for the doctor-patient interaction in family medicine. *J Fam Pract* 1986;3:24–30.
24. McWhinney I. The need for a transformed clinical method. In: Stewart M, Roter D, eds. *Communicating with medical patients.* London: Sage, 1989:25–42.
25. Levenstein JH, Brown JB, Weston WW, et al. Patient centered clinical interviewing. In: Stewart M, Roter D, eds. *Communicating with medical patients.* London: Sage, 1989:107–120.

26. McWhinney I. *An introduction to family medicine.* New York: Oxford University Press, 1981.
27. Rogers CR. *Client-centered therapy.* Boston: Houghton Mifflin, 1951.
28. Engel GL, Greene WL, Reichsman F, et al. A graduate and undergraduate teaching program on the psychological aspects of medicine: a report on the liaison program between medicine and psychiatry at the University of Rochester School of Medicine. *J Med Educ* 1957;32:859–871.
29. Tresolini CP, Pew-Fetzer Task Force. *Health professions education and relationship-centered care.* San Francisco: Pew Health Professions Commission, 1994.
30. Inui TS. What are the sciences of relationship-centered primary care? *J Fam Pract* 1996;42:171–177.
31. Maslow AH. *Toward a psychology of being.* Princeton: Van Nostrand, 1962.
32. Maslow AH. *Motivation and personality.* New York: Harper and Brothers, 1954.
33. Mishler EG. *The discourse of medicine.* Norwood, NJ: Ablex Publishing, 1984.
34. Brody H. *The healer's power.* New Haven: Yale University Press, 1992.
35. Williams GC, Frankel RM, Campbell TL, et al. Research on relationship-centered care and healthcare outcomes from the Rochester Biopsychosocial Program: a self-determination theory integration. *Families, Systems & Health* 2000;18: 79–90.
36. Suchman AL, Matthews DA. What makes the patient-doctor relationship therapeutic? Exploring the connexional dimension of medical care. *Ann Intern Med* 1988;108:125–130.
37. Tanner BL. *The open door.* Orange City, FL: RL Kruse Publishing, 2001.
38. Roter DL, Hall JA, Katz NR. Relations between physicians' behaviors and analogue patients' satisfaction, recall, and impressions. *Med Care* 1987;25: 437–451.
39. Hall JA, Roter DL, Katz NR. Meta-analysis of correlates of provider behavior in medical encounters. *Med Care* 1988;26:657–675.
40. Fletcher RH, Fletcher SW, Wagner EH. *Clinical epidemiology—the essentials,* 3rd ed. Baltimore: Williams & Wilkins, 1996.
41. Sackett DL, Richardson WS, Rosenberg W, et al. *Evidence-based medicine—how to practice and teach EBM.* New York: Churchill Livingstone, 1997.
42. Hart I. Best evidence medical education (BEME). *Medical Teacher* 1999;21: 453–454.
43. Harden RM, Grant J, Buckley G, et al. BEME Guide No. 1: best evidence medical education. *Medical Teacher* 1999;21:553–562.
44. Aspegren K. BEME Guide No. 2: teaching and learning communication skills in medicine—a review with quality grading of articles. *Medical Teacher* 1999;21: 563–570.
45. Steele DJ, Susman JL. Integrated clinical experience: University of Nebraska Medical Center. *Acad Med* 1998;73:41–47.
46. Korsch BM. Current issues in communication research. *Health Commun* 1989; 1:5–9.
47. Smith RC, Lyles JS, Mettler J, et al. The effectiveness of intensive training for residents in interviewing. A randomized, controlled study. *Ann Intern Med* 1998;128:118–126.

48. Beckman HB, Frankel RM. The effect of physician behavior on the collection of data. *Ann Intern Med* 1984;101:692–696.
49. Burack RC, Carpenter RR. The predictive value of the presenting complaint. *J Fam Pract* 1983;16:749–754.
50. Platt FW, McMath JC. Clinical hypocompetence: the interview. *Ann Intern Med* 1979;91:898–902.
51. Roter D. Which facets of communication have strong effects on outcome—a meta-analysis. In: Stewart M, Roter D, eds. *Communicating with medical patients*. London: Sage, 1989:183–196.
52. Bertakis KD, Callahan EJ, Helms LJ, et al. Physician practice styles and patient outcomes—differences between family practice and general internal medicine. *Med Care* 1998;36:879–891.
53. Vacarinno JM. Malpractice—the problem in perspective. *JAMA* 1977;238: 861–863.
54. Huycke LI, Huycke MM. Characteristics of potential plaintiffs in malpractice litigation. *Ann Intern Med* 1994;120:792–798.
55. Levinson W, Roter DL, Mullooly JP, et al. Physician-patient communication—the relationship with malpractice claims among primary care physicians and surgeons. *JAMA* 1997;277:553–559.
56. Kasteler J, Kane RL, Olsen DM, et al. Issues underlying prevalence of "doctor-shopping" behavior. *J Health Soc Behav* 1976;17:328–339.
57. Kaplan SH, Greenfield S, Ware JE. Impact of the doctor–patient relationship on the outcomes of chronic disease. In: Stewart M, Roter D, eds. *Communicating with medical patients*. London: Sage, 1989:228–245.
58. Shear CL, Gipe BT, Mattheis JK, et al. Provider continuity and quality of medical care—a retrospective analysis of prenatal and perinatal outcome. *Med Care* 1983; 21:1204–1210.
59. Egbert LD, Battit GE, Welch CE, et al. Reduction of postoperative pain by encouragement and instruction of patients—a study of doctor-patient rapport. *N Engl J Med* 1964;270:825–827.
60. de Groot KI. The influence of psychological variables on postoperative anxiety and physical complaints in patients undergoing lumbar surgery. *Pain* 1997;69:19–25.
61. Kielcolt-Glaser JK, Page GG. Psychological influences on surgical recovery: perspectives from psychoneuroimmunology. *American Psychologist* 1998;53: 1209–1218.
62. Spiegel D, Bloom JR, Yalom I. Group support for patients with metastatic cancer. *Arch Gen Psychiatry* 1981;38:527–533.
63. Spiegel D, Bloom JR, Kraemer HC, et al. Effect of psychosocial treatments on survival of patients with metastatic breast cancer. *Lancet* 1989;2:888–891.
64. Fawzy IF, Fawzy NW, Arndt LA, et al. Critical review of psychosocial interventions in cancer care. *Arch Gen Psychiatry* 1995;52:100–113.
65. Fawzy IF, Fawzy NW, Hyun CS, et al. Malignant melanoma—effects of an early structured psychiatric intervention, coping, and affective state on recurrence and survival 6 years later. *Arch Gen Psychiatry* 1993;50:681–689.
66. Stewart MA. Effective physician-patient communication and health outcomes: a review. *Can Med Assoc J* 1995;152:1423–1433.

67. Williams S, Weinman J, Dale J. Doctor-patient communication and patient satisfaction: a review. *Fam Pract Res J* 1998;15:480–492.

68. Cox A, Rutter M, Holbrook D. Psychiatric interviewing techniques. V. Experimental study: eliciting factual information. *Br J Psychiatry* 1981;139:29–37.

69. Hennekens CH, Buring JE. *Epidemiology in medicine.* Boston: Little, Brown & Company, 1987.

70. Spilker B. *Guide to clinical trials.* Philadelphia: Lippincott-Raven, 1996.

71. Streiner DL, Norman GR. *Health measurement scales—a practical guide to their development and use,* 2nd ed. Oxford: Oxford University Press, 1995.

72. Cox A, Holbrook D, Rutter M. Psychiatric interviewing techniques. VI. Experimental study: eliciting feelings. *Br J Psychiatry* 1981;139:144–152.

73. Hopkinson K, Cox A, Rutter M. Psychiatric interviewing techniques. III. Naturalistic study: eliciting feelings. *Br J Psychiatry* 1981;138:406–415.

74. Cox A, Rutter M, Holbrook D. Psychiatric interviewing techniques—a second experimental study: eliciting feelings. *Br J Psychiatry* 1988;152:64–72.

75. Feinstein AR. An additional basic science for clinical medicine. I. The constraining fundamental paradigms. *Ann Intern Med* 1983;99:393–397.

76. Odegaard CE. *Dear doctor: a personal letter to a physician.* Menlo Park, CA: Henry J. Kaiser Family Foundation, 1986.

77. Frank AW. Just listening: narrative and deep illness. *Families, Systems & Health* 1998;16:197–212.

78. Levinson W, Roter D. Physicians' psychosocial beliefs correlate with their patient communication skills. *J Gen Int Med* 1995;10:375–379.

79. Bird J, Cohen-Cole SA. The three-function model of the medical interview: an educational device. In: Hale M, ed. *Models of teaching consultation-liaison psychiatry.* Basel: Karger, 1991:65–88.

80. Cohen-Cole SA, Bird J. Interviewing the cardiac patient. II. A practical guide for helping patients cope with their emotions. *Quality of Life and Cardiovascular Care* 1986;3:53–65.

81. Lazare A, Putnam S, Lipkin M. Three functions of the medical interview. In: Lipkin M, Putnam S, Lazare A, eds. *The medical interview.* New York: Springer-Verlag, 1995:3–19.

2 Facilitating Skills

Facilitating skills are the machinery of both patient-centered and doctor-centered interviewing. I present them in detail in this chapter. Once they are learned, synthesis of these skills during integrated interviewing, as presented in Chapters 3 and 5, will fall easily into place. Two categories of facilitating skills—questioning and relationship-building skills—are found and are summarized in Table 2.1. The skills in these two categories are the interviewer's tools on a moment-to-moment basis during the interview.

TABLE 2.1. FACILITATING SKILLS

I. Questioning Skills
- A. Open-ended
  1. Silence[*]
  2. Nonverbal encouragement[*]
  3. Neutral utterances and continuers[*]
  4. Reflection and echoing[†]
  5. Open-ended requests[†]
  6. Summary and paraphrasing[†]
- B. Closed-ended
  1. Yes and no answers
  2. Brief answers

II. Relationship-Building Skills
- A. Emotion-seeking
  1. Direct
  2. Indirect: self-disclosure, impact on life, impact on others, and belief about problem
- B. Emotion-handling
  1. Naming and labeling
  2. Understanding and legitimation
  3. Respecting and praising
  4. Supporting and partnership

[*]Nonfocusing open-ended skills.
[†]Focusing open-ended skills.

Questioning Skills

Open-Ended Skills

Open-ended questions do not encourage one-word answers (yes or no) or short answers. These questions elicit the patient's description, in her or his own words, of symptoms and personal concerns. Open-ended inquiry elicits information from the patient's mind rather than from the student's or the clinician's. When used repeatedly, open-ended skills can generate a story reflecting just the patient (with minimal bias from the interviewer).

The six skills (Table 2.1) are silence, nonverbal encouragement, neutral utterances, reflection, requests, and summarization. The first three "nonfocusing" skills encourage the patient to talk but are not useful for focusing on a particular topic. These are familiar, are easily learned, and are briefly used off and on throughout the patient-centered process. The last three "focusing" skills, on the other hand, not only encourage the patient to talk, but they also focus talk on a particular topic. These more active patient-centered skills focus the patient during much of the patient-centered process of the interview. Focusing skills are the predominant mode of patient-centered interviewing.

Nonfocusing Skills

Silence. Saying nothing while continuing to be attentive signals that the interviewer is listening. Silence prompts the patient to fill the space.

> **PT:** . . . and it rolled down and hit me here (pause)
>
> **DOC:** (attentive but silent for 5 seconds)
>
> **PT:** . . . so I called you, thinking you'd be in, but then . . .

However, sometimes silence can make the patient uncomfortable, which she or he may indicate by shifting about or looking away. If 5 to 10 seconds of silence do not prompt further information, use another skill, especially if the patient appears ill at ease.

Nonverbal Encouragement. Nonverbal encouragement urges patients to talk; it is commonplace in everyday interactions and is much easier to use than silence. Typically, the interviewer gestures with the hand (rotatory motion to continue), makes a sympathetic facial expression (of expectation to continue), or simply indicates by body language (leaning forward) that the patient should continue speaking.

> **PT:** . . . so that it hurt his feelings (pause)
> **DOC:** (leans forward with expectant expression on face)
> **PT:** Well then I felt bad too and . . .

Neutral Utterances, Continuers. Neutral utterances encourage patients to continue talking; they are another example of open-ended skills that we as humans use all the time, particularly in conjunction with nonverbal responses. They are nothing more than brief, noncommittal statements, such as, "Oh," "Uh-huh," "Yes," or "Mmm."

> **PT:** . . . and later the pain went in the front part, right here . . .
> **DOC:** Uh-huh.
> **PT:** Yeah, and it hurt like crazy.
> **DOC:** Mmm.

Focusing Skills

Reflection, Echoing. Reflection (echoing) states what the patient has just said, using the same wording or phrasing. It signals that the interviewer has heard what he or she said and encourages her or him to proceed; it especially focuses the patient on the word or phrase echoed.

> **PT:** After the pain let up, I still couldn't find him.
>
> **DOC:** The pain? (focuses patient on symptom of pain) **OR** Couldn't find him? (focuses patient on personal aspects)

Open-Ended Requests. Open-ended requests can be as general as, "Tell me more" or "Go on." They also can be quite specific by focusing the patient on an already mentioned area that the interviewer wants to expand, such as, "Tell me more about the daughter you mentioned." These directions move patients to deeper levels in their stories.

> **PT:** Then my pain came back because I couldn't afford the medicine.
>
> **DOC:** Go on (encourages patient to continue without additional focusing). **OR** Tell me about not affording it (focuses patient on the personal problem). **OR** Tell me about the pain (focuses patient on physical problem).

Summary and/or Paraphrasing. Instead of echoing only a word or phrase, the interviewer echoes a wider range of talk by summarizing it. Summarizing focuses patients on the material summarized and prompts them to express deeper levels of their stories. It signals that they have been heard and that they should proceed beyond that point.

> **PT:** (tells long story about difficulty getting in to see doctor)
>
> **DOC:** So you had the nausea but couldn't get me on the phone. Then it got worse and your wife still couldn't get ahold of me until today.
>
> **PT:** Yeah, I was really more upset than sick by now.

As the preceding examples show, these skills focus the patient wherever the interviewer chooses to use the focusing skill, whether it is a physical or personal utterance. This gives the student or clinician control of the interview while remaining patient-centered and retaining the ability to develop a narrative thread in the patient's own words. You will be introduced in Chapter 3 to the selective use of these skills for focusing on physical symptom utterances and then to their application to personal or psychosocial utterances. The focusing skills can also be used to select one symptom from a group of physical symptoms or to select one personal statement from among several personal statements.

Closed-Ended Skills

Closed-ended questions are answerable with "yes," "no," or a brief response. They usually are used to focus on specific issues in the student's or clinician's mind. This makes them ideal for the doctor-centered process in which many details have to be obtained and in which the student or clinician takes the lead. Although closed-ended questions enhance the precision of information, they are counterproductive when used alone. They discourage the communication of information originating in the patient's mind by forcing the patient to respond to the doctor's concerns and ideas. Used in isolation, closed-ended skills also can have a deleterious effect on the doctor–patient relationship, can greatly diminish the quantity and quality of data about the patient, and can prove inefficient.

Two types of closed-ended skills, both of which are very familiar and reflexive, are also listed in Table 2.1.

Questions Producing Yes or No Answers. These questions are asked with a specific issue that must be answered.

> **PT:** My pain is right here.
> **DOC:** Is there any shortness of breath? **OR** Does it go out your arm? **OR** Did your wife come with you?
> **PT:** No.
> **DOC:** Did you come into the hospital this morning?
> **PT:** Yes.

Questions Producing Brief Answers. These questions are similar to yes or no questions in type and function.

> **DOC:** How old are you?
> **PT:** 31.
> **DOC:** How high was the fever?
> **PT:** I don't know. **OR** 103°.

Integrating Open-Ended and Closed-Ended Skills

Open-ended and closed-ended skills complement each other. During the patient-centered process, open-ended questions predominate and are used repeatedly, primarily to develop data about symptoms and other concerns. Closed-ended questions are much less prominent but, when used, are primarily for clarification. During the doctor-centered process, open-ended questions are fewer; they are used primarily for brief but repeated scanning, as the bulk of the work is done more effectively with closed-ended questions that pin down details.

Relationship-Building Skills

I must digress briefly so that we can better understand the centrality of the doctor–patient relationship in general because the medical dimensions of the relationship are a focus throughout this book. As nicely summarized by Mitchell (1,2), many scholars reject the primacy of the individual in favor of a relational model as the best theory of how we as humans function. The individual is the product of the relationship. The superordinate need of any individual is not for pleasure or need gratification but rather is for the establishment of relationships and the avoidance of isolation. The story of our lives, in essence, is the nature of our relationships, beginning with the model set by our parents and working and reworking this pattern thereafter. The logical conclusion then is the idea that, as a medical caretaker, one of your central skills in working with human beings is your ability not only to grasp but also to enter the patient's relational world—how is he or she put together, and who are the central players?

   Addressing emotion leads to the strongest doctor–patient relationship and produces the most effective communication (3–7). Relationship-building skills elicit and then address patients' emotions. Expressing needs through emotion antedates language; it is a basic form of human communication (3–5,7–14). Emotions are central to effective decision making (15) and, perhaps, to consciousness itself (16).

A limited, focused understanding of the patient's emotional life often takes temporary precedence over understanding other aspects of the patient in medical situations because of the centrality of emotion to human function and to the doctor–patient relationship (3–5,7–14). Unfortunately, interviewers often ignore patients' emotions and focus instead on a disease diagnosis (17). Even though patients seek and welcome emotional inquiry (17,18), they do not usually spontaneously express emotions; rather, they offer clues that clinicians and students must identify and facilitate (17), as outlined here. As described in the following, we will learn that, as clinicians or students, we do not use these skills until the patient feels comfortable and knows that the interviewing circumstance is a safe setting for addressing emotions. Thus, by addressing emotions, we enhance the doctor–patient relationship (DPR) and achieve the patient-centered benefits of being more scientific, as outlined in Chapter 1.

Emotions can be expressed three ways: acting them out (e.g., crying), nonverbal expression (e.g., depressed facies, slumped shoulders), and verbal statements (e.g., "I was upset"). Although research results vary slightly, four basic emotions have been generally identified: anger, joy, sadness, and fear (3,8,10,14). The many derivative emotional states are listed in Appendix C to give the reader an idea of what constitutes emotion and of how vast this area is; most students are surprised to learn how many different emotions exist.

Emotion-Seeking Skills

Because emotions are so important, I recommend that we, as clinicians and students, actively seek them even when they are not presented or when they are only partially expressed. The emotion-seeking skills serve this purpose. We employ emotion-handling skills, which are subsequently described, once the patient's emotions are clearly present and fully developed.

We use the following methods to seek emotion, often starting in the order now given but subsequently interspersing them freely. Typically, the first suffices to elicit the initial emotion and the second further develops it. The second group also is sometimes required to initiate emotional expression in more reticent patients.

Direct Inquiry. One of the most important questions in interviewing is some variation of, "How did that make you feel?" Directly asking does not mean inserting the hypothesized feeling ("Did you feel angry?"), but instead the patient should identify the specific feeling. The interviewer should ask this question when emotion is suspected from the patient's statement ("She got my job.") or nonverbal behavior (shifts in chair) or when the patient shows no reaction in a situation where emotion is likely (death of spouse). Most respond to this invitation. Some patients may not understand and may respond with how they feel physically ("sick to my stomach"). The interviewer prevents this by asking, "How did you feel emotionally, personally?"

PT: (has just been told he needs surgery)
DOC: So, how's that make you feel, you know, personally?
PT: Surprised, I guess (but looking anxious).
DOC: How are you feeling right now, talking about it?

When patients already are expressing emotion and its nature is obvious (e.g., crying after loss of spouse), the interviewer should not inquire specifically about the feeling but often seeks to develop it further. He or she might say, "I can see you're very sad, can you tell me more about what it's like for you?"

Indirect Inquiry. Emotional expression does not always follow direct inquiry. Because emotions are so important, however, the student or clinician must continue to seek them. Four ways, in no particular order, exist in which we as clinicians encourage the reticent patient or further develop an already expressed emotion.

(a) Self-disclosure may help. (e.g., "I once had a similar experience and I was very upset.") You should avoid loaded emotional terms (anger, depressed) and should use more neutral terms, such as upset, unhappy, or frustrated, for emotions.

(b) Inquiring about how the illness or other situation in question has affected the patient's life also uncovers important information and increases emotional expression. (e.g., "How has your wife's death affected your life?")

(c) Inquiring about how the circumstance has affected others is a more indirect way to encourage emotional expression. (e.g., "How has your wife's death affected your daughter?")

(d) Inquiring about what the patient thinks caused the problem, or what the mechanism of it was, can also elicit emotional expression. (e.g., "Why do you think the cancer got worse?")

PT: (patient has just been told he has leukemia but acknowledges no emotion with direct inquiry)

DOC: That happened to another patient of mine once and she or he was upset. **OR** How's it going to affect your life? **OR** What will your wife say? **OR** Why do you think it happened?

Emotion-Handling Skills (Relationship-Building)

The aptly named emotion-handling skills manage or "handle" emotion once it has been expressed. These are essential to developing a positive doctor–patient relationship and to being patient-centered (19,20). The mnemonic NURS helps recall them: Naming, Understanding, Respecting, and Supporting (i.e., one NURS[es] the emotion). The clinician or student sometimes uses all four skills in this precise order, as shown in the vignette, but more often interviewers use just one or two at a time with the expression of the emotions.

Naming, Labeling the Emotion. In this skill the interviewer names the emotion identified. (e.g., "That sounds sad for you.") As in the preceding, the word should connote less emotion rather than more (i.e., use "frustrated" rather than "angry"). This sends the patient the following message: the interviewer has heard her or him and has properly recognized the emotion.

Understanding, Legitimation. The interviewer acknowledges that the emotional reaction is understandable. (e.g., "Given what happened, it makes sense to me; I can sure understand why.") The emotion is thus legitimized, accepted, and validated. The statement must be genuine, which means that the interviewer must have heard enough about the story to understand it satisfactorily and must also have sufficient experience with the particular issue to be able to understand it. Indeed, we can indicate lack of comparable experiences with equal impact in appropriate circumstances. (For example, when someone has just lost all members of her or his family in an auto accident, the response might be "I've never had that happen, but I can see how deeply it hurts.")

Respecting, Praising. Respecting and/or praising is the most difficult and least natural skill of the NURS quartet. Most interviewers already are behaving respectfully via their nonverbal behaviors and do not understand what else is needed. Verbal respecting statements clearly acknowledge how difficult things have been for the patient (e.g., "You've really been through a lot.") or praise them for their efforts (e.g., "I like the way you've hung in there and kept fighting."). This often involves emphasizing the positive, finding what people have done well, and reinforcing it. Again, one should praise only after having sufficient data to do so legitimately.

Supporting, Partnership. The interviewer indicates that she or he, and perhaps others, are available for support and are "in the soup with you" to do whatever they can to help. Not only is he or she willing to help but he or she is also available to do it as a team with the patient. (e.g., "I'm here to help in any way I can. Together—you and I—we can get to the bottom of this.")

Brief Vignette Using NURS Quartet

PT: (has just indicated feeling lonely since his dog died)

DOC: So, that's been pretty lonesome for you. [Naming]

PT: We were together for a long time. Sounds kind of silly, I know.

DOC: Not at all. I had a dog die a couple years ago. I can really understand. We grieve all our losses—dogs as well as people. It makes sense to me. [Understanding]

PT: He always used to ride in the car with me.

DOC: He meant a lot to you. I can see it's been a difficult time. [Respecting]

PT: It really has.

DOC: Sometimes it helps talking about it. [Supporting]

PT: It does feel better. I was embarrassed to mention it to anyone else.

The interviewer does not have to agree with the emotion for which she or he indicates understanding, respect, or support. Rather, she or he is indicating appreciation of the patient's point of view and circumstance. To an abusive parent one might say "I understand how all her crying upset you," or "It's really been hard on you," or "I'm here to help you do what's best"—without condoning or reinforcing abusive behavior.

Addressing emotions provokes anxiety in some interviewers, who may raise fears about harming patients or of being intrusive, for example. Although understandable, these common fears are groundless; indeed, the truth is quite the opposite, as our research has shown (21–25) (Appendix A). Another fear of some students and clinicians is that the emotional expression will get out of control. Patients, however, easily control how far they want to go, and the interviewer always controls how far she or he wants to proceed. Thus, patients can be allowed and encouraged to express emotion. Interviewers must guard against the impulse to shut them off or to change the subject. Many find this new area to be difficult.

Integrating All Facilitating Skills

The facilitating skills (questioning skills, relationship-building skills) are not intended for isolated use. Rather, you should dynamically integrate them, as is illustrated in the following discussion and in Fig. 2.1. When the clinician or student masters this incorporation of the facilitating skills, she or he will have mastered patient-centered interviewing. Chapter 3 merely provides structure and guidance for how clinicians use these facilitating skills, which are directly incorporated as Steps 3 and 4 in the next chapter.

I am now going to outline an exercise to demonstrate the integrated use of the facilitating skills. Essentially, after starting with an open-ended beginning question, we often use the skills in the order presented earlier in the chapter: nonfocusing → focusing → emotion-seeking → emotion-handling; using a few closed-ended questions for needed clarification of data is appropriate. The process is continuous—we spend the suggested amount of time with each skill category (using all skills within interchangeably) and then continue directly to the next. **Your charge is as follows: master the following exercise, the centerpiece of the patient-centered interview and the key to being most scientific.**

1. Begin with an open-ended question like, "How are you doing?"

Facilitating Skills: Patient-Centered

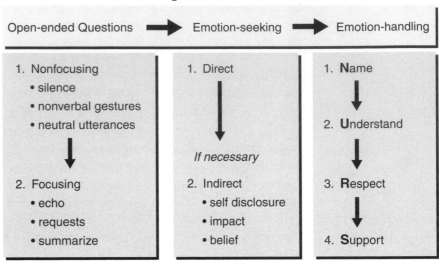

Figure 2.1. Dynamic use of Facilitating Skills.

2. Continue directly without breaking. Use *nonfocusing open-ended skills* alone for *15 to 30 seconds*. Basically, this means that you should be quiet (silence) and should use encouraging nonverbal gestures and neutral utterances; however, you should not just sit and listen attentively for too long because the patient will become uncomfortable.

3. Continue without a break and change to a more active style by responding verbally to exactly what the patient already said; use the *focusing open-ended skills* to encourage additional conversation. For approximately *2 minutes,* intersperse echoing, requests, and summaries to draw out the patient's now evolving story. Simply "follow your nose" and apply the skills to whatever the patient says, whether the topic is vision problems, chest pain, a job-related issue, or the family pet. You do not have to work hard in order to figure out what to say; rather, simply follow the patient's lead using focusing skills. This will generate some sort of story, which can be medical, personal, or both.

4. Without breaking, you should now change from focusing skills to find what emotion attends the story you have elicited. To do so, you can use *direct emotion-seeking skills.* (e.g., "So, how does all that make

you feel emotionally?") These will produce some emotion, such as fear (of cancer) or worry (about job), which you then develop a little further with an open-ended request (going back to the focusing skills). ("Tell me more about that [fear of cancer; worry about losing job].") Continue to use the focusing open-ended skills until you can understand the situation well enough to say genuinely that you understand it (the next step)—this process usually takes *1 to 2 minutes.*

5. Proceed directly without breaking and switch to *emotion-handling skills;* you should use these for *1 minute.* To help yourself learn these skills, you should use all four of them in the order given (NURS). However, once you have learned them, you will use one or two at a time.

6. You could continue the practice at this point, or you could stop. Continuing is easy because using NURS generates additional information from the patient. You then return to the focusing skills and elicit what becomes the second chapter of the patient's story. This is followed by another round of emotion-seeking and, in turn, by emotion-handling skills to complete the second chapter. You can elicit as many chapters as you wish to develop by simply continuing to use this sequence of skills.

7. You should also practice a situation where the patient gives no emotion so that you have to learn to use the indirect emotion-seeking skills.

Patient-Centered and Doctor-Centered Interviewing Further Defined and Illustrated

Patient-centered interviewing means addressing open-ended skills, emotion-seeking skills, and emotion-handling skills to material that has already been introduced by the patient. Indeed, with many of these skills, we as interviewers cannot do otherwise. (Neutral utterances, echoing, summarizing, naming, and understanding can be applied only after the patient introduces material to which they can be addressed.) These skills encourage the patient's direction by focusing on material already introduced. We, however, can refocus the patient on an important topic that may have slipped by too quickly. Often patients mention a loaded topic, such as death, but rapidly move away from it.

We can return to the topic by saying, "You mentioned death a minute ago, tell me more about that," for example. Because the patient initially introduced the topic of death, this action is patient-centered even though it does interrupt the immediate thread of conversation. On the other hand, to be the most patient-centered, we should avoid shifting the conversation away from important personal topics back to physical symptoms already mentioned. When we address these skills to the material that has already been introduced by the patient, we obtain a story that originates more completely from the patient's mind and that is less "contaminated" by our thoughts and actions. Viewing each individual bit of new information, whether from the interviewer or patient, as being placed on a table between them is a useful metaphor. Patient-centered interviewers place no new bits of information on the table. Certainly, we do always influence and affect the conversation, but a patient-centered approach minimizes our impact and precludes the gross contamination of conversation that occurs during a doctor-centered approach.

Open-ended requests (one of the focusing open-ended skills) and emotion-seeking skills, in addition to closed-ended skills, also can be used to focus on a topic that has not yet been introduced by the patient. Such action is not patient-centered; that is, when "health" or "wife" have not been mentioned or alluded to by the patient, saying "Tell me about your health." (an open-ended request) or "What are your feelings about your wife?" (direct emotion-seeking) is not patient-centered. Inquiry that introduces new information contaminates the conversation with the interviewer's ideas and is, by definition, doctor-centered—that is, the doctor determines the content of conversation. Such inquiry is appropriate during the doctor-centered process where we frequently must introduce ideas and concepts that have not yet been mentioned by the patient; to do so, we use open-ended requests (frequently), emotion-seeking skills (rarely), and closed-ended skills (primarily).

I have presented general guidelines to distinguish patient-centered from doctor-centered interviewing. We seldom can rigidly adhere to them; rather, we try simply to be predominantly patient-centered. For example, we often insert new information, by using clarifying closed-ended questions, into a patient-centered conversation. For example, when the interviewer is confused by a patient who begins telling her or his problem without a timeline, the interviewer should ask, "Wait a minute, when did all this happen?" The warning for us is not to continue inserting new information; therefore, once the confusion has cleared, we should return to being patient-centered. Also, the astute reader will have already recognized that the use of indirect emotion-seeking skills does insert new information into the conversation. That is the intent—to suggest emotion—but only when patients do not offer it spontaneously or following our direct inquiry. Again, this is not a problem as long as we quickly return to the patient-centered approach.

SUMMARY

The facilitating skills described in this chapter are the tools for all interviewing. As Chapters 3 and 5 describe more fully, they are integrated in both patient-centered and doctor-centered processes, but they are used in different balances and for different purposes. The relationship-building skills, because of their close link to patients' emotional lives, are the key elements in eliciting information efficiently and in establishing a relationship. Open-ended skills, emotion-seeking skills, and emotion-handling skills are the tools for implementing a patient-centered approach. Open-ended requests, along with closed-ended skills, can also be used in a doctor-centered approach where the student appropriately introduces new data and determines the content of the conversation.

More importantly, the facilitating skills are dynamically integrated, often in this order: nonfocusing → focusing → emotion-seeking → emotion-handling. We typically repeat this sequence to obtain multiple chapters of the story. Mastery of this integrated process leads to mastery of patient-centered interviewing. In Chapter 3, we will see that this sequence of skills is used repeatedly; it is the core of the patient-centered process (Steps 3 and 4).

We are ready to learn the actual interview. In Chapter 3, I detail the patient-centered process; and, in Chapter 5, the doctor-centered process is explained. Let us begin!

LEARNING EXERCISES

1. Define open-endedness. Name the skills associated with this technique.
2. Define emotion-seeking. Name the skills associated with this technique.
3. Define emotion-handling. Name the skills associated with this technique.
4. Why are emotions important? What do they have to do with being scientific?*
5. When would you use all four emotion-handling skills together?
6. Describe how and when you would use indirect inquiry to elicit emotions.
7. When might using an open-ended skill not be patient-centered? Explain.
8. Describe how the facilitating skills often are integrated into the interview process.*

*Good test questions.

PRACTICE EXERCISES

1. In role-play, practice individual facilitating skills for 5 to 10 minutes.
2. Now practice integrating all facilitating skills in role-play or with a simulated patient as outlined in the text and summarized in Fig. 2.1. Use the book initially, but, **before proceeding, you should be able to integrate the facilitating skills without aids.** This takes a little practice and requires good feedback from teachers and colleagues. You can often master this in one teaching session, but follow-up at a later date does help.
3. Do the same exercise again but have the person in the patient role give no emotion when asked. The challenge is then to use the indirect emotion-seeking skills to elicit some emotion.

References

1. Mitchell SA. *Relational concepts in psychoanalysis—an integration.* Cambridge: Harvard University Press, 1988.
2. Mitchell SA. *Relationality.* Hillsdale, NJ: The Analytic Press, 2000.
3. Sternberg EM. *The balance within—the science connecting health and emotions.* New York: WH Freeman, 2000.
4. Vaughan SC. *The talking cure: the science behind psychotherapy.* New York: Grosset-Putnam, Putnam's Sons, 1997.
5. Pennebaker JW. *Opening up—the healing power of expressing emotions.* New York: Guilford Press, 1997.
6. Smith RC, Hoppe RB. The patient's story: integrating the patient- and physician-centered approaches to interviewing. *Ann Intern Med* 1991;115:470–477.
7. Holmes J. Attachment theory: a biological basis for psychotherapy? *Br J Psychiatry* 1993;163:430–438.
8. Damasio AR. *The feeling of what happens—body and emotion in the making of consciousness.* New York: Harcourt Brace, 2000.
9. Sternberg E. Emotions and disease: a balance of molecules. In: Conlan R, ed. *States of mind—new discoveries about how our brains make us who we are.* New York: John Wiley & Sons, 1999:103–122.
10. LeDoux J. The power of emotions. In: Conlan R, ed. *States of mind—new discoveries about how our brains make us who we are.* New York: John Wiley & Sons, 1999:123–149.
11. Darwin C. *The expression of the emotions in man and animals.* Chicago: University of Chicago Press, 1965. (Reprinted from the authorized edition of D. Appleton and Company, New York.)
12. Engel GL. *Psychological development in health and disease.* Philadelphia: WB Saunders, 1962.
13. Damasio AR. *Descartes' error.* New York: GP Putnam's Sons, 1994.

14. Plutchik R. *The psychology and biology of emotion.* New York: Harper Collins College Publishers, 1994.

15. Bechara A, Damasio H, Tranel D, et al. Deciding advantageously before knowing the advantageous strategy. *Science* 1997;275:1293–1294.

16. Eccles JC. *Evolution of the brain: creation of the self.* London: Routledge, 1989.

17. Suchman AL, Markakis K, Beckman HB, et al. A model of empathic communication in the medical interview. *JAMA* 1997;277:678–682.

18. Brody DS, Khaliq AA, Thompson II TL. Patients' perspectives on the management of emotional distress in primary care settings. *J Gen Int Med* 1997;12:403–406.

19. Platt FW, Keller VF. Empathic communication. *J Gen Intern Med* 1994;9:222–226.

20. Platt FW, Gaspar DL, Coulehan JL, et al. Tell me about yourself: the patient-centered interview. *Ann Intern Med* 2001;134:1079–1085.

21. Smith RC, Lyles JS, Mettler J, et al. The effectiveness of intensive training for residents in interviewing. A randomized, controlled study. *Ann Intern Med* 1998;128:118–126.

22. Smith RC, Lyles JS, Mettler JA, et al. A strategy for improving patient satisfaction by the intensive training of residents in psychosocial medicine: a controlled, randomized study. *Acad Med* 1995;70:729–732.

23. Smith RC, Mettler JA, Stoffelmayr BE, et al. Improving residents' confidence in using psychosocial skills. *J Gen Intern Med* 1995;10:315–320.

24. Smith RC, Dorsey AM, Lyles JS, et al. Teaching self-awareness enhances learning about patient-centered interviewing. *Acad Med* 1999;74:1242–1248.

25. Smith RC, Marshall-Dorsey AA, Osborn GG, et al. Evidence-based guidelines for teaching patient-centered interviewing. *Patient Educ Counsel* 2000;39:27–36.

3

Patient-Centered Interviewing

Because patient-centered interviewing has often seemed confusing, my colleagues and I developed a user-friendly and complete method. The evidence-based method that I will present has been effective in both our and many others' hands during the last 10 years, as our research confirms (1–5). **The most difficult learning occurs at the outset when one learns the five steps and 21 substeps.** I urge the reader to **learn these thoroughly to the point that they become reflexive,** which is easily accomplished by first studying them and then using them in practice. Just as you, as a student, learned the intricacies of the Krebs cycle and cardiac physiology, learning these steps is your major task in mastering the most important clinical skill you must have. Once you know and can use the steps and substeps, you will have no problem. Using these steps and substeps will make you a more scientific and more humanistic physician, and your patients will benefit (see the Rationale section of Chapter 1). To assist you, a videotape that demonstrates the same skills described here has also been developed (6) (see Preface).

I recommend that, when first learning these skills, you use them in the order outlined, primarily as a way to learn them. As you become more comfortable with the interview, I recommend varying the steps and substeps to experiment, as well as to adapt to specific occasions and needs. Not infrequently, some substeps can be omitted; and, in other instances, you may want to change the order in which you use them. The steps and substeps are simply signposts and guidelines to lead you through the interview; using them flexibly enhances the individuality of both you and your patient.

This chapter describes and demonstrates the 5-step method. The method describes, step by step, exactly what to do. The five steps in the patient-centered process enhance the patient's lead and ability to express what is most important to her or him. As part of text material, an ongoing interview with "Mrs. Jones" is introduced to demonstrate each step; this and other examples used are derived from real people and situations but are masked to protect confidentiality.

To begin, I first address some patient-centered skills that have not yet been introduced: setting the stage for the interview (Step 1) and determining the agenda (includes the chief complaint) for the interview (Step 2). These steps are not, strictly speaking, patient-centered because they may insert new information into the interaction, but they do serve a patient-centered purpose as they are preparatory or staging areas for the true patient-centered process that occurs in Steps 3 and 4, which are where the facilitating skills learned in Chapter 2 are incorporated.

Setting the Stage for the Interview (Step 1)

Step 1 skills are sometimes overlooked courtesies that ensure a patient-centered atmosphere. Table 3.1 lists these substeps in their usual order of use at the first meeting with a patient; appropriate adjustments are made when the interviewer already knows the patient. These rapport-building skills enhance the relationship, establish or reaffirm participants' identities, and set the stage for the patient-centered process in Steps 3 and 4; they *should take no more than 1 to 2 minutes* (7–9).

TABLE 3.1. SETTING THE STAGE FOR THE INTERVIEW (STEP 1)

1. Welcome the patient.
2. Use the patient's name.
3. Introduce yourself and identify your specific role.
4. Ensure patient readiness and privacy.
5. Remove barriers to communication.
6. Ensure comfort and put patient at ease.

Welcome the Patient

The patient must feel valued and welcome. Simple statements, such as "Welcome to the clinic," or, in a hospital setting, "Sorry to see you're sick but I am glad you came to see us," suffice. This sets the proper tone for a patient-centered interaction. The clinician or student should always try to shake hands with the patient, although sometimes this is not possible with very ill patients; in this scenario, a friendly pat on the hand or arm is equally beneficial to the relationship. He or she can develop some important initial nonverbal impressions about the patient from the handshake (e.g., the hearty handshake of a confident person, the cold sweaty palm of an anxious person, and the feeble handshake of someone who is very ill).

Use the Patient's Name

This can be done efficiently by combining one courtesy with another, such as "You're Mrs. Garcia aren't you? Welcome to the clinic." The interviewer should use the patient's last name unless the patient volunteers the use of another name. If the patient has a difficult name, he or she may need to ask how to pronounce it.

Introduce Self and Identify Specific Role

Although first names are permissible, the interviewer usually begins by using her or his last name and also by noting her or his official role with the patient. Introductions can be combined with other patient-centered gestures, for example, by saying, "How do you do, Mrs. Garcia? I'm Ms./Mr. Burns, the [medical student/physician/etc.] who will be part of the team looking after you." A student also can use the term 'student doctor' or 'student physician' to designate herself or himself, particularly when she or he is in a clerkship (10). Many believe that applying the label 'doctor' prior to graduation is inappropriate and, furthermore, is counter to the patient's wishes (10,11). Occasionally at the beginning, but more often after the relationship has matured, a first name relationship develops. The student or physician should carefully match identity terms and, thereby, avoid suggesting an unequal relationship. In other words, both the interviewer and patient are on a last name basis, or they are on a first-name basis (e.g., the interviewer should not say, "Hi, George. I'm Dr. Smith" or "Welcome, Mr. Brown. I'm Betty.").

Introductions can be difficult. A student often feels torn between misrepresenting herself or himself as a doctor and not wanting to appear inept by conveying a perceived lack of expertise (e.g., "I'm not a real doctor.") (10). However, if you are a student in this situation, honestly portraying your circumstances goes a long way toward developing a sense of professional identity, particularly as patients repeatedly accept your professional role (8,10,12). In addition to noting that you are a student doctor, you might say,

"I am part of the team taking care of you. I'll be getting much of the information about you and will be (one of) your major contact person(s)." Apologizing or otherwise devaluing yourself is not necessary (e.g., "I'm just a student, thanks for letting me talk to you."). Nor should the patient's acceptance of a student working with them be an item for questioning—the preceptor should have established this with the patient beforehand (10). As a student, you must understand and confidently convey that you are indeed a key part of the patient's care. The annals of medicine are replete with stories of students' contributions to care and with stories of patients deferring to students' opinions (e.g., when the resident or faculty makes a recommendation directly to the patient, the patient says, "I'll have to ask Ms. Burns [the student].").

Ensure Patient Readiness and Privacy

Initially and especially in hospital settings and with acutely ill patients, as an interviewer, you should ascertain if the time is convenient for the patient. Sometimes, postponing the interview is necessary (e.g., the patient is eating dinner; relatives are visiting; patient is vomiting from recent chemotherapy treatment). Severe pain, severe nausea, need for a medication, and a soiled bed, for example, are other physical problems that must be addressed before the patient is ready for an interview. Postponement is less of an issue with outpatients because outpatients generally are healthier and are on scheduled visits. Nevertheless, you should also monitor patients' circumstances for nonphysical, potentially interfering problems (e.g., a patient may have lost her or his car keys in the waiting room, may have just received a disturbing telephone call, or may be worried that the babysitter will have to leave before she or he can get home). With all patients, you should determine if pressing needs might require a brief delay in the interview (e.g., the need to use the bathroom or to get a drink of water). These courtesies not only help the patient directly, but they also enhance the patient's acceptance of you as a caring professional. Once the patient is ready, some obvious actions improve the patient's readiness and privacy, including shutting a door or respectfully excusing a curious laboratory technician.

Remove Barriers to Communication

You may have to turn off a noisy air conditioner or TV set or make efforts that require more insight, such as recognizing that the patient hears best out of one ear or that she or he needs to be able to see your mouth directly in order to lip read. If any question exists in your mind, you should inquire, "Can you hear me and see me ok?" Strategies for addressing specific communication problems are outlined in Chapter 6.

Ensure Comfort and Put the Patient at Ease

When interviewing, you should determine if anything at the immediate time is interfering with the patient's comfort. Questions like "Is that a comfortable chair (bed) for you?" "Is the light bothering your eyes?" or "Can I raise the head of the bed?" are essential. In turn, you must continue to monitor the patient's state as the interview proceeds. Our task as clinicians is to put the patient as much at ease as we can. Attention to these problems not only helps the patient and allows her or his subsequent full attention but also bespeaks our professionalism and concern.

When, as is normal, no such interfering problems need to be addressed, conducting a light conversation to put the patient at ease is appropriate, as the preceding discussions would have done for patients with some problems. You may be ready to start; but the patient often is not, and he or she still does not know much about the interviewer. This conversation should have a patient focus (e.g., "I hope you got your car parked ok with all the construction going on around here."). With an inpatient, you might inquire about the care or the food. Whatever is appropriate to the patient's situation can be briefly discussed. This helps the patient get used to talking and also allows her or him to learn what you are like. A caring, friendly atmosphere is established.

Obtaining the Agenda (Chief Complaint and Other Current Concerns) (Step 2)

In Step 2, the interviewer takes charge and focuses the patient on the agenda, just as he or she did in setting the stage for the interview. Although it is interviewer-originated, the action is patient-centered because it establishes a patient-centered atmosphere. Research shows that doctors often do not elicit the expectations that patients have for their visits (13,14), typically because they begin to explore a problem in detail before hearing all the patient's concerns (15). Agenda setting takes little time, improves efficiency, and yields increased data (15). However, it is not as easy as Step 1, and serious pitfalls arise if it is conducted improperly. *It usually takes no more than 1 minute, but it can take longer if many problems are present.* The following substeps, summarized in Table 3.2, are usually performed in the order in which they are given.

TABLE 3.2. CHIEF COMPLAINT AND AGENDA SETTING (STEP 2)

1. Indicate time available.
2. Indicate own needs.
3. Obtain list of all issues patient wants to discuss (e.g., specific symptoms, requests, expectations, understanding).
4. Summarize and finalize the agenda; negotiate specifics if too many items on the agenda.

Indicate Time Available

Begin by indicating how much time is available for the interaction, although setting limits often is difficult for interviewers. Doing so lets the patient know whether she or he has 10 minutes or 60 minutes and helps her or him gauge what and how much to say (16).

Indicate Own Needs

As an interviewer, you should also indicate your own professional demands, such as whether you need to ask many questions to get a full history and to perform a physical examination with a new patient or if you need to follow up on a recent cholesterol test in a return patient.

Obtain a List of All Issues the Patient Wants to Discuss

Most importantly, you as an interviewer must obtain a list of all the issues that your patient wants to discuss (17,18). You can begin, for example, by covering the preceding two items and then can start on this one with a new clinic patient by saying, "We've got about 40 minutes today, and I need to ask a lot of questions and do an examination. But, more importantly, I'd like to know what you want to cover."

You want the patient to enumerate all his or her problems. Then they won't arise at the end when time has already run out (15,16,19). If too many issues are raised for this visit, you and the patient can prioritize which ones are most important (these are not always the first ones that are given) (20).

Enumeration should go beyond symptoms and should include the patient's requests (e.g., prescription for a sedative), expectations (e.g., get sick leave), and understanding about what the interaction is supposed to accomplish (e.g., perform a treadmill test). Asking once is not sufficient (21); rather, you should carefully probe for additional issues of concern and should try to learn what is most important to the patient and why he or she came at this particular time. You need to ask, "What else?" "Anything else?" "How did you hope I could help?" or "What would a good result from this visit today look like?" For patients to have just one issue is unusual; more likely, they will have three to five. Careful agenda setting forestalls the common patient complaint that he or she didn't get to talk about all his or her concerns, as well as the common physician complaint that the patient voiced his or her most serious concern at the end of the appointment.

Although I have discussed the content of agenda setting, we must next consider how to perform it. At this point, as an interveiwer, you want a list. Indeed, you should avoid details of any particular problem until the list is completed. This can be difficult because patients, understandably, often want to go right into details. When this happens, you must respectfully interrupt the patient and refocus on the list. Holding up your fingers prominently and counting the problems identified can help. For example, while holding up one finger to signify the first problem given, you might say, "Sorry to interrupt; we'll get back to the leg pain. First, I need to know if there is a second problem you'd like to talk about. I want to be certain we know what all your concerns are." You often have to do this several times as patients may give many problems and may want to discuss each as it arises.

You should encourage further discussion while setting the agenda only if the patient has raised highly charged emotional material (e.g., if the patient is acutely distraught about a recent death in the family or about a recent cancer diagnosis). Even in most emotionally charged situations, however, the agenda usually can be set and the emotional material can be delayed briefly.

Summarize and Finalize Agenda

Usually, covering all problems is possible; in that case, they would be simply summarized. This also is a good time to determine which complaint is most important, if you do not already know. Doing this identifies the chief complaint. When too many issues have been raised for just one visit, you and the patient negotiate and agree on what will be addressed and when you will consider the deferred issues.

We will now follow Mrs. Joanne Jones through her initial visit by providing a continuous transcript for each step. Later, as noted, some areas are shortened for space considerations.

Vignette of Mrs. Jones

Step 1

DOC: (enters examining room and shakes hands) Welcome to the clinic, Mrs. Jones. I'm Ms. White, the medical student who will be working with you along with Dr. Black. I'll be getting much of the information about you and will be in close contact with you about our findings and your subsequent care.

[The student welcomed the patient, used her name, and identified herself and her role.]

PT: Hi. This is my first time here.

DOC: If it's ok with you, I'll close this door so we can hear each other better and have some privacy.

[The student ensured readiness for the interview and established as much privacy as possible.]

PT: Sure, that's fine.

DOC: Anything I can help with before we get started?

PT: Well, they didn't give my registration card back to me. I don't want to lose it.

DOC: We'll give that back when we're finished today. They always keep them. Anything else?

PT: No.

DOC: You may want to sit in that chair. It's more comfortable than the examining table.

[The student has noticed no barriers to communication and now ensures comfort and puts the patient at ease.]

PT: Sure. Thanks. (She moves.)

DOC: Well, I'm glad to see you made it despite the snow. I thought spring was here last week.

PT: I guess not. My kids have been home the last 2 days. I'm ready to get them back to school! I'm getting spoiled with them both in school.

DOC: People have had all kinds of trouble getting in here for their appointments since the snow. It's no fun.

PT: You're telling me. I don't even ski!

[The student has set the stage, a light conversation has occurred, and the patient is joking.]

Step 2

DOC: (laughs) Well, we've got about 40 minutes today, and I know I've got a lot of questions to ask and that we need to do a physical exam. Before we get started, though, it's most important to find out what you wanted to cover today. You know, so we're sure everything gets covered.

[The student has given her agenda in one statement. Doing this, she first models the more difficult task to follow: obtaining the patient's agenda.]

PT: It's these headaches. They start behind my eye and then I get sick to my stomach so I can't even work. My boss is really getting upset with me. He thinks that I don't have anything wrong with me and says he's going to report me. Well, he's not really my boss, but rather is . . . (student interrupts)

DOC: That sounds difficult and really important. Before we get into the details, though, I'd like to find out if there are any other problems you'd like to look at today, so we can be certain to cover everything you want. We'll get back to the headache and your boss after that. That's two things (holding up two fingers). Is there anything else?

PT: Well, I wanted to find out about this cold that doesn't seem to go away. I've been coughing for 3 weeks.

DOC: (holding up three fingers now) Anything else you want to look at today?

PT: No. Well, I did want to find out if I need any medicine for my colitis. That's doing ok now but I've had real trouble in the past. My parents were very upset about that. It started bothering me way back in 1982 and I've had trouble off and on. I used to take cortisone and . . . (student interrupts)

[The student has now interrupted her twice in order to complete the list of complaints. Done respectfully, this was necessary to complete the agenda in a timely way.]

DOC: (holding up five fingers) So there are two more problems we can look into, the colitis and the medications. We'll get back to all these soon; they're all important. To make sure we get all your questions covered, though, is there anything else?

PT: No. The headache is the main thing.

DOC: So, we want to cover the headaches and the problem they cause at work, cough, colitis, and the medications for the colitis. Is that right?

[Here, the patient and interviewer would negotiate what to cover at this visit if the interviewer determined that the patient had raised too many issues to cover on this visit.]

PT: That's about it.

DOC: And, do I understand correctly that the headache is the worst problem?

[Mrs. Jones' headache was her most bothersome complaint, which we defined earlier as the chief complaint.]

PT: Yes.

Opening the History of the Present Illness (Step 3)

After setting the stage (Step 1) and obtaining the agenda (Step 2), we, as interviewers, now become truly patient-centered and incorporate the facilitating skills learned in the last chapter to begin the History of the Present Illness (HPI). As was reviewed in Chapter 1, the HPI is the most important component of the interview because it reflects the patient's current problem in its personal and medical totality. The HPI begins during the patient-centered process and continues as the first part of the doctor-centered process, as relevant details are clarified.

Step 3, summarized in Table 3.3, is quite brief; it establishes an easy flow of talk from the patient, conveys that the doctor will listen, and gives a feel for "what the patient is like." Ordinarily, *this step lasts no more that 15 to 30 seconds, during which the interviewer listens attentively,* using the following substeps.

TABLE 3.3. OPENING THE HISTORY OF PRESENT ILLNESS (STEP 3)

1. Ask an open-ended beginning question.
2. Use "nonfocusing" open-ended skills (attentive listening): silence, neutral utterances, nonverbal encouragement.
3. Obtain additional data from nonverbal sources: nonverbal cues, physical characteristics, autonomic changes, accouterments, and environment.

Open-Ended Beginning Question

Immediately after summarizing the agenda, you, as an interviewer, should use an open-ended beginning question, such as "Given what you've told me, how are you doing?" "How are things going?" or "Now, tell me some more." You should link the question to the agenda to start developing the patient's story. When she or he has raised strong but deferred emotional material during the agenda-setting, you should specifically direct the patient back to it (e.g., "Now, you mentioned that you're upset about your daughter moving."). A good beginning question, as is befitting to its nonfocusing intent, allows the patient to go anywhere, from past to present to future, and can concern anybody or anything.

You should initially avoid framing the question in a way that specifies the patient's problem (e.g., "Now, what about the chest pain?" or "What about the trouble with your wife?"). Only if the patient continues to ask (e.g., to clarify the question), should you provide such instruction. For example, in response to the query, "What do you mean?" or "You mean about my chest pain?", the interviewer can initially reply "Whatever you like" or "Whatever is most important to you." The intent of the patient-centered interview is to allow free discussion, but, at the same time, you do not want to puzzle the patient or to make her or him uncomfortable.

This open-ended beginning question is not always necessary. Once the agenda has been completed, especially if only one or a few related items need to be covered, many patients continue spontaneously.

"Nonfocusing" Open-Ended Skills (Attentive Listening)

As an interviewer, you encourage a continued free flow of information after asking the open-ended beginning question by using the nonfocusing open-ended skills described in Chapter 2. Silence, nonverbal gestures (eye contact, attentive behavior, hand gestures), and neutral utterances ("Uh-huh", "Mmm") encourage the patient. If the patient does not talk freely, you can use the focusing open-ended skills (echoing, request, summary) to promote a free flow of information (i.e., you should not continue just to sit in silence and to appear attentive with a patient who is not talking). If focusing open-ended skills are not effective, closed-ended questions about the patient's problem can be used to get a dialog going; this is rare.

Obtain Additional Data From Nonverbal Sources

Although you are passive verbally during the brief Step 3, you should be very active mentally; you should be thinking about what the information means. You also observe the patient for nonverbal cues, reviewed further in Chapter 7 (e.g, depressed facies, arms folded across chest, tapping toes nervously). You will note clues in the following areas that will give additional information about the patient (22,23): (a) *physical characteristics*: general health, skin and hair color and odor, deformities, and habitus (e.g., emaciated and disheveled, "uremic" breath, jaundice, amputated leg, kyphoscoliosis); (b) *autonomic changes*: heart rate, skin color, pupil size, skin moisture, and skin temperature (e.g., rapid pulsation of the carotid artery observed in the neck, handshake reveals cold and moist palms, pupils constricted but then dilate when relaxed, sweating at outset of interview); (c) *accouterments:* clothing, jewelry, eyeglasses, and make-up (e.g., expensive suit and jewelry, thick eyeglasses, no make-up); (d) *environment:* decorations, greeting cards, flowers, and photographs (e.g., in a hospital setting—several paintings by a grandchild, photograph of spouse, no greeting cards or flowers).

Patients seldom show emotion in this early period, but, if it is strongly expressed, you address it as explained later. Otherwise, you simply observe where the patient is going and how the emotion fits with the rest of the evolving material. The type of data that is produced makes no difference. As long as a good flow of information occurs, either symptoms (of possible disease) or personal data are acceptable.

Continuation of Vignette of Mrs. Jones

(immediately continuous with the previous vignette)

PT: Yes.

DOC: So, that's a lot going on. How are you doing with it?

[A good open-ended beginning that is linked to the agenda allows the patient to go anywhere she wants.]

PT: Oh, ok I guess.

DOC: (silence)

PT: At least now.

DOC: (sits forward slightly) Uh huh.

PT: Things weren't so good last week, though, when I made the appointment.

DOC: Mmmm.

PT: That's when my boss really got on me. Well, he's kind of uptight anyway, but he was saying how I was upsetting the whole office operation because I was off so much. And someone had to cover for me. I'm the lead attorney.

DOC: I see.

PT: These headaches are right here (points at right temple) and just throb and throb. And I get sick to my stomach and just don't feel good. All I want to do is go home and go to bed.

[A good open-ended beginning, briefly followed by several 'nonfocusing' open-ended skills, resulted in a good flow of symptoms and personal data without any focusing activity by the student.]

Continuing the Patient-Centered History of Present Illness (Step 4)

The much longer Step 4—*it usually takes between 5 and 10 minutes*—is summarized in Table 3.4 and follows immediately after Step 3. The intent changes from simply establishing a flow of information to focusing very actively on the most important story theme(s). In general, clinicians and students usually obtain first a description of the *physical* symptoms; second, the patient's *personal* but nonemotional reactions attending the physical symptoms; and, third, the patient's *emotional* reactions to both.

TABLE 3.4. CONTINUING THE PATIENT-CENTERED HISTORY OF PRESENT ILLNESS (STEP 4)

A. **Physical Symptom Story**
1. Obtain description of the physical symptoms (focusing open-ended skills).
B. **Personal Story**
2. Develop the more general personal/psychosocial context of the physical symptoms (focusing open-ended skills).
C. **Emotional Story**
3. Develop an emotional focus (emotion-seeking skills).
4. Address the emotion(s) (emotion-handling skills).
D. **Expand Story**
5. Expand the story to new chapters (focused open-ended skills, emotion-seeking skills, emotion-handling skills).

As clinicians and students, we use the focusing open-ended skills, emotion-seeking skills, and emotion-handling skills outlined in the last chapter to identify the story theme(s) and, occasionally, the closed-ended skills for clarification. We are much more active and participatory in our verbal interaction and are often figuratively on the edge of our seat during the give-and-take interaction between ourselves and the patient. The new learner may find that this step is the most difficult of the entire interview. To help in her or his understanding, I have broken Step 4 into five substeps, which will now be considered in their usual sequence. These substeps produce the overarching story themes, which are physical, personal, and emotional.

Physical Symptom Story

Obtain a Description of the Physical Symptoms

In a medical setting, patients typically present their physical symptoms mixed with their personal context. Because most patients expect the following, I recommend an initial focus on physical symptoms while you are learning these skills; later, you can experiment with a different order. You should concentrate on the symptoms, using the focusing open-ended skills (echoing, open-ended requests, summarizing). This produces a description in the patient's own words of the immediate context in which the physical symptoms occurred. As an example, we pick up Mrs. Jones' interview again.

Continuation of Vignette of Mrs. Jones

PT: . . . All I want to do is go home and go to bed.

DOC: Say more about the headaches.

[An open-ended request, one of the focusing open-ended skills, to learn more about the headaches]

PT: Well, I never had any trouble until I got here.

[Comment about the present context of her symptom and how long it has been present]

DOC: How long has that been?

[Appropriate closed-ended question for clarification]

PT: Only 4 months. The headaches started about 3 months ago.

DOC: Tell me more.

[Keeps the focus on the headaches]

PT: Well, they just throb and throb and it seems like every time I see my boss, I get one of these headaches. I sometimes just get a little nauseated and can't concentrate because of the pain.

[The student learns much more of the description of the symptom and, also, that her boss seems to precipitate the symptom.]

DOC: Your boss.

[Echoing puts the focus on how her boss relates to the headache.]

PT: Well, I have no trouble at all when he's not there. He was gone for 2 weeks and I didn't have any. But he's there a lot, although I don't have to be around him all the time.

[The relationship between Mrs. Jones' headaches and her boss is becoming clearer.]

DOC: Not around him?

[Echoing, a focusing open-ended skill, maintains the focus.]

PT: I'm on the road a lot. No trouble then either, I guess. Except once when he called me.

[The student has a good description of the physical symptom, knows when it began, has heard some associated symptoms, and knows that it occurs in the setting of her boss. In less than a minute, she has learned how the personal and physical interact by facilitating (encouraging) the patient's spontaneous narration. The description of the pain in this vignette has considerable diagnostic value (for migraine headaches) and also raises some considerations for treatment (e.g., avoiding her boss). Such unique data often do not arise during isolated doctor-centered interviewing. Although the reference to her boss is psychosocial material, which I focus on more in the next substep, it also is directly related to the symptom and provides its immediate context. The next substep shows that the psychosocial data no longer directly relate to the physical symptoms.]

This detailed, personal description of symptoms and their immediate context is what you, as the interviewer, want at the outset of Step 4, and it seldom takes more than a minute. In the example, the student now understands, in the patient's own words, much of the chronology of symptoms and their descriptive terms (throbbing headache and nausea) that she will expand later in the doctor-centered process, in addition to the unique personal context in which the symptoms occur. She knows that she needs more diagnostic data about a possible underlying disease (e.g., any head injury, fever, or prior investigation?), but that would insert new information, and besides, she will do just that in 5 to 10 minutes when she switches to the doctor-centered process. By avoiding a focus on the symptoms that inserts information that was not introduced by the patient or on other diagnostic data via the use of closed-ended questions (e.g., "Did you ever have a head injury?" or "How does the headache affect your vision?"), the student has learned who else is involved, what the patient thinks, and generally what is going on in the patient's life. She already has an explanation for her headaches and knows what is most bothersome to Mrs. Jones.

Although the beginning student may not be aware of this, others will realize that the physical symptom data given by Mrs. Jones are quite suggestive of migraine headaches (i.e., they are throbbing, periodic, and associated with nausea). **Highly diagnostic data for the patient's underlying disease almost always arise during the detailed description of symptoms (24).** Indeed, the great diagnostic yield here was what reportedly led Sir William Osler to say, "Listen to the patient, he is telling you the diagnosis" (25). **Research has also shown that, occasionally, data diagnostic of a disease arise here that do** *not* **arise in later doctor-centered interviewing (24).** On the other hand, even when symptom data are not diagnostic, the interviewer obtains in this step a good overview of the problem, one that does not need to be repeated when he or she switches to the doctor-centered process.

The symptoms are treated in the same way if only psychological complaints are seen (i.e., no physical symptoms are presented). In the above case, the interviewer should determine the personal description and immediate context of these symptoms with open-ended queries if Mrs. Jones complains of anxiety or feeling blue instead of the headaches.

In this step, the interviewer thus hears the patient's own description of the symptom data. Here the initial integration of symptoms and personal factors occurs; this represents the first view of the patient's mind–body connection. This integration is the core of the interview and of the patient-centered process. Most subsequent information in the HPI links to this core.

Personal Story

Develop the More General Personal and Psychosocial Context of the Physical Symptoms

As an interviewer, you should next learn about the patient and her or his illness in its broader personal and psychosocial context. This material relates less to the symptoms and may be of less diagnostic value for disease but is nevertheless important for an understanding of the illness. In general, the longer the interview is, the less the personal data relate to symptoms and the more they reflect the patient's general life situation. Nonetheless, important diagnostic data about actual diseases can still arise (e.g., clues to occupational or to drug or alcohol problems). These data directly influence treatment and prevention programs. You should continue to rely on focusing open-ended skills, directing them to the patient's personal statements that seem most important to understanding the personal story; in our example, Mrs. Jones' stressful job situation would be considered worthy of this exploration.

Direct Continuation of Vignette of Mrs. Jones

PT: I'm on the road a lot. No trouble then either, except one time when he called me.

DOC: Tell me more about your boss.

[The interviewer is encouraging discussion of an important personal issue rather than just keeping the focus on physical symptoms such as headache or nausea; she also could have focused on the job itself and accomplished the same goal of obtaining more personal data. Rather than making an open-ended request, she alternatively could have focused the patient by echoing ('he called you') or summarizing the personal aspects—any of the focusing open-ended skills could be used as they all lead to the same theme.]

PT: Well, he's been there a long time and I've replaced him in every way there is, except he is still in charge, at least in his title. He yells at everybody. Nobody likes him and he doesn't do much. That's why they got me in there, the Board, so something would get done. These headaches have all come since I got this job—right here. They throb behind my eye and . . .

[Note the corroboration of earlier data: the job is linked to the headaches, but Mrs. Jones is now giving additional personal information about her situation that helps the interviewer better understand this connection.]

DOC: Wait a second, I'm not following you. You say he's in charge, but you are the lead attorney?

[The student interrupted respectfully and then summarized personal issues to refocus on the job because the patient was getting away from personal data and was going back to physical symptoms that have already been discussed; also, she plans to address symptom details about 5 to 10 minutes from this point during the doctor-centered process.]

PT: Yeah, they are phasing him out but he's still there in the meantime. Who knows how long it'll take? I hope I last.

[She is further expanding the story to personal issues that are less directly related to symptoms, allowing the student to begin to appreciate the nuances and depth of how her job and headaches interact.]

DOC: Hope you last?

[Echoing maintains the focus in this personal and psychosocial area. Note how focusing open-ended skills are used repeatedly to focus the patient and that they can be applied to the patient's immediately preceding utterances. The interviewer can also interrupt the patient to focus on others that were previously mentioned, but she or he should never introduce new data to the conversation.]

PT: I'm not sure how much of this I can take. They said there wouldn't be any problem with him and that he would be helpful. Actually, I kind of liked him at first but then all . . .

DOC: They said? Who are they?

[The student interrupted to focus on a bit of information mentioned just before and to redirect her to that with echoing; if she had wanted her to simply proceed, an open-ended request, such as 'Go on,' would have sufficed.]

PT: The Board, they run the company. It's not real big, but it's a good chance for someone young like me to get experience in corporate stuff.

[This adds a new layer of data that is not directly related to her headache but that provides a deeper understanding of the context.]

DOC: Sounds like the Board told you one thing, that you liked him at first, but then he changed, and you're left with a problem?

[The student summarizes what is becoming a free flow of personal data. This was abbreviated for space reasons, but she ordinarily would further develop this with more focusing open-ended inquiry.]

Patients do not always refer to stressful events in their lives, as Mrs. Jones did in this example; but they often have personal concerns about the symptom itself. Although no disease explanation is found for 20% to 75% of physical symptoms (26,27), patients exhibit several personal concerns around their physical symptoms with high rates of frequency: 67% worry about serious illness, 72% expect medications, 67% want testing, 53% expect referral, and 62% indicate interference with routine activities. Although 47%, like Mrs. Jones, describe stress and about 20% recognize depression and anxiety, only 1% consider the problem psychiatric (28). Usually, doctors view symptoms as far less serious than the patients themselves do; therefore, not surprisingly, residual unaddressed concerns account for most patient dissatisfaction (28). Other concerns include disbelief or distrust of the medical system, grief and other losses, becoming independent (young people) or dependent (older or seriously ill people), retirement, family or job problems, and administrative issues (e.g., insurance forms). **As clinicians, we want to understand these personal concerns, which are the context of our patients' physical symptoms.** In general, whether stress or disease worries, a personal focus is easily established as we move into the broader personal context of the patient's illness. A sense of the patient's personal situation has begun to develop.

To maintain the personal focus, as the interviewer, you should avoid focusing back on previously discussed physical symptoms. You will focus on physical symptoms when moving to the doctor-centered interview in the next 5 to 10 minutes. First, however, you want to expand your understanding of the patient as a person.

Patients occasionally give their story without much facilitation. Usually, however, they give small bits of personal information, one at a time, as though testing the water to see if you are interested, comfortable, and willing to follow them into what is often new material. Because of this step-by-step unfolding of the story, you must use the focusing open-ended skills repeatedly to draw out the underlying narrative thread.

Early on, you should focus on and facilitate whatever bits of personal data appear to be of most interest to both the patient and you. Once you have identified the narrative thread of the patient's story and its apparent meaning and significance, you should stay with this line. If the patient gets away from this theme, you should interrupt with focusing open-ended skills and should refocus on the main story thread. Such refocusing often helps because patients wander back to previously discussed physical symptoms (or other diagnostic or therapeutic data).

After no more than a few minutes, you usually have a good sense of the broader personal story—and you have further enhanced the doctor–patient relationship by addressing features of central importance to the patient's life. If emotions become evident during these early stages, you often should address them.

Emotional Story

Develop an Emotional Focus

Just as you seek to understand the personal context of the symptoms, you should now explore the emotional context of the personal and physical symptom information. This further deepens the story and makes apparent a three-way interaction among the symptom, personal, and emotional dimensions. **The mind–body link and biopsychosocial description come into full focus when we as clinicians include the emotions, an event thereby of scientific as well as humanistic significance.**

In developing an emotional focus, you should always monitor the patient's readiness to engage in this sometimes more stressful discussion by observing how well he or she has responded to the process so far and for any untoward responses to inquiries about emotion (e.g., changing the subject after the interviewer asks about them).

As an interviewer, you must first change the style of inquiry to establish an emotional focus (29). Emotion-seeking skills, both direct and indirect, temporarily supplement the focusing open-ended skills. By starting with direct inquiry about how a patient feels concerning the personal situation that she or he has so far described (e.g., "How'd that make you feel?"), you can fully and actively explore the emotional domain. Sometimes, you must make several efforts before emotion can be expressed. As I have noted, you should avoid making the patient uncomfortable. Indirect questioning using self-disclosure and inquiry methods about the patient's beliefs and their impact also may be necessary; this is used when direct inquiry does not reveal emotional content.

In addition, you should continue to expand your understanding of the emotions, once they have been identified, by using focusing open-ended skills. You do this until you feel that you have a reasonable understanding of the emotion and what produced it.

You do not need to use emotion-seeking skills when the patient is already showing or expressing emotions, as some do spontaneously following open-ended inquiry alone.

Continuation of Vignette of Mrs. Jones

DOC: Sounds like the Board told you one thing, that you liked him at first, but then he changed, and you're left with a problem?

PT: Yeah, sounds kind of bad, huh?

DOC: How do you feel about that?

[Direct emotion-seeking]

PT: Oh, I don't know. The headache is what bothers me.

DOC: But how do you feel, you know personally, your emotions?

[The patient did not give any emotion the first time, and so the interviewer uses direct emotion-seeking inquiry again. To "push" like this can be appropriate as long as you are always monitoring the patient's response and readiness to engage at an emotional level.]

PT: Oh, nothing really bothers me that much. We were taught to turn the other cheek.

DOC: You know, an old boss of mine once put me in a bind like this. It took me quite awhile but I finally realized I was very upset.

[The interviewer changes her strategy and pushes further using self-disclosure, which, of course, must be accurate and genuine.]

PT: Well, yeah, I guess I am too, now that you mention it.

DOC: What is the feeling?

[The patient has acknowledged her emotion, but the interviewer, pushing further to get the full picture, returns to a direct emotion-seeking question about feeling.]

PT: Well, I just want to throw something at him. He makes me so mad. I didn't do anything against him. I work really hard there, and things are going much better since I've been there. It's when I get mad that the headaches come. The nausea is even worse, and then sometimes I get these spots in my eyes and . . .

[A more precise direct link to headaches, now not just to her job situation but more specifically to being angry. Note the value of pushing for emotion: the patient is now expressing it.]

DOC: So you get mad when he gets on you?

[The student is interspersing open-ended skills, which is appropriate, as she summarizes to continue on this focus.]

Address the Emotion

When emotions have been expressed, either spontaneously during open-ended inquiry or via the interviewer's use of emotion-seeking skills, and the interviewer understands them, yet another set of skills becomes more important temporarily. As was discussed in Chapter 2, the emotion-handling skills consist of Naming, Understanding, Respecting, and Supporting and are recalled by the mnemonic NURS.

To address an emotion, as an interviewer, you should convey that you have recognized it by naming it, that you understand it, that you respect the patient's plight (or joy), and that you are available to help in any way possible. These skills often are needed several times during the course of an interview as people may take considerable time to work through strong emotional reactions. Using these skills once is seldom enough.

Occasionally, you will use all four emotion-handling skills together in the order given. Usually, however, you will use only one or two skills at one time. You should use them selectively and should fit them smoothly and unobtrusively into the conversation because excessive use will stand out and will strike the patient as peculiar or manipulative.

Emotion-handling skills are used only after you have heard enough to understand the emotion adequately. For example, when someone expresses sadness over loss of a spouse, you cannot immediately say that you understand and appreciate how difficult the situation is. You must first listen to enough of the story open-endedly to be able to make these emotion-handling statements legitimately. On the other hand, with reticent patients, you may have to use emotion-handling skills with much less emotional information than you would normally consider desirable. For instance, you would still use the NURS quartet actively with a very reticent patient who has lost her or his job and who only acknowledges being "slightly upset."

Some interviewers resist the use of emotion-seeking and emotion-handling skills, usually because of unfamiliarity. They remark that **these skills seem forced and false** at first. For those who respond this way, **I recommend only that they try** and that they **review the compelling scientific rationale for using them** that was presented in Chapter 2 (see "Relationship-Building Skills"). Their use will indeed feel awkward and phony at first for some; however, as interviewers overcome their self-consciousness, gain confidence, and observe the benefit to their patients, they often become rapid converts. They also recognize that they themselves feel progressively more comfortable with the process, and that their responses begin to feel quite genuine. Many experienced clinicians have had to overcome these same reservations. Because emotions are a basic means of human expression (see Chapter 2), effective relationships with patients are more likely when emotion-seeking and emotion-handling skills are used, as my work and that of others has shown (1,4,29–31).

Continuation of Vignette of Mrs. Jones

DOC: So you get mad when he gets on you?

PT: Yeah, he really gets me mad. I just get so furious I could scream sometimes. (clenches fist and strikes table firmly)

DOC: It sure makes sense. It seems like you've done so much there to help, and all you get is grief from him. I appreciate the way you're able to talk about it. He sure gets you mad.

[The student briefly expressed her understanding and spent more time expressing respect for her by acknowledging that she had been through a lot and that she was successful at work and in praising her for talking about her emotions. Finally, the student again names the emotion; she continues to use Mrs. Jones' term—'mad'—rather than 'anger' or another more loaded term.]

PT: He sure does. Just talking about it gets me upset and gives me a headache, right now.

[This further demonstrates the association between the headaches and emotional upset; it is now occurring as a result of anger-laden material in the interview.]

DOC: I can imagine. You've put up with a lot.

[Naming 'mad' again is unnecessary because the emotion is obvious, but the interviewer again indicated understanding and made a respecting statement.]

PT: You know, I think I'm even madder at that damn Board. They didn't tell me any of this and said everything would be ok. Who needs all this?

[As a result of addressing her emotions, the patient is now presenting new personal data and its associated emotional material; that is, the story is deepening.]

DOC: That's a tough situation.

[Interviewer again demonstrated respect.]

The first part of Figure 3.1 summarizes the critical dimensions of the first chapter of the patient's story we have just reviewed in Step 4: we begin with a physical symptom focus and then proceed to a personal, nonemotional focus and, finally, we elicit and address the patient's emotion. As you will learn next, subsequent chapters of the patient's story, also shown in Figure 3.1, usually do not include a somatic focus and, rather, concern just the personal and emotional aspects of the story.

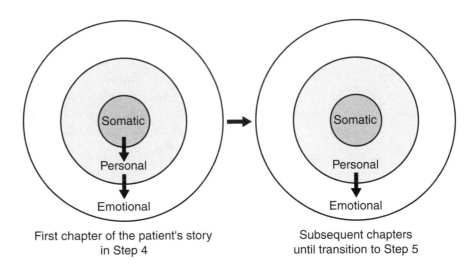

FIGURE 3.1. Somatic, personal, and emotional relationships of chapters of the patient's story in Step 4.

Expand the Story

Expand the Story to New Chapters

We now review the sequence of skills that have been outlined so far in Step 4: focusing open-ended skills, followed by emotion-seeking skills, followed by emotion-handling skills. This typically produces the beginning of the story, but it is still incomplete. To develop the story further requires the repetitive, cyclic use of this sequence of facilitating skills. Each cycle produces a deeper level of the story (i.e., another chapter). Personal data and their associated emotions evolve in parallel, and neither is more important than the other. **This deepening of the narrative thread occurs because emotion-handling skills have a powerful facilitative effect on the patient's subsequent expression of new nonemotional, personal information.** The interviewer can then return to open-ended inquiry to develop the newly evolving, deeper thread of the story for a while; later, he or she returns to emotion-seeking and emotion-handling skills to develop the emotional dimension of the new data. This continues until she or he is satisfied with the depth of the story. This self-reinforcing effect of patients' psychological statements and emotions is key for obtaining the full psychological and emotional story. The interviewer cannot focus on just the psychological or just the emotional aspect. One supplies the context for the other, and both are developed nearly simultaneously in a progressive unfolding of the narrative theme. **However, the interviewer does not usually return to a physical focus;** rather, he or she prefers to remain in the personal, emotional realm to develop these areas better.

The story develops spontaneously as the interviewer repeatedly cycles among focusing open-ended, emotion-seeking, and emotion-handling skills. As the patient becomes comfortable in expressing emotion, fewer of the emotion-seeking skills are needed; at this stage, emotion-handling and focusing open-ended skills are alternately used, taking the patient quickly to progressively deeper levels of her or his story (see Figure 3-1).

In developing the story, you as the interviewer always will have ideas (hypotheses) about what it implies. However, paradoxically and distinct from the doctor-centered process, you do not ask directly about a hypothesis until it has first been mentioned by the patient. For example, if you think a patient's story about disliking a woman who "looks like my wife" means that the patient dislikes his wife, you cannot ask directly, "Do you not like your wife?" because that question inserts new data (dislike of wife) into the conversation. Rather, you must get the patient to raise this issue himself (e.g., by saying, "Tell me more about your wife."). The hypothesis-testing process is analogous to dancing. Although the patient leads the dance, once the patient has led the conversation to a specific place, you can maintain a focus on that spot. This is how we as interviewers test specific hypotheses: we focus, first open-endedly and then emotionally, on the area where the answer to the hypothesis lies.

Continuation of Vignette of Mrs. Jones

DOC: . . . That's a tough situation.

PT: You know the head of the Board even told me my boss is a good guy who was looking forward to me coming so he could retire!

DOC: The head of the Board?

[The interviewer shifts away from emotion handling to focusing open-ended inquiry with echoing to get what appears to be new information about the situation. This will start a new cycle of active open-ended, emotion-seeking, and emotion-handling skills.]

PT: She's the one who recruited me here. I could have gone to a couple other places but came here because she convinced me it was such a good chance for me.

DOC: Sounds like you didn't get a full picture of this place?

[The student uses focusing open-ended summary and is still trying to learn more new information.]

PT: Yeah, it's not really fair.

DOC: How's that make you feel?

[Now she is back to emotion with a direct emotion-seeking inquiry.]

PT: Well, I must sound kind of stupid, and I feel kind of sheepish. But mostly I'm just mad.

DOC: It makes sense to me, but I don't understand why you feel sheepish. You did everything that you could.

[She moves back to emotion-handling skills with an understanding statement and a respect statement. Notice how open-ended and relationship-building skills are interwoven to generate both nonemotional data and emotions. Notice also that the interviewer can indicate lack of understanding and can ask for clarification.]

PT: Yeah, I guess, but I still feel kind of dumb.

DOC: Dumb?

[She uses echoing. An obvious story is already present, but she is exploring further by again moving away from emotion.]

PT: That's what my mother used to say, that I was smart but dumb. You know what I mean?

DOC: Smart with books but not so much with people?

[She uses a combination of a summary and an educated guess.]

PT: Yeah, maybe she's right.

DOC: How'd that feel, when she'd say that?

[She moves back to emotion with direct emotion-seeking.]

PT: Mad! Seems like a pattern, huh? And I used to get headaches as a kid too when she'd get on me. I'd forgotten that.

[This is additional supportive data about the association of headaches and anger.]

DOC: So that made you mad too. I'm impressed at how you're able to talk about it and put this together.

[The student uses a naming and a respecting statement. Depending on the length of time available, she could further address another obvious clue, the patient's mother, perhaps with an open-ended request, such as, "Tell me more about your mother." Note in this vignette that another cycle of focusing open-ended, emotion-seeking, and emotion-handling skills has been used to continue development of the story.]

PT: Well, I appreciate your saying that. Actually, it feels kind of good talking.

[A positive response to this interaction]

DOC: Say more about that.

[An open-ended request]

PT: Well, I just haven't talked much about it. My husband doesn't want to talk about it.

DOC: He doesn't want to talk?

[Echoing]

> **PT:** No. I think he feels bad because he thought this was the best place for me to come.
>
> **DOC:** I'm glad it's been helpful here. You've really been open.
>
> [A support statement that is followed by a respect statement. An obvious new area for further discussion, the patient's husband, has been introduced, and this could be pursued further if time allows. The patient also has referred positively to their present interaction; this often would be addressed further. Simply acknowledging it, as the student did in this case, is also appropriate. The patient's comment confirms their good relationship.]
>
> **PT:** Thanks. My headache's better now. It does help.

Because of the importance of the provider–patient relationship, the interviewer should often check with the patient to see how he or she feels the interaction is going. As an interviewer, you may inquire directly by saying something like, "So, how are we doing so far?" If you have been patient-centered, the response will usually be positive; you can simply acknowledge this (e.g., "Good. It seemed like things were going ok to me, but I wanted to check."). When the patient introduces the topic, as Mrs. Jones did in this example, this provides the answer about the relationship; a simple acknowledgment is adequate. Of course, if the patient raises problems with the interaction, you should address these (e.g., the patient indicates that he or she is becoming tired).

If an urgent personal problem exists, which can be easily determined in 5 to 10 minutes, the patient may require additional time or even immediate action. **In the absence of an urgent problem, as is the usual situation, the interviewer should begin to conclude this portion of the interview when she or he has an understanding—not of the entire story, but of the most salient, immediate aspects of the patient's story (i.e., the first few chapters).** Certainly, Mrs. Jones' story has more to it, but, given time constraints and lack of urgency, these areas can be explored another time, if they need to be at all. The student has a good understanding, and, more importantly, the patient feels understood, which is the essence of a good relationship (30).

The student still has not explored Mrs. Jones' colitis and recent cough. Usually, this is done later in the past medical history (PMH) unless the problem is urgent or is related to the chief complaint. During this portion of the interview, the student will obtain a personal description of these complaints and will address their broader personal context, just as she did with the headaches. Usually, however, no more than a few minutes are needed because these are less pressing and troubling.

Transition to the Doctor-Centered Process (Step 5)

At this point, the interviewer, realizing that she or he will soon enter a more doctor-controlled process, anticipates ending this section on a positive, supportive note. As an interviewer, you can weave the emotion-handling skills into the summary (substep 1) and can check the accuracy of the story (substep 2). Even in the most desperate situations, you can usually find something positive and supportive about the patient's situation and can provide some hope, even if it is only your personal support and availability.

TABLE 3.5. TRANSITION TO THE DOCTOR-CENTERED PROCESS (STEP 5)

1. Summarize briefly.
2. Check accuracy.
3. Indicate that both content and style of inquiry will change if the patient is ready.

Step 5 is summarized in Table 3.5; it *usually takes no more than 30 seconds*. In this step, the clinician warns the patient that the content and, more importantly, the patient-centered style of the interview are about to change (substep 3). Otherwise, the patient might be confused or taken aback by the doctor taking control in the doctor-centered style that follows.

Continuation of Vignette with Mrs. Jones

PT: Thanks. My headache's better now. It does help.

DOC: So, you're in a new job that hasn't worked out quite like you were led to believe and that has caused you to be somewhat upset with at least a couple people and to have quite bad headaches. Do you want to add anything?

[The interviewer summarizes nicely. A positive tone to the interaction already exists and nothing further is needed; if the patient were distraught or upset, she could highlight her and others' support.]

PT: No. I think you've pretty much got it.

DOC: If it's ok then, I'd like to shift gears and ask you some different types of questions about your headaches and colitis. I'll be asking a lot more questions about specifics.

[She is checking to make sure that it is satisfactory to change the subject; she is indicating what is going to occur.]

PT: Sure, that's what I came in for.

(Mrs. Jones' story continues in Chapter 5.)

Beyond Basic Interviewing

Using the techniques presented in this chapter, we as interviewers have already begun to develop a clear understanding of the patient as a complex, unique person. Focusing open-ended skills, emotion-seeking skills, and emotion-handling skills are essential vehicles for eliciting the required data, but they are just a few of the many tools in the experienced interviewer's armamentarium. Prejudices, time pressures, and preoccupation with other issues, for example, can interfere with hearing the patient's story. We, however, can offset these influences: we prepare for the interview by clearing ourselves, much as an athlete or musician might prepare for a performance (32). The student who is just learning should take care of pressing personal or professional issues beforehand, should relax and clear other issues from her or his mind, and should focus on the patient. This is especially important if he or she wants to listen at multiple levels (32,33), a skill that can be acquired over time as the basics described in this text become reflexive. Attention to multiple levels means that she or he goes beyond the obvious content and emotion presented by the patient to consider how the patient says something, what is left unsaid, and what is implied. To be able to do so requires attention to the subtleties of grammar, syntax, verb tense, changes of subject, nonverbal cues, incongruity in verbal and emotional content, and understanding of metaphors (32,34). Changes in these areas can then be addressed using the same basic skills (e.g., "What do you mean when you keep saying 'my daughter's father?'" or "I've noticed you often say, 'You can't win for losing.'") .

SUMMARY

The five steps and 21 substeps of the patient-centered process of integrated interviewing have been presented. Two preparatory steps, setting the stage (Step 1) and identifying the chief complaint and agenda (Step 2), exist. The truly patient-centered parts of the interview are opening the HPI (Step 3) and continuing the patient-centered HPI (Step 4), where almost all interaction occurs in the latter. The transition (Step 5) prepares the patient for the doctor-centered interview to follow. In conducting the more difficult Steps 3 and 4, the interviewer orchestrates (32) the patient's personal story using the following tools: nonfocusing and focusing open-ended inquiry, occasional closed-ended questions, emotion-seeking and emotion-handling skills, and hypothesis testing. The cyclic, integrated use of these facilitating skills produces successful patient-centered interviewing and constitutes all of the longest and most important step, Step 4. These are the tools that allow the interviewer to begin to understand the depths of the human condition.

Figure 3.2 summarizes the major events in the patient-centered interview. Usually, preparing the patient takes 1 to 2 minutes, eliciting the story (physical symptoms, personal data, and emotional data) takes 5 to 10 minutes, and making the transition takes 1 minute. The 5 to 10 minutes spent in the patient-centered process just described are easily learned and lead to the remarkable advantages described in Chapter 1 (see the "Rationale"), including improved patient satisfaction, decreased lawsuits, and improved health outcomes with problems such as diabetes and hypertension.

The student or clinician has conducted the most difficult part of the interview. The data generated are easily understood, and they usually describe the primary symptoms and their personal context. The mind–body connection is established, data that will lead to an integrated biopsychosocial story have begun to emerge, and, most importantly, the patient feels understood.

Overarching View of the Patient-Centered Interview

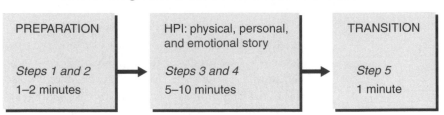

FIGURE 3.2. Overarching view of the patient-centered interview.

LEARNING EXERCISES

1. What is the truly patient-centered part of the 5-step method? What function do Steps 1 and 2 serve?
2. When is interrupting the patient appropriate?*
3. What types of concerns do patients with physical complaints have?
4. What skills are used almost entirely in the very brief Step 3?
5. Under what circumstances would you be likely not to address physical symptoms as the first order of business in Step 4?
6. What is the patient's personal and emotional response when a good relationship occurs?*

*Good test questions.

PRACTICE EXERCISES (LIKELY SPREAD OVER SEVERAL SESSIONS)

1. Practice Steps 1 and 2 together in role-play until you can do them and their six and four substeps, respectively, without looking at the book for recall. Work on simple opening statements for each step, including ways to incorporate several substeps in one sentence or so. See the vignette of Ms. Jones and the demonstration videotape (6).

2. When question #1 is mastered, practice Steps 1 to 5, covering all 21 substeps, together in role-play. Conduct the entire patient-centered interview in 15 minutes, spending about 1 minute each in Steps 1 to 3 and 5 and from 10 to 12 minutes in Step 4.

3. After you can complete all steps and substeps in role-play, conduct the same exercise with a real or simulated patient.

4. Watch for the following problems:
   a. Hurrying into the interview rather than engaging in some small talk to let the patient become accustomed to the setting.
   b. Allowing inefficient agenda-setting and omitting repeated 'what else' statements until you know all items the patient wants to discuss.
   c. Spending excessive time in Step 3, a 30- to 60-second step where you should simply listen attentively after an initial open-ended question.
   d. Not touching the key bases in Step 4: physical symptoms, personal concerns, and emotions.
   e. Not engaging in enough emotion-seeking.
   f. Not displaying enough NURS.
   g. Not signaling the transition adequately.

5. With time and practice, you will notice the following markers of success:
   a. Smooth, seamless flow of data.
   b. Understanding of mind–body links.
   c. An ability to focus wherever you wish.
   d. The ability to interrupt effectively and respectfully.
   e. Control of the interview.
   f. Skill in critiquing your own and others' interviews.
   g. Efficiency in the interview. Once facile with the five steps and 21 substeps, you will be able to conduct the patient-centered process in 5 to 10 minutes. With further mastery, you will be able to be equally effective in 3 to 5 minutes.

References

1. Smith RC, Lyles JS, Mettler J, et al. The effectiveness of intensive training for residents in interviewing. A randomized, controlled study. *Ann Intern Med* 1998; 128:118–126.
2. Smith RC, Mettler JA, Stoffelmayr BE, et al. Improving residents' confidence in using psychosocial skills. *J Gen Intern Med* 1995;10:315–320.
3. Smith RC, Lyles JS, Mettler JA, et al. A strategy for improving patient satisfaction by the intensive training of residents in psychosocial medicine: a controlled, randomized study. *Acad Med* 1995;70:729–732.
4. Smith RC, Dorsey AM, Lyles JS, et al. Teaching self-awareness enhances learning about patient-centered interviewing. *Acad Med* 1999;74:1242–1248.
5. Smith RC, Marshall-Dorsey AA, Osborn GG, et al. Evidence-based guidelines for teaching patient-centered interviewing. *Patient Educ Counsel* 2000;39:27–36.
6. Smith RC. Videotape of Evidence-Based Interviewing: (1) Patient-Centered Interviewing and (2) Doctor-Centered Interviewing. Marketing Division, Instructional Media Center, Michigan State University. Contact information: PO Box 710, East Lansing, MI 48824; 517-353-9229 (tel); 517-432-2650 (fax); http://www.msu-vmall.msu.edu/imc.
7. Smith RC, Hoppe RB. The patient's story: integrating the patient- and physician-centered approaches to interviewing. *Ann Intern Med* 1991;115:470–477.
8. Morgan WL, Engel GL. *The clinical approach to the patient.* Philadelphia: WB Saunders, 1969.
9. Lipkin JM, Frankel R, Beckman H, et al. Performing the interview. In: Lipkin M, Putnam M, Lazare A, eds. *The medical interview.* New York: Springer-Verlag, 1995:65–82.
10. Marracino RK, Orr RD. Entitling the student doctor—defining the student's role in patient care. *J Gen Intern Med* 1998;13:266–270.
11. Silver-Isenstadt A, Ubel PA. Erosion of medical students' attitudes about telling patients they are students. *J Gen Int Med* 1999;14:481–487.
12. Stern DT. The development of professional character in medical students. *Hastings Center Report* 2000;30(4):s26–s29.
13. Kravitz RL. Patients' expectations for medical care: an expanded formulation based on review of the literature. *Med Care Res Rev* 1996;53:3–27.
14. Kravitz RL, Callahan EJ, Paterniti D, et al. Prevalence and sources of patients' unmet expectations for care. *Ann Int Med* 1996;125:730–737.
15. Marvel MK, Epstein RM, Flowers K, et al. Soliciting the patient's agenda—have we improved? *JAMA* 1999;281:283–287.
16. White J, Levinson W, Roter D. "Oh, by the way . . .": the closing moments of the medical visit. *J Gen Intern Med* 1994;9:24–28.
17. Barrows HS, Pickell GC. *Developing clinical problem-solving skills. A guide to more effective diagnosis and treatment.* New York: WW Norton, 1991.
18. Kravitz RL, Cope DW, Bhrany V, et al. Internal medicine patients' expectations for care during office visits. *J Gen Intern Med* 1994;9:75–81.
19. Platt FW. *Conversation failure: case studies in doctor–patient communication.* Tacoma, WA: Life Sciences Press, 1992.

20. Beckman HB, Frankel RM. The effect of physician behavior on the collection of data. *Ann Intern Med* 1984;101:692–696.
21. Kravitz RL, Callahan EJ. Patients' perceptions of omitted examinations and tests—a qualitative analysis. *J Gen Int Med* 2000;15:38–45.
22. Carson CA. *A course in nonverbal communication for medical education.* Rochester, NY: Cecile A. Carson, The Genesee Hospital, 1988.
23. Levinson D. *A guide to the clinical interview.* Philadelphia: WB Saunders, 1987.
24. Cox A, Rutter M, Holbrook D. Psychiatric interviewing techniques V. Experimental study: eliciting factual information. *Br J Psychiatry* 1981;139:29–37.
25. Jackson SW. The listening healer in the history of psychological healing. *Am J Psychiatry* 1992;149:1623–1632.
26. Kroenke K, Mangelsdorff AD. Common symptoms in ambulatory care: incidence, evaluation, therapy, and outcome. *Am J Med* 1989;86:262–266.
27. Kroenke K, Price RK. Symptoms in the community—prevalence, classification, and psychiatric comorbidity. *Arch Intern Med* 1993;153:2474–2480.
28. Marple RL, Kroenke K, Lucey CR, et al. Concerns and expectations in patients presenting with physical complaints—frequency, physician perceptions and actions, and 2-week outcome. *Arch Intern Med* 1997;157:1482–1488.
29. Platt FW, Gaspar DL, Coulehan JL, et al. Tell me about yourself: the patient-centered interview. *Ann Intern Med* 2001;134:1079–1085.
30. Suchman AL, Markakis K, Beckman HB, et al. A model of empathic communication in the medical interview. *JAMA* 1997;277:678–682.
31. Brody DS, Khaliq AA, Thompson II TL. Patients' perspectives on the management of emotional distress in primary care settings. *J Gen Int Med* 1997;12:403–406.
32. Lipkin M. The medical interview and related skills. In: Branch WT, ed. *Office practice of medicine.* Philadelphia: WB Saunders, 1987:1287–1306.
33. Reik T. *Listening with the third ear: the inner experience of a psychoanalyst.* New York: Farrar, Straus and Giroux, 1948.
34. Feldman SS. *Mannerisms of speech and gestures in everyday life.* New York: International Universities Press, 1959.

4 Symptom-Defining Skills

With the patient-centered process of integrated interviewing now complete, the interview begins a major transition with the shift to the doctor-centered process. Before discussing specifically how to conduct this portion, however, the new skills required for it must be addressed. These are considered individually in this chapter and are synthesized in Chapter 5 as the doctor-centered interviewing process.

During doctor-centered interviewing, multiple bits of information are processed by the interviewer and are briefly addressed with open-ended requests (focused on a specific topic); then diagnostic details are pinned down with many closed-ended questions. This coning-down process occurs repeatedly until all the multiple areas within the history of present illness (HPI), other current active problems (OCAP), health issues (HI), past medical history (PMH), family history (FH), social history (SH), and review of systems (ROS) have been covered. Many of the required details that the student must elicit relate to the patient's symptoms, which are the focus in this chapter. The student focuses the coning-down process on two categories: (a) developing a common language of symptoms and (b) further refining these symptoms into more precise data. The symptom-defining skills presented in this chapter describe this process. I illustrate them with vignettes that do not involve Mrs. Jones. We will see her again in Chapter 5 when the doctor-centered interview is discussed.

Developing a Common Language for All Symptoms

The System Review (Review of Systems) Lists the Symptoms of Most Diseases

The system review, the original purpose of which is explained in the next chapter, is significant at this point because it lists and organizes the symptoms for most diseases, as Table 4.1 shows. Symptoms are important because they are the common language through which, in large part, the student converts a patient's complaints to a disease diagnosis. Table 4.1 lists isolated symptoms according to the body system with which they are associated, although many do occur in more than one system. The system review listing is not exhaustive. Those readers who are preclinical students should not worry if they do not understand what symptoms signify which underlying diseases. The possible disease explanations given in parentheses for each symptom are not diagnostic of the disease but are rather examples of frequent associations that occur. Diseases can be identified only after enough data have been obtained and synthesized by the student. Medical terminology for some symptoms is also noted in italics (within parentheses). Preclinical students are urged to learn all 14 categories and a few symptoms in each. Clinical level students will learn and develop an understanding of all symptoms during clinical rotations. At this point, they are urged to memorize all symptoms in each category, which is a necessary prerequisite for effective doctor-centered interviewing (1). The clinician must know and understand the language into which she or he translates the patient's complaints—it is the basis for diagnosis and treatment.

Distinguishing Closely Related Material from Symptoms

Patients directly experience symptoms; therefore, they are the only authorities on their own symptoms and no verification is necessary (e.g., abdominal pain and diarrhea). This defines so-called primary data (2). However, away from a patient's direct experiences, data are less reliable and more in need of verification (e.g., "The doctor said it was appendicitis."). Thus, nonsymptom disease information obtained from the patient (e.g., a diagnosis, treatment, procedure, medication, cause of the problem, or a laboratory test) differs from the patient's actual symptoms. Although these secondary data are less important (2), they often guide the student or clinician to areas that require verification and additional information. Incorporation of secondary data into the interview is described in Chapter 5.

Symptoms are distinguished from "signs" in medicine. The patient complains about a symptom (chest pain, dyspnea) while a clinician, student, or patient observes a sign on physical examination (tender ribs, heart murmur). Symptoms and signs may rarely overlap, as in the case of a patient who complains of "yellow jaundice" and the student or clinician who observes that the patient is jaundiced. Students learn about signs in physical diagnosis courses and on clinical rotations.

TABLE 4.1. THE SYSTEM REVIEW (REVIEW OF SYSTEMS) WITH EXAMPLES OF SOME SYMPTOMS*

A. General
1. Poor appetite (cancer, hepatitis, AIDS, medications, depression)
2. Excessive appetite (uncontrolled diabetes, hyperthyroidism, depression)
3. Weight loss (AIDS, cancer, emphysema, chronic infection, depression)
4. Weight gain (overeating, hypothyroidism, fluid retention)
5. Fever, chills, sweats (infection)
6. No enjoyment of life (*anhedonia*) (depression)
7. Pain (many causes)
8. Fatigue, lack of energy (many causes)

B. Integumentary
1. Sores and skin ulcers (infection, trauma, vascular insufficiency, diabetes, self-induced lesions)
2. Itching (*pruritis*) (bites, allergy, medications, dry skin, anxiety)
3. Rash (medications, measles, German measles, chicken pox)
4. Change in size or color of moles (malignant melanoma)
5. Abnormal hair growth (adrenal tumor, steroid medications)
6. Changes in nails (infection, iron deficiency, hypoxia, nail-biting)

C. Hematopoietic
1. Enlarged glands (*lymphadenopathy*) (infection, leukemia, infectious mononucleosis, lymphoma)
2. Lumps anywhere (lipoma, trauma, metastatic or primary cancer)
3. Urge to eat dirt (*pica*) or ice (iron deficiency, psychosis)
4. Abnormal bleeding or excessive bruising (liver disease, leukemia, idiopathic thrombocytopenic purpura, medications)
5. Frequent or unusual infections (AIDS, diabetes, immunologic deficiency, self-induced)

D. Endocrine
1. Heat intolerance (hyperthyroidism, excessive thyroid medication)
2. Cold intolerance (hypothyroidism, weight loss)
3. Decreased sexual drive (*libido*) (hypogonadism, medications, depression)
4. Salt craving (adrenocortical insufficiency, salt loss)
5. Enlarging glove and hat size (acromegaly)
6. Excessive thirst (*polydipsia*) (uncontrolled diabetes, water loss)

E. Musculoskeletal
1. Frequent fractures (osteoporosis, osteogenesis imperfecta, metastatic cancer, trauma)
2. Muscular weakness (polymyositis, old polio or stroke, electrolyte imbalance)
3. Painful muscles (trichinosis, polymyalgia rheumatica, muscle strain)
4. Joint pain and swelling (osteoarthritis, rheumatoid arthritis, gout)
5. Low back pain (psychogenic cause, herniated disc, muscle strain, infection, tumor)
6. Paralysis (stroke, polio, head injury)
7. Movement difficulty (Parkinson disease, medications)
8. Pain in calf with walking (*intermittent claudication*) (vascular insufficiency, muscle strain)
9. Swollen leg (trauma, varicosities, venous stasis, thrombophlebitis, infection, chronic dependent positioning)

F. Eyes, ears, nose, and throat
1. Change in vision (aging, diabetes, glaucoma, foreign body, stroke, brain tumor)
2. Bright flashes of light (vitreous or retinal detachment)
3. Image of light with jagged, shimmering appearance (*scintillating scotomata*) (migraine)

(Table continued)

TABLE 4.1. *continued.*

4. Spots in visual field (migraine, glaucoma)
5. Double vision (*diplopia*) (brain tumor, stroke)
6. Loss of hearing (aging, ear wax, tumor)
7. Ringing in the ears (*tinnitus*) (Ménière disease, tumor, aging)
8. Drainage from nose (common cold, cerebrospinal fluid rhinorrhea, allergy)
9. Decreased or altered sense of smell (brain tumor, rhinitis)
10. Bloody nose (*epistaxis*) (trauma, tumor, infection)
11. Sore throat (bacterial or viral infection, psychogenic, medication-induced)
12. Impaired speech (stroke, tumor, cleft lip or palate, psychogenic cause)
13. Painful tooth (cavity [caries], abscess, trauma)
14. Hoarseness (laryngeal cancer, voice abuse, polyps)

G. Head and neck
  1. Headache (tension, migraine, brain tumor, medications)
  2. Dizzy (*vertigo*) (labyrinthitis, tumor, vertebral-basilar insufficiency, medications)
  3. Lightheadedness (psychogenic cause, anemia, fluid/electrolyte disturbance, rapid standing [orthostatic])
  4. Loss of consciousness (*syncope*) (orthostatic origin, aortic stenosis, rapid bleeding, cardiac arrhythmia, cerebrovascular accident, trauma, stress)
  5. Stiff neck (arthritis, muscle strain, cervical disc)

H. Breasts
  1. Lump or mass (cancer, fibrocystic disease, abscess, trauma)
  2. Discharge (cancer, medications, lactation)
  3. Tenderness (menstruation, medications)

I. Cardiovascular and pulmonary
  1. Chest pain (pneumonia, muscular strain, coronary artery disease, pulmonary embolus, psychogenic cause, pericarditis, pleurisy)
  2. Shortness of breath (*dyspnea*) (see most of chest pain; also heart failure, anemia)
  3. Shortness of breath when lying down; needs to sit to breathe (*orthopnea*) (heart failure, emphysema, pneumonia)
  4. Wakening at night with dyspnea (*paroxysmal nocturnal dyspnea*) (heart failure, emphysema, sleep apnea)
  5. Wheezing (asthma, heart failure, pulmonary embolus, cancer, foreign body, upper airway obstruction)
  6. Cough (see most of the preceding)
  7. Yellow or green sputum (bronchitis, pneumonia)
  8. Clear sputum (heart failure, asthma)
  9. Bloody sputum (*hemoptysis*) (pneumonia, pulmonary embolus, heart failure, cancer)
  10. Pounding sensation in chest (*palpitations*) (arrhythmias, ventricular hypertrophy, tachycardia)
  11. Peripheral arterial and venous insufficiency (see Integumentary and Extremities)

J. Gastrointestinal
  1. Appetite and weight changes (see General)
  2. Sticking sensation in throat (*globus hystericus*) (stress, foreign body, infection)
  3. Difficulty swallowing (*dysphagia*) (achalasia, cancer, esophagitis, foreign body)
  4. Heartburn (esophagitis, medications, cancer)
  5. Upper abdominal pain (gastritis, peptic ulcer disease, medications, psychogenic cause, gall bladder disease, pancreatitis, abdominal wall pain)
  6. Mid-lower abdominal pain (appendicitis, diverticulitis, irritable bowel syndrome, cancer, vascular insufficiency, Meckel diverticulum, regional enteritis, ulcerative colitis)
  7. Nausea (many of the preceding, medications, hepatitis, migraine)

(Table continued)

TABLE 4.1. *continued.*

8. Nonbloody vomiting (*emesis*) (many of the preceding)
9. Bloody emesis (*hematemesis*) (upper gastrointestinal bleeding—esophatitis, gastritis, ulcer, cancer)
10. Black stools (*melena*) (upper gastrointestinal bleeding)
11. Bloody stools (*hematochezia*) (rapid upper gastrointestinal bleeding or lower gastrointestinal bleeding—hemorrhoids, cancer, vascular insufficiency, diverticulitis, vascular anomalies, ulcerative colitis)
12. Difficult or infrequent bowel movements (*constipation*) (cancer, hypothyroidism, medications, diverticulitis, low-fiber diet)
13. Loose or frequent bowel movements (*diarrhea*) (infection, diverticulitis, cancer, medications, ulcerative colitis, excessive dietary fiber)
14. Yellow discoloration of sclerae and skin (*jaundice*) (hepatitis, biliary obstruction, medications, hemolytic anemias)
15. Dark urine that is the color of tea or a cola drink (see jaundice, excluding obstruction)
16. Excessive upper (*belching or eructation*) or lower (*flatus*) bowel gas (many of the preceding, swallowing air when eating fast, high-fiber diet)
17. Rectal pain (*proctalgia*), discharge, or itching (*pruritis ani*) (psychogenic cause, hygienic origin, hemorrhoids, fissure, infection [gonorrhea or pinworm])
18. Lump in groin or scrotum (hernia, lymphadenopathy)

K. Urinary
1. Increased urinary frequency (*polyuria*) (infection, bladder neck obstruction, excessive water intake, diabetes)
2. Burning with urination (dysuria) (infection)
3. Getting up more than once during the night to void (*nocturia*) (infection, bladder neck obstruction, excessive fluid intake)
4. Need to urinate suddenly and urgently (*urgency*) (infection)
5. Loss of urinary control (*incontinence*) (brain or spinal cord lesion, infection, stress incontinence)
6. Bloody urine (*hematuria*) (infection, cancer, kidney stone, bladder polyps)
7. Particulate matter in urine (stones, small stony debris [gravel], sloughed renal papillae)
8. Slow to get urinary stream started (*hesitancy*) (bladder neck obstruction)

L. Genital, male
1. Urethral discharge (gonorrhea and other infections)
2. Penile sores or growths (syphilis and other infections, cancer)
3. Painful or swollen testicle (cancer, epididymitis, orchitis, trauma, hernia, hydrocele, spermatocele)
4. Impotence (psychogenic origin, diabetes, vascular disease, medications)
5. Bloody ejaculation (*hematospermia*) (prostatitis, tumor)
6. Retrograde ejaculation into bladder (diabetes, autonomic dysfunction)
7. Premature ejaculation (psychogenic cause, prostatitis)
8. Decreased libido (psychogenic origin, chronic illness, medications)

M. Genital, female
1. Vaginal discharge or itching (gonorrhea or other infection, foreign body, fistula, irritant)
2. Sores or lumps (syphilis or other infection, cancer, abscess)
3. Painful menses (*dysmenorrhea*) (pelvic inflammatory disease, endometriosis, cancer)
4. Absence of menses (*amenorrhea*) (pregnancy, lactation, malnutrition, menopause, medications, endocrine)
5. Irregular, heavy menses (*menometrorrhagia*) (medications, endocrine, endometriosis, pelvic inflammatory disease)
6. Hot flashes (menopause, ovarian failure)
7. Decreased libido (see Endocrine in the preceding)

(Table continued)

TABLE 4.1. *continued.*

8. Painful intercourse (*dyspareunia*) (endometriosis, pelvic inflammatory disease)
9. Nonorgasmic (chronic illness, psychogenic cause)

N. Neuropsychiatric

1. Cranial nerves (see Head and Eyes, Ears, Nose, and Throat).
2. Motor (see Musculoskeletal).
3. Numb, tingling sensation in extremities (*paresthesia*) (neuritis, tumor, disc)
4. Decreased (*hypesthesia*) or absent (*anesthesia*) sensation (neuritis, disc, tumor)
5. Tremor (Parkinson disease, anxiety, tumor, medications)
6. Loss of balance (labyrinthine disease, tumor, stroke, visual cause, infection)
7. Difficulty walking (*ataxia*) (Parkinson disease, stroke, tumor, neuritis, head injury)
8. Seizures (epilepsy, tumor, stroke, medications, infection, vitamin deficiency)
9. Bizarre, unrealistic thoughts (*intrusive thoughts*) (psychosis, head injury, medications or street drugs, drug–alcohol withdrawal, depression, dementia)
10. Bizarre, unrealistic perceptions (*hallucinations*) (see 9)
11. Depression (psychiatric origin, chronic disease, medications)
12. Mania (manic-depressive, medications, hyperthyroidism)
13. Poor judgment, orientation, memory, attention, and concentration (see 9, psychogenic origin)
14. Inability to get to sleep or to stay asleep (*insomnia*) (depression, psychogenic cause, sleep apnea, medications, drug–alcohol use and withdrawal, nocturnal myoclonus, chronic disease)
15. Hypersomnolence (depression, sleep apnea, narcolepsy, medications, insufficient sleep, tumor, infection, head injury, chronic diseases)
16. Nightmares (depression, severe stress, medications)
17. Anhedonia (see General)
18. Suicidal (depression, other psychiatric causes, medications, chronic disease)
19. Anxiety, nervousness (stress, depression, hyperthyroidism, medications or drugs, panic disorder)
20. Symptoms without an explanation (*somatization*) (normal variant, personality disorder)

---

* Many of these symptoms can occur in systems other than those where they are listed; in addition to those listed, many other diseases and disorders can cause these symptoms. Italicized terms listed in the first set of parentheses immediately following a term are synonyms for that term.

Translating Complaints into Specific Medical Symptoms Is Sometimes Necessary

Patients often speak in nonmedical terms (Table 4.2) that must be converted to medically meaningful terms in the review of systems (ROS). When the student or clinician hears that the patient has the "blahs," a "wrung-out feeling," or "bad blood," he or she must ask himself or herself, "What does that mean and how is the information to be used medically?" As is shown in the following example, a brief, open-ended question (focused on the symptom) is followed by enough closed-ended questions so that the interviewer can adequately understand.

TABLE 4.2. SOME COMMON COMPLAINTS NEEDING CONVERSION TO SYMPTOMS IN THE SYSTEM REVIEW

A. Blahs
B. Dragged-out
C. Bad blood
D. I've got a "bunch"
E. Really weird
F. Funny smelling urine
G. Wrung-out
H. Mid-life crisis
I. Menopause
J. Old age
K. Terrible twos
L. A rod in my head
M. Wigged-out
N. Sun troubles
O. Chronic fatigue syndrome
P. Heart murmur
Q. Indigestion
R. The flu
S. Dizzy
T. Allergies

DOC: Say more about what you mean by the blahs.

[A focused, open-ended request]

PT: Well, you know, the nausea all the time and no appetite.

[Nausea and no appetite are medically meaningful symptoms (see GI System in ROS)]

DOC: Any vomiting?

[Closed-ended question]

PT: No.

DOC: How has your weight been?

[The interviewer will continue to pursue this to define better what the patient calls the blahs but has already identified at least two commonly understood medical symptoms in the ROS.]

Likewise, certain medical terms are ambiguous or are used by patients in an unconventional way. For example, "dizzy" generally means vertigo or a sensation of whirling as though a person has just gotten off a merry-go-round or has had too much to drink. However, some physicians and many lay people use the term dizziness to mean a faint or light-headed feeling that is unattended by vertigo. This distinction is important because a clinician approaches the patient with vertigo differently from the patient who is light-headed.

> **DOC:** Tell me what you mean by dizzy.
>
> [Focused, open-ended request; this could also be phrased as a question like "What do you mean by dizzy?"]
>
> **PT:** I get wobbly on my feet.
>
> [Still not very specific]
>
> **DOC:** Do you get a sensation of whirling about, like you just stepped off a merry-go-round?
>
> [Closed-ended question to get necessary details]
>
> **PT:** Yeah, that's it. I feel like I'm going around the room.
>
> **DOC:** Do you feel lightheaded, like you might faint, or have to put your head down between your knees to get relief?
>
> [Closed-ended inquiry for more details]
>
> **PT:** No, that makes it worse to put my head down.
>
> [The interviewer has identified the medical symptom vertigo as the meaning of the complaint of dizziness, although many more questions remain about associated symptoms and the other details of the problem.]

Refining Individual Symptoms into More Precise Data

Once a medical symptom is identified, interviewers can make the symptom descriptions more precise to improve their meaningfulness for diagnosing diseases. Greater specificity derives from the set of descriptors outlined here and usually requires mostly closed-ended inquiry. As I already indicated, the examples given in this text are not exhaustive and more data are needed to make a final diagnosis.

The following descriptors, summarized in Table 4.3, should be sought to the fullest extent that is possible for each individual symptom. These descriptors reflect the "classic seven" dimensions of symptoms: body location, quality, quantification, chronology and timing, setting, moderating factors (aggravating or alleviating), and associated symptoms (3,4); nonpain symptoms usually do not require all seven descriptors.

TABLE 4.3.   THE SEVEN DESCRIPTORS OF SYMPTOMS

A. Location and radiation
   1. Precise location
   2. Deep or superficial
   3. Specific or diffuse
B. Quality
   1. Usual descriptors
   2. Unusual descriptors
C. Quantification
   1. Type of onset
   2. Intensity or severity
   3. Impairment or disability
   4. Numerical description
      a. Number of events
      b. Size
      c. Volume
D. Chronology and timing—course of individual symptom over time
   1. Time of onset of symptom and intervals between its occurrence
   2. Duration of symptom
   3. Periodicity and frequency of symptom
   4. Course of symptom
      a. Short-term
      b. Long-term
E. Setting
F. Moderating factors
   1. Precipitants or aggravating factors
   2. Relieving factors
G. Associated symptoms

Location of the Symptom and Its Radiation

Precise locations of symptoms should be given when possible. Both the location and the area of radiation of the symptom can have diagnostic significance (e.g., headache without radiation [nonspecific]; substernal pain radiating into the neck, jaw, and left arm [angina, esophagitis]; low back pain radiating into the left buttock and posterior thigh with extension into the lateral aspect of the calf and over the dorsum of the foot into the great toe [L5-S1 nerve root impingement from a herniated lumbar disc]). If they do not do so automatically, patients should be asked to point to their area of discomfort (e.g., numbness on the ulnar portions of the hand suggests irritation in a C8-T1 nerve root distribution).

Does the patient feel the distress deep or on the surface? Is it specific in location or more diffuse (e.g., left temporal headache localized to the region of the temporal artery that was located by the patient as "on the surface" [temporal arteritis, skin problem])? These questions should also be asked if they are not already indicated by the patient.

The student begins this inquiry with a focused, open-ended request, which can be phrased as a question, such as, "Can you describe the location for me?" Closed-ended inquiry is often needed to get sufficient specificity.

DOC: So, as part of the blahs you've got this stomach pain. Can you describe its location for me?

[A focused open-ended request, phrased as a question; this will be followed by several closed-ended questions]

PT: It's in my stomach.

DOC: Where exactly is it? Point at it, if you can.

[Always be as specific as possible]

PT: (points to upper mid-abdomen, the epigastrium)

DOC: How big an area? Can you draw a circle around it?

PT: (draws an outline) This big.

DOC: Does it move anywhere else like your back or chest?

[Giving examples is helpful as long as the answer is not suggested]

PT: No.

DOC: Is it deep down or does it feel more like it is right on the surface?

PT: Down inside.

Quality of the Symptom

Additional diagnostic specificity sometimes is derived from knowing what the symptoms feel like (e.g., aching [nonspecific], burning [gastritis or ulcer disease when substernal or epigastric], sharp [nonspecific], dull [nonspecific], crushing [coronary insufficiency when substernal], throbbing [migraine when in head, localized infection anywhere], or cramping [disorder of a hollow organ such as the ureter, intestine, or uterus]).

Unusual descriptions can signify psychological problems or stress and can sometimes be understood metaphorically (5). For example, psychotic people have said things such as "it feels like my intestines have grown shut" or "it feels like they left an instrument in there." Similarly, comments like "it's pushing up through my soul and tearing my heart out" are extraordinary; they can suggest the presence of some associated psychological issues.

The interviewer learns the quality of the symptom by starting with a focused, open-ended request, such as "Tell me what the pain is like." As before, more closed-ended inquiry may be necessary to pin down details.

> **DOC:** What does it feel like?
>
> [A focused open-ended request, again phrased as a question]
>
> **PT:** Pretty bad.
>
> **DOC:** Well, how would you describe it? Aching? Sharp? Dull?
>
> [Giving examples is appropriate, if necessary, as long as an answer is not suggested.]
>
> **PT:** Kind of burning, like hot or on fire.

Quantify the Symptom

Further precision and specificity for disease diagnosis can be gained by quantifying the symptom in the following four ways.

Type of Onset

Whether the symptom began gradually or appeared suddenly has diagnostic significance; the latter suggests an acute, but not necessarily more important, disease process. A clinician or student might hear, for example, that "the weakness just gradually developed in my shoulders and thighs over a couple months" [polymyositis] or that "the shortness of breath had been kind of gradual over that day, but the chest pain and coughing blood came all of a sudden" [pulmonary embolus, heart failure].

Focused open-ended inquiry often suffices, although patients sometimes benefit from being given examples (e.g., "Would you tell me how this began?").

> **DOC:** How did this begin?
> **PT:** What do you mean?
> **DOC:** You know, slow or all of a sudden.
> **PT:** Gradual, a little bit at a time.

Intensity

The interviewer should obtain a measure of intensity or severity by asking for comparisons to prior experiences (e.g., a toothache or delivering a baby) or getting a rating on a 1 to 10 scale where a 10 rating is the worst ever. In general, the more severe the symptoms are, the more serious the problem. Lower grade pain, however, does not necessarily signify that a problem is unimportant (e.g., angina pectoris reflects serious disease but the pain is not always severe). In addition, certain pains are characteristically more severe than others (e.g., testicular injury, renal calculus, labor pains).

The clinician or student should begin open-endedly with a question like, "Give me an idea of how bad it was." Usually, however, closed-ended questions are necessary to get the needed details.

> **DOC:** Tell me how severe it is.
> **PT:** Well, it wasn't too bad.
> **DOC:** On a 1 to 10 scale where 10 is the worst ever, how would you rate it?

> **PT:** Not so bad, really. I guess a 3.
>
> **DOC:** How is it compared to a toothache?
>
> **PT:** Not that bad.

Impairment or Disability Resulting from the Symptom

Another measure of severity is how the complaint has affected the patient on a daily basis. For example, a minor episode of hoarseness could cause severe hardship for an opera singer or public speaker, whereas it would be of little consequence to a writer or night watchman.

The student or clinician again begins with a focused, open-ended request, such as, "What effect is this having on your life?" Closed-ended questions are used for detail. Specific inquiries about what the patient is no longer able to do helps to clarify the situation (e.g., "Since the chest pain started, what have you had to give up?"). Comparing the patient's daily activities both before and after the symptom further clarifies this. Many of these data will have been obtained during the patient-centered process; if so, they are not repeated.

> **DOC:** How is this affecting what you do?
>
> **PT:** Well, it's caused a lot of problems.
>
> **DOC:** Is it keeping you off work or anything?
>
> [Note the continued need for closed-ended questions to get accurate details.]
>
> **PT:** No, nothing like that really. I haven't missed a day of work. I'm just getting tired of it.

Obtain Numerical Data Where Possible

The total number of occurrences of the symptom usually can be identified or closely estimated by the interviewer. For instance, she or he might discover that the patient has had about 20 such episodes of chest pain in the last week after no more than one weekly during the preceding year. Precisely quantifying the symptoms in other ways when applicable can also be necessary (e.g., "It swells to the size of a softball at times but then goes back down to like a golf ball." [inguinal hernia] or "I only passed about a glassful of urine all day." [bladder neck obstruction, dehydration]). Patients seldom respond with precise numbers and prefer to answer with "quite a bit" or "not too much" instead of with precise quantities. The interviewer's job is to find these out without alienating the patient.

These data are obtained almost entirely by closed-ended inquiry. The interviewer often has to follow up on answers that are not precise enough. If, on being asked how many times a pain occurs, the patient answers "a lot," the student or clinician might respond by saying, "Can you be more specific? You know, how many times in a day?" as in the following example.

DOC: How many times a day do you have the pain?

PT: Oh, three or four or five.

DOC: What's the most you've had?

PT: Seven or eight times.

DOC: And the least?

PT: One or even none sometimes.

Chronology and Timing: Course of Individual Symptom Over Time

The student must learn the precise sequence of symptoms and other events to be effective diagnostically. In this portion, the interviewer focuses on the chronology and timing of individual symptoms; these data will be integrated into the overall chronology of all symptoms and other data in Chapter 5.

Time of Onset of the Symptom and Intervals Between Its Occurrence

The time of onset of the symptom and the time intervals between occurrences of the symptom have considerable diagnostic significance—the onset of a cough 6 months earlier that recurs at intervals of 1 to 2 days suggests a chronic pulmonary problem, such as cancer or tuberculosis, whereas the on-set of a cough 2 days prior to the visit that is continuous suggests an acute process, such as bronchitis or pneumonia. Recalling Mrs. Jones from the last chapter, migraine headaches characteristically have specific times of onset and pain-free intervals of days to weeks, as contrasted to daily and nonremit-ting headaches from a brain tumor or tension.

Duration of Symptom

The duration of a symptom is also of diagnostic significance. Precise under-standing is essential (e.g., a few seconds, 5 minutes, 2 hours, 10 days, 3 years). Typical substernal crushing pain of coronary disease lasting only 5 to 10 min-utes suggests angina pectoris without myocardial infarction (heart attack), whereas a similar pain lasting an hour or so suggests myocardial infarction. Migraine headaches typically last from 1 to 12 hours, which contrasts, as be-fore, with the more constant headaches of a brain tumor or from tension.

Periodicity and Frequency of the Symptom

Symptoms often have patterns that reflect the underlying disease process and are of diagnostic importance. For example, the symptoms of different types of malaria occur at distinctive and sometimes diagnostic frequencies. Body cy-cles also can affect symptoms (e.g., premenstrual syndrome focuses around menses and nocturnal myoclonus occurs during nonrapid eye movement sleep). In addition, external influences can have a cyclic impact (e.g., regular stressful events; disorders, such as allergies and acid peptic disease, that have a seasonal association).

Course of the Symptom

The course of the symptom over an individual episode and its pattern of oc-currence over a longer period are essential diagnostic data. The individual course of pain stemming from obstruction of a hollow organ is that of a pro-gressive increase in pain followed by apparent relief, often described as cramping, only to be followed at varying intervals by a recurrence of the same pattern (e.g., labor pains, ureteral colic). A migraine headache, on the other hand, typically pursues a slow but progressive build-up of a constant throb-bing pain.

The overall course of a symptom is equally important, and it will be de-scribed more extensively in the next chapter. A patient with headaches that are of 20 years duration and that are unchanged will seldom have a brain tumor, whereas a headache that progressively worsens over several months is more suggestive of a tumor or other intracerebral disease process.

The following chronological description is obtained almost entirely with closed-ended questions.

DOC: When did the burning in the stomach begin?

PT: About a year ago.

[Onset]

DOC: Do you have pain every day?

PT: No, sometimes it will be gone for weeks at a time.

[Intervals between symptom]

DOC: And how long do they last each time?

PT: Quite a while.

DOC: How long is that? I need a little more detail.

PT: Oh, I don't know. Maybe a couple of hours.

DOC: What's the shortest that they might last and the longest?

PT: Well, some of them are gone in just a few minutes. But most are about an hour, I guess.

DOC: What's the longest?

PT: The worst one I ever had lasted from supper until just before bedtime, about 4 hours.

[Longest and shortest duration of symptom]

DOC: What seems to determine that?

PT: I don't know, but it's always worse in the spring; and it's not there on weekends when I'm not working.

[Frequency and periodicity]

DOC: What's the course of the pain with each episode?

PT: It just gradually comes on and then gets a little worse.

[Short-term course of symptom]

> **DOC:** Overall, how is the pain doing?
>
> **PT:** It seems worse to me.
>
> **DOC:** How's that?
>
> **PT:** Well, it's not more pain, but it's more often. It used to be just once every day or so but now it's four or five times a day.
>
> [Overall course of symptom]

Setting

If the setting in which the symptoms occur is not obtained during the patient-centered process, it usually is described as part of obtaining the patient's chronological descriptions or as part of learning her or his functional impairment from the symptoms. Here, the interviewer should determine it with questions like, "Where were you?" "Who else was present?" "What were you doing?" or "Where was this?"

This interviewer should begin open-endedly with questions like, "Can you tell me the background of the symptom? You know, what you were doing at the time and who was there?" If this does not suffice, closed-ended inquiry can help.

> **DOC:** Can you give me some of the background for the pain, like who is around and where you are when it happens?
>
> **PT:** Almost always at work—there's been a lot of stress lately.
>
> **DOC:** Not at home?
>
> **PT:** Never. Isn't that funny?
>
> **DOC:** Who's around at work?
>
> **PT:** Well, it's just since I transferred to the parts department.
>
> [If these data have not been produced during the patient-centered process as part of the personal dimension of the illness, they should be developed here.]

Moderating Factors

To this point, the interviewer has addressed just the symptom per se, but she or he now considers some external influences that are of diagnostic value: precipitants of the problem, aggravations of it once it is present, and substances that provide relief. For example, aspirin, alcohol, tobacco, spicy foods, and caffeine all are known both to precipitate and to aggravate gastritis or acid peptic disease, whereas relief is typically obtained by drinking milk, eating bland food, and using antacids. Similarly, angina is precipitated and aggravated by exertion, mental stress, or cold air blowing in the face, whereas it is relieved, usually in less than 10 minutes, by rest and the use of nitroglycerin.

Although the interviewer begins open-endedly, most of this information is elicited through closed-ended questioning, the specific content of which reflects the clinician's or student's knowledge of individual diseases.

> **DOC:** Tell me about anything that seems to aggravate or to bring on these pains.
>
> **PT:** Well, coffee does sometimes.
>
> **DOC:** What about aspirin, does that cause it?
>
> [The interviewer would continue, closed-endedly, to ask about what she or he knows causes epigastric burning: other medications, tea, alcohol, tobacco, spicy foods.]
>
> **DOC:** (continuing after completing the preceding inquiry) Have you noticed anything that helps, you know that relieves it?
>
> **PT:** Eating almost anything, especially milk.
>
> **DOC:** What about antacids?
>
> **PT:** Yeah, they help a lot.

Often the patient is unable to describe moderating factors but is able to say what she or he does (or avoids) during the symptoms (e.g., walks about, lies down, quits eating).

Associated Symptoms

Having only one symptom with an underlying disease is uncommon. Rather, several symptoms often occur that are specific to the disease; in addition, secondary symptoms that reflect the general impact of the disease may be found (e.g., in a patient with pneumonia, cough and chest pain are likely specific symptoms from the pneumonia, whereas fatigue and irritability are nonspecific symptoms owing to the general effect of the pneumonia on the body). Associated symptoms are important because different combinations have diagnostic importance (e.g., in a patient with weight loss, a good appetite often suggests diabetes mellitus or hyperthyroidism, whereas a poor appetite might suggest infection or cancer).

The interviewer detects associated symptoms by beginning with open-ended questioning, such as, "Tell me any other symptoms that go along with this." Closed-ended questions usually are required, however, for him or her to pin down important details about the presence or absence of symptoms that might be expected in association with the presenting symptom; this is outlined in the next chapter (e.g., in a patient with chest pain, the clinician or student should always ask if they currently have or have had shortness of breath).

DOC: Tell me any other symptoms that go with this burning pain.

PT: Well, a little diarrhea when it's bad.

[This new symptom and its descriptors would be fully developed just as was already done for the epigastric burning pain.]

DOC: Any other symptoms with it?

PT: Not really.

DOC: Any nausea?

[After the patient gives no additional symptoms, the interviewer uses her or his knowledge of common associations to make further specific inquiry, which will be expanded on in Chapter 5.]

SUMMARY

Clinicians and students use open-ended and closed-ended skills to establish a common, medical understanding of the individual symptom and then to refine it. They use seven descriptors to enhance its diagnostic specificity; however, individual symptoms are of little value in making a disease diagnosis. The integration of multiple symptoms and a description of the entire clinical problem in a way that points to an underlying disease are addressed in Chapter 5.

LEARNING EXERCISES

1. What does coning-down mean when it is applied to interviewing skills?
2. Define primary and secondary data and distinguish them from 'signs' of disease.*
3. Describe at least two functions of doctor-centered interviewing.
4. Describe the function of the system review or review of systems (ROS).
5. List all 14 body systems and at least three different symptoms within each system. For clinical level students, list all symptoms within each system.*

*Good test questions.

PRACTICE EXERCISES

1. Each member of the group reads about a specific disease in a standard textbook (6) with pain as a major symptom (e.g., low back pain in sciatica, headache in migraine, flank pain in renal colic, chest pain in angina pectoris, abdominal pain in intestinal obstruction, and headache in temporal arteritis).
2. This member should then act as the 'patient' in a role-play and should portray the pain problem he or she just read about to another group member who must elicit the seven classic descriptors of pain.
3. Elicit the symptoms and their descriptors from a real or simulated patient.

References

1. Barrows HS, Pickell GC. *Developing clinical problem-solving skills: a guide to more effective diagnosis and treatment.* New York: WW Norton, 1991.
2. Platt FW. *Conversation failure: case studies in doctor–patient communication.* Tacoma, WA: Life Sciences Press, 1992.
3. Morgan WL, Engel GL. *The clinical approach to the patient.* Philadelphia: WB Saunders, 1969.
4. Bates B. *A guide to physical examination—and history taking,* 5th ed. Philadelphia: JB Lippincott, 1991.
5. Melzack R. *Pain measurement and assessment.* New York: Raven Press, 1983.
6. Humes HD, DuPont HL, Gardner LB, et al, eds. *Kelley's textbook of internal medicine,* 4th ed. Philadelphia: Lippincott Williams & Wilkins, 2000.

5 Doctor-Centered Interviewing

This chapter describes step-by-step how the student or clinician conducts the doctor-centered interviewing process. This involves the latter part of the history of the present illness (HPI) and other current active problems (OCAP), continuing directly from the patient-centered HPI, and the entire health issues (HI), past medical history (PMH), social history (SH), family history (FH), and review of systems (ROS).

The patient-centered process appropriately produced much raw information—the patient's personal description and knowledge of her or his symptoms and, more generally, her or his personal experience. Most symptoms, however, require further clarification for diagnostic and therapeutic purposes. Therefore, the student or clinician must take the lead to guide what becomes a doctor-centered process by definition. Although as interviewers we assiduously avoided symptom-defining skills (see Chapter 4) during the patient-centered process, in the doctor-centered process we actively use these skills to synthesize raw patient-centered symptom data into a meaningful, chronological story that identifies or suggests an underlying disease. The doctor-centered process also provides the extensive, routine database that we need. Nevertheless, we do switch back to a patient-centered process when pertinent personal data or emotions arise, as they often do (Fig. 5.1).

Recall our progress to this point. During the patient-centered process of the HPI (Steps 1 to 5), the interviewer set the stage; obtained the chief complaint and agenda; identified the physical, personal, and emotional aspects of the data; and made a transition to the doctor-centered process of the HPI, the point at which we now find ourselves. Seven additional steps (Steps 6 to 12) are part of the doctor-centered process to complete the interview and are labeled in Fig. 5.1. We continue to follow Mrs. Jones to illustrate each step.

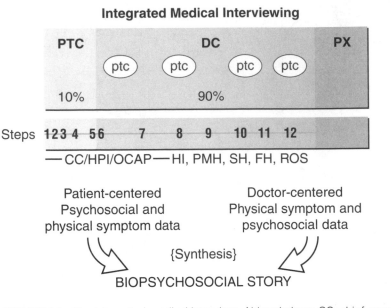

FIGURE 5.1. The integrated medical interview. Abbreviations: CC, chief complaint; DC, doctor-centered; FH, family history; HI, health issues; HPI, history of the present illness; OCAP, other current active problems; PMH, past medical history; PTC, patient-centered; PX, physical examination; ROS, review of systems; SH, social history.

Continuing the History of the Present Illness and Other Current Active Problems: General Overview (Step 6)

In many instances, a satisfactory overview will have occurred during Steps 2 to 4, in which case the interviewer will summarize and will proceed directly

TABLE 5.1. CONTINUING THE HISTORY OF PRESENT ILLNESS AND OTHER CURRENT ACTIVE PROBLEMS

I. Step 6. General overview
II. Step 7. Chronological description of all primary and secondary data
  A. Scan and describe data without interpreting them
    1. Describing symptoms already introduced by the patient
    2. Describing symptoms not yet introduced in the already identified body system (or general health symptoms)
  B. Interpret data while obtaining them: testing hypotheses about the possible disease meaning of symptoms*

*Only clinical-level students are expected to be proficient with this style of inquiry.

to Step 7. If not, the overview is developed at this point (Table 5.1). An overview of the major symptoms, when they began, and the most pressing current issue is essential; it requires both open-ended and closed-ended skills. The problem usually concerns physical symptoms. In the dialogue in my example, a physical focus is assumed with the understanding that severe psychological symptoms could also be addressed, which is considered at the end of this discussion of the HPI. In our continuing vignette of Mrs. Jones, the interviewer picks up at the end of Step 5 and completes an overview of the patient's problem that has already been initiated.

Direct Continuation of Vignette of Mrs. Jones

(This continues from the end of Chapter 3, in which the student learned that Mrs. Jones' headache occurred in the context of a distressing work situation.)

PT: Sure, that's what I came in for.

[Responding to student's inquiry about changing the conversation to her headaches, cough, and colitis from the patient-centered process that was just ending.]

DOC: I know the headache is the biggest problem now. (Chief Complaint)

[The student starts generally and summarizes the primary physical complaint in an open-ended way; shortly, she will ask specific closed-ended questions for the details. If the student somehow had not yet heard about the headache and other physical problems, she now obtains a detailed description in the patient's own words. Ordinarily, this will have occurred during the patient-centered process, as in Mrs. Jones' situation, and thus, Step 6 is very brief.]

PT: Yeah, it sure is.

DOC: When exactly did it begin?

[The interviewer wants to reaffirm the time frame of the headaches, so she uses a closed-ended question.]

PT: Oh, just a few weeks after I got here. That's about 4 months ago now, so the headaches have been about 3 months.

DOC: The nausea?

[Pinning down this unknown detail with another closed-ended question.]

PT: Oh, that was later, a month or so after when they got worse.

DOC: And the colitis started in 1982 you said. How long has the cough been going on?

PT: Just the last couple of weeks.

[The student has now summarized Mrs. Jones' problems, has established which is most important, and has discovered when each began. A good overview provides a general map of where the student needs to focus for details. Notice the increase in closed-ended questions and how they provide necessary details.]

Continuing the History of the Present Illness and Other Current Active Problems: Chronological Description of All Primary and Secondary Data (Step 7)

Step 7 (Table 5.1) is the most important and most difficult part of the doctor-centered process. The symptoms and secondary data that point to the patient's disease story are further developed and clarified. By the end of this step, we, as clinicians, are often able to make a disease diagnosis or, if not, we can greatly narrow the range of possible disease explanations for the symptom(s). This guides what we look for most carefully on the physical examination and during the subsequent laboratory evaluation, if any. The companion videotape demonstrates what I now describe (1) (see Preface).

As the preceding chapter presented, the interviewer converts each complaint to a standard symptom in the System Review (Review of Systems) and then further identifies it according to the seven descriptors (location, quality, quantification, chronology and timing, setting, moderating factors, and associated symptoms). However, symptoms do not occur in isolation or at just one point in time. In a continuation of what was introduced briefly in the last chapter (see "Associated Symptoms" and "Long-term Course of Symptoms"), I now consider more extensively how to group symptoms and to put all data in chronological order; this serves as the database for eventually making a disease diagnosis.

Research has shown that learners, as well as seasoned clinicians, make diagnoses of diseases by testing hypotheses during the course of the interview (2), using both decision rules and experience (3). We first generate a hypothesis about a specific disease diagnosis, such as angina or migraine, and then deductively test it by eliciting specific symptoms that do or do not support the hypothesized diagnosis (4). Experts are faster, more efficient, and more accurate because of their greater knowledge and experience, which allow them to supplement their hypothesis-testing approach with pattern recognition and seasoned intuition (2).

Preclinical and beginning clinical students are understandably much less effective in making diagnoses by hypothesis testing because they have less experience and knowledge. To offset this, beginners often need to scan patients extensively for relevant symptoms and then simply to describe their findings without hypothesizing a diagnosis, which is an inductive process. Students then use these data to form hypotheses for subsequent testing (e.g., in a later interview) after they have had time to read about the problems they have described so that they can formulate hypotheses. Beginning level students still test hypotheses during the interview but have this additional source of data from which they often can generate better and more hypotheses (4). These students scan only in relevant areas, do not ask the same questions of every patient, and do not simply elicit all known symptoms from the entire System Review (4). As students acquire clinical experience and their knowledge base grows, hypothesis testing becomes more prominent and scanning less so; nevertheless, even seasoned clinicians scan when hypothesis testing is ineffective (4).

Preclinical and beginning clinical students can generate a surprisingly relevant database with the purely "descriptive" or scanning approach that I now present. After discussing this, I then briefly consider how the learner can integrate the hypothesis-testing approach.

Scanning and Describing Data Without Interpreting It: For Preclinical and Beginning Clinical Students

Symptoms and secondary data are grouped in two general categories: (a) data introduced by the patient and (b) data not yet introduced that are in the same body system (as those already mentioned) or that pertain to general health.

Describing Symptoms Already Introduced by the Patient

The student begins with the problem most important to the patient and identifies all symptoms and secondary data starting from the beginning. Complaints are aggregated by common times of occurrence and are each translated into a symptom as it arises; the symptom is then refined using the seven descriptors. At times, obtaining the patient's symptoms first and then filling in the secondary data is easier. In either case, as interviewers, we make use of repeated queries for temporal connections, such as, "Then what?" or "What happened after that?" or "And then?" The patient sometimes will not introduce secondary data, and the interviewer must then ask about treatment, procedures, diagnoses, and other secondary information. Alternatively, the patient may present a host of secondary data from which the clinician or student must sift out the symptoms.

The pattern of all data over time must be clearly understood. No time interval during the course of the illness can remain unaccounted for. Calendar dates and exact times are used when possible and should always be indicated for recent or acute problems. More remote problems often can be marked by weeks, months, or even years.

Closed-ended inquiry is applied to elicit most information, as the vignette that follows notes. Periodic supportive remarks are appropriate, and a patient-centered atmosphere of warmth and understanding should be continued.

Continuation of Vignette of Mrs. Jones

PT: Just the last couple of weeks.

DOC: Well, let's look more at the headaches when they began 3 months ago.

[*Time of onset* is already known. The student is starting at the beginning of the most important problem with a focused open-ended request.]

PT: The headaches started one day at work when I'd had a bad time with my boss. You know, that time I told you about.

[Mrs. Jones is referring to the earlier patient-centered process during which she told about the personal events associated with her headache. No need for going into this personal description again exists.]

DOC: Tell me more about the headache.

[This focused open-ended request does not help much; the student proceeds to closed-ended inquiry.]

PT: Well, like what?

DOC: You said it was in the right temple, can you point at it for me? Is it always in the same spot?

[She is closed-endedly focusing away from the personal dimension and the symptom itself and is now getting the precise *location.*]

PT: (puts hand over much of right side of head) It's all over here, sometimes larger than others.

[Sounds like it is more diffuse than specifically in one location.]

DOC: Does it move any place else?

[Another of what will be many closed-ended questions as the student continues to develop the seven descriptors of illness. Note that she is introducing new material into the conversation, which is appropriate for the doctor-centered process. She is also leading the interaction.]

PT: No, it stays right there.

[No *radiation.*]

DOC: Does it feel like inside your head or outside on the surface; you know, does it hurt to comb your hair or touch it?

PT: No, it doesn't hurt to touch it. It's down inside I think.

[A deep rather than superficial pain.]

DOC: Could you give me a description of what it feels like; you know, aching, burning, or however you'd describe it?

[Giving examples, if necessary, is appropriate as long as an answer is not suggested.]

PT: Oh, it's more throbbing or pounding, like you feel each pulse beat.

[*Quality* of the pain identified; no bizarre description.]

DOC: How do they begin, gradual or all of a sudden?

PT: Oh, pretty much out of the blue.

[The *type of onset* is sudden.]

DOC: How severe are they?

PT: Well, sometimes they're worse than having a baby! Especially when they get bad. And I've missed work a few days but not very often.

[Severe level of *intensity* at times and some *disability.*]

DOC: Wow, that's pretty bad. You've really had a lot of trouble with this! How long does each headache last, the shortest and longest they might last?

[Empathetic comments and behaviors are continued during the doctor-centered process.]

PT: At least a couple of hours. When they get bad, they'll last up to 12 hours or so.

[*Duration* identified.]

DOC: What happens to the symptom during the time it's there?

PT: Well, it's not so bad at first but it just keeps getting worse and then the nausea comes.

[*Course of individual symptom.*]

DOC: How many do you have in a week or a month?

PT: I can have 2 or 3 a week when they're bad. You know, every 2 or 3 days.

[*Symptom frequency and intervals.*]

DOC: How long have they been that often?

PT: Since things got bad in the last month, especially the last couple of weeks. Before that they were only once or twice a week.

[*Total number* can be calculated if important.]

DOC: Do you know of anything that brings them on?

[The student is not inquiring about the *setting* because she already knows that from the patient-centered process.]

PT: Well, just what I've told you, getting upset. Once or twice it seemed like having some wine did it but I was stressed then too.

[Perhaps another *precipitant*.]

DOC: Anything that worsens them once they've begun?

PT: No, they're bad enough already! Well, bright lights sure do, now that I think about it.

[An *aggravating event* identified.]

DOC: They sure have been bad. What seems to help them once they occur?

PT: Just lying down in a dark room, and an ice bag on my head. Well, the narcotic shot they gave me in the emergency room took it away too.

[*Relief measures* developed. Also, *secondary data,* the narcotic and the emergency room visit, are introduced by the patient.]

DOC: What about the nausea?

[With a full description of the headache symptom, she now is moving to define better an *associated symptom,* staying with primary data for the moment. Notice that a nonpain symptom has fewer appropriate descriptors; for example, the interviewer usually does not try to identify location or radiation of nausea.]

PT: That's when the headaches are bad.

DOC: Help me understand a little better what the nausea is like.

[A focused open-ended request.]

PT: Like I'm sick to my stomach and could vomit if it got worse.

[Quality of nausea.]

DOC: And how does it begin?

[A closed-ended question, as many of the subsequent inquiries will be.]

PT: Oh, it just kind of gradually comes on after the pain has been there awhile.

[Gradual onset.]

DOC: How bad is it, how severe?

PT: It's minor compared to the pain. It's never really been the problem the pain is.

[Not additionally severe or disabling.]

DOC: How often does the nausea occur?

PT: Just when the pain gets bad. I've probably had it each time with the headache in the last month; that's when the pain has been worse.

[Number of episodes identified.]

DOC: You said this began about a month after the pain, so that means the nausea has been there about 2 months?

[Mrs. Jones has previously indicated the time of onset.]

PT: Yeah, but it's been worse in the last month.

DOC: How long does the nausea last once it begins?

PT: Oh, about a couple hours, until the headache finally goes away.

[Duration of nausea and relieving factor.]

DOC: Anything else that relieves it?

PT: Not that I know of. I tried some antacid, but it made me worse.

[Other aggravating and relieving factors explored. Secondary data are also introduced (antacid).]

DOC: And what's the time between each episode?

PT: Same as the headaches, you know, every couple of days.

[Intervals identified. Course of symptom and setting can be inferred from what Mrs. Jones has said already because the nausea is linked to headaches.]

DOC: Ever throw-up with them?

PT: Just once. That's when I went to the emergency room.

[Associated symptom.]

DOC: How much did you vomit?

PT: Oh, just enough to soak a hankie.

[The student has obtained pertinent descriptions of the nausea and now has discovered another symptom, vomiting, which would now be similarly explored. Complicated patients, unlike Mrs. Jones, can take considerable time in obtaining appropriate details of each symptom.]

DOC/PT: [Not recounted here. The student and the patient now develop details of the patient's vomiting. **As students gain experience, they begin to recognize that headache, nausea, and vomiting go together. This recognition allows them to develop the symptoms simultaneously and to avoid the repetition noted in the preceding.**]

DOC: It sounds like you went to the emergency room once when it was bad. What's been the *course* of the headaches and nausea; you know, better, worse, or about the same?

PT: They are getting worse. They last longer and are more often in the last 2 weeks.

[The overall course of the primary data is learned.]

DOC: Who've you seen for them?

[A good description of the symptoms and their course to the present has been obtained, and the student is beginning to move away from symptoms to associated secondary data.]

PT: Nobody, except the emergency room a week ago. I thought the aspirin would help.

DOC: Have you taken anything else?

PT: Nothing except that one shot; a narcotic of some sort, I think.

DOC: Did they do any tests on you in the emergency room?

PT: Yeah, they did a blood count and a urine test.

DOC: Any scans or x-rays of your head?

[Recent inquiry is aimed at understanding pertinent *secondary data.* Notice the repeated use of closed-ended questions to obtain a more precise description of the symptoms.]

PT: No.

Describing Symptoms Not Yet Introduced in the Already Identified Body System (or General Health Symptoms)

To this point, the interviewer has addressed symptoms volunteered by the patient (and related secondary data). But often, other pertinent symptoms are significant, either by their presence or absence; the absence of a symptom can be just as important diagnostically as its presence. The student thus needs to develop a more complete profile of the patient's problem.

Other pertinent data include the presence or absence of other symptoms in the body system that has already been identified as symptomatic. As clinicians, we can often assume that symptoms in the same system are related to the same underlying disease process. We know what the patient's major complaints are and therefore can identify the body system of likely disease involvement from the System Review; for example, hesitancy and increased urinary frequency suggest that some disease is affecting the urinary system. At times, however, a symptom can suggest more than one system as a source of disease; for example, substernal pain can reflect disease in the gastrointestinal system (esophagitis) or the cardiopulmonary system (angina). When any question exists, both systems should be considered as areas of possible involvement.

Using closed-ended inquiry, we determine the presence or absence of each symptom possibility in the system(s) involved. In the two examples from the previous paragraph, inquiry about all other possible urinary symptoms would occur in the first instance (dysuria, bloody urine, particulate matter in the urine, etc. until all possible urinary symptoms in the System Review had been screened); and questioning about all possible cardiopulmonary and gastrointestinal symptoms would take place in the second (hemoptysis, orthopnea, vomiting, diarrhea, etc.).

Inquiry often reveals the presence of symptoms that the patient has forgotten or has not thought were important, and it can, at times, provide crucial diagnostic information. For example, in the preceding patient with urinary complaints, discovering the periodic presence of particulate matter in the urine in association with bloody urine suggests renal calculi. Frequently, however, this inquiry indicates the absence of most symptoms on the list, a fact that is of diagnostic importance; therefore, the absence of hematuria in this patient weighs against renal calculi, as well as against some bladder or renal diseases.

Inquiring about symptoms of general health (see the System Review) fills out the symptom profile. Questions about appetite, weight, general feeling of well being, pain, and fever are germane in most patients, no matter what system is symptomatic. Many diseases, especially more serious ones, exhibit one or more of these general symptoms. In our vignette, predominantly closed-ended inquiry continues to be relied on, and supportive remarks continue to be interspersed.

Continuation of Vignette of Mrs. Jones

DOC: Any other symptoms you might have had?

[A focused, open-ended request, phrased as a question.]

PT: Well, nothing that I can think of.

DOC: Ever had problems with dizziness or lightheadedness?

[Because the patient's major symptom, headaches, is a neuropsychiatric system symptom, the student is beginning to inquire closed-endedly about other possible symptoms in the neurologic aspects of the Neuropsychiatric System, as well as about relevant neurological symptoms listed primarily in Head, Neck, Eyes, Ears, Nose, and Throat.]

PT: Not now. I used to get carsick as a kid and did a couple of times then.

DOC: Ever had a fainting spell?

PT: No.

DOC: Stiff neck?

PT: No.

DOC: Any problems with your vision?

PT: No. I don't even use glasses.

DOC: Any double vision?

PT: No.

DOC: Difficulty hearing?

PT: No.

DOC: Any change in your sense of taste or smell?

PT: No.

DOC: Any pain in the face?

PT: No.

[The student continues to explore all remaining symptoms in the preceding systems of the ROS: facial paralysis; difficulty swallowing or with speech; difficulty elevating the shoulders; muscle weakness or movement difficulty; extremity numbness, tingling, decreased sensation, or paralysis; the shakes or tremor; difficulty with balance or walking; and seizures.]

DOC: Besides the nausea and vomiting once, have you had any other digestive problems?

[A focused, open-ended question starts a new area of inquiry. The student now obtains a complete profile of the patient's other major symptom, nausea.]

PT: There haven't been any.

DOC: [Even though the patient indicates that none was present, the student would now closed-endedly go through the symptoms in the Gastrointestinal System that have not already been addressed: appetite, weight, heartburn, abdominal pain, vomiting blood (hematemesis), bloody or black stools, constipation or diarrhea, dark urine or jaundice, and rectal pain or excessive gas. The student then shifts to general symptoms.]

DOC: You've told me a lot already about this, but how've you been in general?

[A focused open-ended question introduces a new area of inquiry, her general health. Information about appetite and weight already have been obtained during the inquiry about gastrointestinal symptoms.]

PT: Great, except all these things.

DOC: What do you enjoy in your life, you know for recreation or fun?

[Another focused open-ended question for information about general health.]

PT: Well, my painting is my true love. I like to do that every day, come rain or shine. It really helps get my mind off of things.

[Active outside interests weigh against anhedonia and its frequent concomitant, depression.]

DOC: That's great. I'm impressed how you do so many things. Any problem with fevers or chills?

[The student continues to make supportive comments and asks a closed-ended question.]

PT: No.

[Therefore, no problem exists with general health symptoms of appetite, weight, fever, chills, or anhedonia.]

With experience, the interviewer bases the extent of this review of symptoms on clinical acumen; it almost always can be considerably shortened. An experienced clinician might already be comfortable with a diagnosis of migraine and may inquire only about "ever have anything like a stroke or any head injuries or fevers?" For beginning students, however, learning to go systematically through all the possibilities is essential.

Interpreting Data While Obtaining It: Testing Hypotheses About the Possible Disease Meaning of Symptoms: For Clinical Students and Graduates

The preclinical student now has a complete profile and chronology of symptoms from the scanning and describing interview; however, they have not been interpreted or grouped in a way that points to the specific diseases that could cause them. Just recounting symptoms usually does not identify a disease. Nor has the preclinical interviewer accounted for potentially significant symptoms in other systems. Moreover, simply inquiring about all symptoms outside those involved is not feasible—it would take too long and it is intellectually unsound and boring (4).

The beginning clinical student may initially need to obtain much data by the scanning or descriptive approach. However, the student will learn to test hypotheses actively during the interview in order to increase the diagnostic value of the interview. This requires incorporating knowledge of diseases, their unique symptom constellations, and other diagnostic features, learned from standard textbooks (5) and clinical experience, into the interaction.

Chest pain, for example, has well over 20 possible disease causes, each with its unique symptoms, other diagnostic features, and, often, different associated symptom patterns (e.g., angina pectoris, myocardial infarction, esophagitis, pneumonia, rib fracture, pulmonary embolus, or pericarditis).

How does the interviewer test hypotheses during the interview? He or she ranks or orders disease possibilities in her or his mind very early in the interview based on unique symptom(s) characteristics and secondary data that suggest one diagnosis over others and on knowledge of what diseases are most common (2,4,6). The interviewer then seeks additional diagnostic data (primary and secondary) to support the current best choice, almost always via extensive closed-ended questioning. If complete data have already been obtained descriptively, the new data will be largely outside the involved system. If the first hypothesis is not supported, another disease hypothesis becomes the best choice ("next best choice") to explain the symptom(s) and is similarly explored. By following this process of testing multiple, ever-changing hypotheses, she or he eventually arrives at the best diagnostic possibility, or the "current best hypothesis"—the best fit of our patient's primary (and secondary, if available) data with a known disease. To start with one disease hypothesis (angina) and, based on symptom descriptors and associated symptoms, to end with a quite different one (esophagitis) is not uncommon. For example, because of substernal chest pain radiating into the arms, the interviewer's first hypothesis may be angina; but, she or he knows that esophagitis is also a possible cause of chest pain radiating to the arms and so asks about descriptors and other symptoms associated with this diagnosis. When these were present (precipitation of pain by coffee; relief by belching and antacids; poor appetite) and others expected with angina were not (no relationship of pain to exertion), she or he can then make a diagnosis. When a hypothesis is well supported, it becomes a "diagnosis." A diagnosis can derive from the history alone (e.g., angina), but sometimes additional data from the physical examination (e.g., enlarged liver) or the laboratory (e.g., low hemoglobin) are needed before the clinician or student can establish a diagnosis (4).

The more knowledge and experience that the interviewer has, the more facile and efficient she or he becomes in formulating the diagnosis and in knowing the proper questions to ask during an interview rather than in a subsequent interview. Nevertheless, virtually all beginning clinical students will find themselves fully synthesizing the diagnosis only after the interview—when they have read about the problem, have talked again with the patient to clarify issues that they overlooked, and have discussed the problem with faculty and residents. Although this vast topic of clinical diagnostics (2,4,6–10) is outside the province of this text, the process of clinical problem solving is well illustrated in Table 5.2, which shows how the student tests hypotheses while obtaining the HPI.

TABLE 5.2. AN EXAMPLE OF CLINICAL PROBLEM-SOLVING

Clinicians proceed, much as Sherlock Holmes, by first obtaining a few bits of presenting data (e.g., nonradiating chest pain, fever, shortness of breath, and a swollen left leg in a 70-year-old man) to generate the current best hypothesis (e.g., pulmonary embolus); they then ask specific questions (e.g., hemoptysis, which means coughing-up blood) that would further support or detract from this hypothesis. In this example, the clinician introduces the previously unmentioned hemoptysis because her or his first hypothesis was pulmonary embolus and this symptom is pertinent to its diagnosis. Let us say that hemoptysis was not present but that the clinician pursued the hypothesis further by inquiring if the leg swelling was recent or if any immobility of the leg had occurred recently, which are common findings of some diagnostic value in pulmonary embolism. We'll suppose that the symptoms began following a 12-hour car ride just 3 days ago, so the clinician became more confident of pulmonary embolus as a possible diagnosis.

Even though the diagnosis may be likely, the interviewer tests alternative hypotheses among the other most likely diseases causing this patient's chest pain. For example, the advanced student also would consider distinguishing questions supporting myocardial infarction (substernal location of pain, crushing pain, diaphoresis), pneumonia (fever, cough, chills), rib fracture (injury), pericarditis (pain relieved by sitting up and leaning forward, and aggravated by lying supine), lung cancer (weight loss, cigarette or asbestos exposure), and a host of other possibilities as long as they reflected reasonable possible causes of the patient's chest pain and other symptoms. Notice that none of these symptoms had been mentioned previously; that the clinician introduced them closed-endedly; that, if left to a simple scanning/descriptive approach and subsequent routine inquiry, many would have been completely dissociated from the history of present illness (chest trauma and cigarette use are asked about in the past medical history usually); and that some may never have arisen without a hypothesis-driven inquiry (relief of pain from sitting up is not a routine question).

The clinician in this case would of course proceed to obtain a complete history and physical examination and appropriate laboratory data to clarify her or his hypotheses and, hopefully, to establish a diagnosis.

Elstein AS. Psychological research on diagnostic reasoning. In: Lipkin M, Putnam SM, Lazare A, eds. *The medical interview*. New York: Springer-Verlag, 1995:504–510.

Barrows HS, Pickell GC. *Developing clinical problem-solving skills. A guide to more effective diagnosis and treatment*. New York: WW Norton Medical Books, 1991.

Elstein AS, Kagan N, Shulman LS, et al. Methods and theory in the study of medical inquiry. *J Med Educ* 1972;47:85–92.

Continuation of Vignette of Mrs. Jones

DOC: Ever had problems with swelling or pains in your joints?

[The student has hypothesized that vasculitis might be causing the headaches and has found that this diagnosis is sometimes associated with arthritis. She is thus inquiring closed-endedly about specific primary data outside the system involved to support this hypothesis.]

PT: No.

DOC: Ever had any dancing or bright, shimmering lights in your vision with the headaches?

[The student has learned that this symptom (scintillating scotomata) is of diagnostic value with migraine and properly is inquiring specifically about it as a way to build support for the hypothesis of migraine headaches.]

PT: No.

DOC: Because these could be vascular headaches, you know like migraine, I need to ask you some specifics about that. Do you use birth control pills or other hormones?

[The student is beginning to formulate diagnostic hypotheses about what has caused the headaches. She suspects migraine from the clinical story and from reading about headaches. Accordingly, obtaining additional supporting diagnostic data—hence, the question about birth control pills—is appropriate. In addition, because head injuries also can cause headaches, the interviewer will ask about that as an alternative hypothesis. Indeed, any of the possible causes that have been entertained could be further addressed in this way. (If the student were suspicious of meningitis from the story, perhaps because of intermittent fever and stiff neck, additional questions to support or to refute that hypothesis would be in order: any rashes, exposure, and whatever else the student considered important in supporting a diagnosis of meningitis.)]

PT: Yeah, I've been on them for the last 6 years.

[The student should pursue the type, doses, and experience with these later in the PMH.]

DOC: Any family history of migraine?

[These questions are included here rather than in the FH because a positive family history supports the hypothesis of migraine.]

PT: One of my aunts had what they called "sick headaches" when she was young but they cleared up when she got a lot older.

DOC: By the way, have you ever had any head injuries?

[The student is testing another nonmigraine hypothesis for the headache.]

PT: No.

DOC: Have you ever been unconscious for any reason?

PT: No.

DOC: Any neck injuries or problems there?

[Neck problems also can cause headaches, and the student is exploring this hypothesis.]

PT: Nope.

DOC: Well, we need to change to some other questions now, about your colitis, cough, and past medical history, if you feel finished talking about this. Anything else we need to cover, before we go on?

[When mentioning transitions in this section of the interview, checking whether the patient is finished and seeing if she or he has anything further to add to the topic at hand continues to be important.]

PT: That's fine. You've covered everything, I think.

[This evaluation, performed by a beginning clinical level student, shows how the new interviewer first obtains data in the involved system to help develop hypotheses and then tests the hypotheses with selective questions designed to support or to refute them.]

Procedural Issues

When more than one problem has been raised, the student evaluates it in the same way. For example, Mrs. Jones also has had colitis and a recent cough. These now could be systematically explored. However, if these are not currently active health problems, they also can be explored as part of the PMH. They are included in the PMH portion of the written report when they do not contribute to the current problems as in Mrs. Jones' situation. When they are contributing to current problems, they are included as OCAP at the end of the HPI.

This is a lot for the student to assimilate, and to do so requires much practice. Review of the demonstration videotape will also help (1) (see Preface). Students can be reassured by the knowledge that, once the symptoms in the System Review and the symptom-defining skills are learned in their clinical context, this process becomes quite reflexive. Nor does it take the seasoned clinician very long to obtain diagnostic and therapeutic information. Most can conduct a full HPI/OCAP, HI, PMH, SH, FH, and ROS with a patient like Mrs. Jones in 30 to 40 minutes. **With advancing skills and knowledge of diseases, the student learns which are the most pertinent questions and how to ask them efficiently instead of needing to ask all of them.** (See the end of Chapter 6 for a discussion of how much time the beginning clinical student will need to spend with the patient.)

Much of the interview occurs by predominantly closed-ended inquiry, which raises the following two important issues. (a) A poorly conducted closed-ended inquiry can lead to considerable bias of the data. Table 5.3 lists important ways to avoid this. (b) Because the interviewer is now in the doctor-centered process, she or he can ask direct questions that insert new information into the conversation where necessary. This is especially helpful for testing hypotheses. (In a patient with a chronic cough, introducing the fol-

---

TABLE 5.3. TO MINIMIZE BIAS FROM CLOSED-ENDED QUESTIONING

A. Proceed from general to specific. Start with an open-ended question in each major area.

B. Use single questions. Avoid a question such as, "Have you ever had headaches, fainting, loss of vision, blurred vision, poor memory, or a stroke?" Rather, one might ask, "Have you ever had headaches?"

C. Do not suggest a response by the way the question is framed. Avoid questions like, "You haven't had any blood in the urine have you?"

D. Give equal weight to alternative answers. An advised way to ask is, "It sounds like there is some pain with exertion, but what about when you're not exerting?"

E. Do not interpret data while collecting them. Avoid saying, "Must be hemorrhoids. Ever had any nausea or vomiting?"

F. Give balanced attention to all aspects. An appropriate way to do so is, "We've talked a lot about your constipation, but not much yet about the chest pain."

G. Do not confuse the patient with rapid shifts or technical language. Do not ask, "Did they do an ERCP or another endoscopy; were any lesions found?"

H. Ensure that the conversation is congruent with the patient's experience.

Abbreviation: ERCP, endoscopic retrograde cholangiopancreatography.

lowing material is perfectly appropriate: "Are you a cigarette smoker?" or "Have you lost weight?")

The HPI/OCAP concludes when all presenting symptoms have been addressed. The clinician, but perhaps not the beginning clinical student, understands the problem and has the best possible disease explanation in mind, if he or she has not actually made the diagnosis. This determines what corroboration she or he will look for on the physical examination and in the laboratory evaluation. Interviewers also more fully recognize the close interaction of symptoms and secondary data with the personal data that was obtained during the patient-centered process.

The interviewer should then make a statement about changing the conversation to some material that "we haven't yet covered about your past medical history," as the student did with Mrs. Jones. At this point, she or he should ask the patient if she or he thinks her or his story has been completely discussed, should summarize what has happened thus far, and should see if the patient has anything further to add.

Addressing a Predominantly Psychological Problem

The personal, contextual data obtained during the patient-centered process usually are not sufficient for complete evaluation in patients with psychiatric diseases or other serious psychological problems. Steps 1 through 5 are just the beginning. In the doctor-centered HPI, the interviewer pins down details about the psychological problem, just as she or he would with a physical disease problem. The clinician or student elicits the patient's symptoms and tests hypotheses about the underlying diagnosis by selectively testing different diagnostic possibilities. For example, a patient's depression may have been apparent during Steps 1 to 5, but the interviewer's task is now to explore its possible disease causes, potential complications, and treatment options. Using scanning open-ended inquiry followed by closed-ended inquiry, he or she can differentiate the actual cause of the depression from among the possible culprits, such as major depression, bipolar disorder, schizophrenia, drugs, and medical diseases. Just as a student will gain more experience with the diagnosis of medical diseases during clinical clerkships, she or he will learn much more about psychological diagnoses during clinical clerkships and during psychiatry rotations.

On the other hand, most medical patients are like Mrs. Jones and have no apparent overriding psychological problem or diagnosis. That statement might surprise some readers after all that they have heard about Mrs. Jones' job stresses and interpersonal conflicts. Although understanding the patient is important to the interviewer, such conflict does not necessarily bespeak disease. Indeed, this type of problem defines our personal lives and is not outside the realm of normal. Additional personal details for patients like Mrs. Jones, who has minimal psychological problems, usually are obtained in the SH.

General Comments About the Process to Follow

We now have completed the most important part of doctor-centered interviewing. Step 7 is where you will spend most of your time. **The remaining steps (Steps 8 to 12) are very straightforward.** The interviewer simply asks and the patient answers many questions, **often guided by a questionnaire that has been previously completed by the patient.** Most hypothesis testing should be complete, but as an interviewer you should continue to be on the lookout for items that could be clues to hypotheses.

The reader will note that the questions are extensive; to ask and answer all of them could literally take several hours! I present all of this material so that the student has an idea of the magnitude of the information about the patient that can potentially be important and about what can be necessary for understanding her or him fully. Note, however, that the experienced clinician rarely obtains all of this information, certainly not at one sitting; pertinent but nonurgent information often is obtained over many visits. Rather, **the information in Steps 8 to 12 is gathered selectively according to the individual patient's needs.** As the clinician or student proceeds through these steps, he or she considers those that might be more important for a certain type of patient, such as the older patient, women, men, children, crisis situations, and high-risk patients. Beginning clinical level students, however, are advised initially to obtain complete information in all areas as a way of learning the categories and of beginning to appreciate the rich diversity of patients. When they have learned the categories, then they also can become more selective.

Although much of the information in Steps 8 to 12 is quite routine, the interviewer should continue to watch the patient's response and should particularly look for fatigue and impatience with a long process. She or he should periodically inquire about comfort and should ask if the patient needs a break or if continuing at a later time would be appropriate. At the other extreme, although these may appear to be very routine questions, they often strike an emotional chord in patients and therefore returning to patient-centered inquiry, particularly emotion-handling, may be necessary (e.g., when asking a spouse's age, a patient becomes sad because of a recent divorce). In this more routine part of the history, as an interviewer, maintaining the respectful, patient-centered atmosphere that we have previously established and not becoming hurried are essential. Finally, **repeating often to patients that the questions are indeed routine and that the questions do not bespeak something you have recognized or suspected about them is useful** (e.g., asking some patients about drug use might be insulting if the reason for asking is not explained).

Health Issues (Step 8)

Health issues (HI) include important information that is often omitted from the database but that, nonetheless, is essential to understand and help the patient best. Health issues involve ethical-social-spiritual issues, functional status, health-promoting and health-maintenance habits, and potential health hazards (11–17).

Each major HI area in Table 5.4 is initiated with a focused open-ended request or question (e.g., "Tell me what you do to stay healthy.") and is followed by enough closed-ended questions to get the necessary details. The in-

---

TABLE 5.4. HEALTH ISSUES (STEP 8)

A. Cover ethical-social-spiritual issues: advance directives, power of attorney, whom to contact if the patient cannot speak for herself or himself, and spiritual practices.

B. Discuss functional status: dressing, bathing, feeding, transferring, walking, shopping, using the toilet, using a telephone, cooking, cleaning, driving, taking medications, managing finances, and cognitive function; extent of interference with normal life.

C. Inquire about health-promoting and health-maintenance activities.
   1. Health-promoting habits: diet, seat belts, use of a helmet with bicycle or motorcycle, protection of self and others from poisonous substances (including medications) and dangerous circumstances at home and work, exercise, relaxation, recreation.
   2. Health screening: periodic health exams, mammograms, Pap smear, sigmoidoscopy, stools for occult blood, cholesterol, blood sugar, serologic test for syphilis, tuberculosis skin testing, HIV testing, prostatic evaluation, dental check, audiograms, eye exam, tonometry; self-examination (breasts, genitals, and skin).
   3. Disease prophylaxis: diphtheria, pertussis, tetanus, polio, measles, German measles, hepatitis, influenza, vaccine for pneumococcal pneumonia, for diseases in areas of foreign travel.

D. Ask about health hazards.
   1. Use of addicting substances: caffeine, tobacco, alcohol, street drugs, prescription medications.
   2. Sexual practices: activity, preferences, diseases, abuse, risky habits, contraception, satisfaction.
   3. Abuse: sexual, physical, verbal, psychological, other.

terviewer must be especially careful to be patient, courteous, and understanding as a way of ensuring continuation of the patient-centered atmosphere as health issues concern many sensitive areas. Patients often are reassured by the fact that the questions are routine and that they are asked of everyone. Tension-laden areas must be addressed delicately with considerable use of open-ended and emotion-handling skills (i.e., the interviewer may need to resume the patient-centered process described earlier). The interviewing strategy for obtaining very sensitive material (e.g., sexual or drug abuse history) is expanded in Chapter 6.

Ethical-Social-Spiritual Issues

In the severely ill, disabled, or elderly patient and with many others, the interviewer especially needs to inquire about advance directives (e.g., "do not resuscitate" wishes, living will, use of a respirator to sustain life), power of attorney, and whom to contact in the event of serious health problems. These data are essential for any patient who may become seriously ill and unable to speak for herself or himself. Research data show that addressing advance directives improves the satisfaction of elderly patients (18). Research shows also that, in addition to knowing what to say, a patient-centered approach is the most effective way to determine it (19).

Information that is rarely addressed but that is essential, especially in times of crises, are patients' spiritual affiliations and beliefs, whether they are attached to a formal religion or not (20). Some data indicate an association between spirituality and good health (17). The interviewer should try to understand what is ultimately meaningful for patients, how this relates to their suffering, what their beliefs and faith are, who and what they love, their meditation or prayer practices, their orientation to giving and forgiving, and the patient's actual worship practices (i.e., the integration of mind, body, and spirit) (12).

Functional Status

Especially in the elderly and in those with disabling problems, the student or clinician needs to know what the patient's functional status is in several areas. These can include how well she or he can dress herself or himself, walk, shop, use the toilet, and keep track of her or his bank account. Indeed, the American College of Physicians has asked that patient histories be standardized to include routine functional status and well being assessments (13). In addition, the interviewer must make an assessment of how much a disability interferes with the patient's life and wishes. (She or he may no longer be able to climb stairs, but this may not interfere with what the patient wants to do; alternatively, the same disability may cause a great hardship for another patient because it prevents her or him from attending baseball games.)

Health-Promoting and Health-Maintenance Habits

In this section, the interviewer asks what the patient thinks of her or his own health status and then inquires specifically about health-promoting habits. Does the patient partake of a low-salt and low-fat diet with healthy protein and calorie content? use a seat belt and have airbags? use a helmet while riding a bicycle or motorcycle? have a smoke detector? have all poisonous substances (including medications) safe from their children's reach? have safeguards against toxic exposure and dangerous situations at home and at work? exercise at least three times weekly? take satisfactory amounts of time for relaxation and to enjoy outside recreational activities? Much more attention is now given to injury prevention, including how weapons in the home are handled and stored, than in the past (15).

A number of recommended health-screening procedures, which vary by age, circumstance, and gender, that the interviewer should ensure are up to date do exist, including periodic health examination, mammograms, Pap smear, sigmoidoscopy, stools for occult blood, cholesterol, blood sugar, serologic test for syphilis, tuberculosis skin testing, HIV testing, prostatic evaluation, dental check, audiograms, eye examination, and tonometry. Preventive health services are crucial to health care, although differences of opinion are found in some recommendations (16). To know if patients are performing self-examination of the breasts, testes, penis, and skin is also important; with these, a significant disease often can be detected early when it is less advanced and more amenable to treatment.

Finally, the interviewer should determine the patient's level of disease prophylaxis with regard to the following: diphtheria, pertussis, tetanus, polio, measles, German measles, hepatitis, influenza, pneumococcal pneumonia, and diseases unique to areas of intended foreign travel.

Health Hazzards

Use of Addicting Substances

Patients often minimize this material, particularly drug and alcohol usage, and inquiry can produce tension for the interviewer and patient alike. The interviewer should ask about duration, amount, and type of addicting substance used (e.g., drinks three beers daily, except on weekends when it is six or seven per day, and started this 11 years ago; smoked two packages of cigarettes daily for 8 years [16 pack-years]). Data about alcohol problems can be obtained using the CAGE questionnaire. CAGE is an acronym for the following four highlighted areas (21): (a) Have you ever tried to Cut down? (b) Do you get Angry when people talk to you about your drinking? (c) Do you feel Guilty about your drinking? (d) Do you ever take an Eye opener? In addition, the student or clinician should inquire about whether the patients have had problems from using addicting substances (e.g., divorce, job loss, delirium tremens with alcohol withdrawal, emphysema from cigarettes), if they have attempted to quit or to decrease the habit, why they were or were not successful in stopping, and if they are interested in getting help abstaining. As well, problems with the legal system, with sharing drug equipment, and with other substance abuse problems in the patient's life are essential data. Finally, particularly with drug and alcohol abuse, the interviewer looks for the psychiatric issues that commonly accompany these problems (e.g., anxiety and depression). Indeed, **full primary and secondary data are elicited for any perceived drug-alcohol problem. When alcohol or drug abuse exists, it often belongs in the HPI** because it frequently relates to the major problem the patient has and it almost always has a major impact on the patient's health (e.g., a patient presents with chest pain suggesting angina and also a history suggesting alcoholism). Students will learn the details of drug and alcohol abuse evaluation during clinical work.

Sexual Practices

Although sexual activity per se is not hazardous, many hazardous situations occur as a result of patients' sexual habits (22). A good history requires the following information: heterosexual, homosexual, or bisexual orientation; current sexual activity (type, amount, and number of partners); past sexual activity (type, amount, and number of partners); risky sexual habits; condom usage; sexual satisfaction and pleasure; contraceptive measures; sexually transmitted diseases; impotence; nonorgasm; and any sexual concerns. With prominent sexual disorder, attendant psychiatric disease, such as depression and anxiety, is common and must be clarified. The history is not complete until the student or clinician also learns about the patient's relationship with a partner(s), especially about their communication pattern.

Abuse

Abuse is increasingly prominent in many areas of patients' lives, and the student or clinician should inquire specifically about sexual, physical, verbal, and psychological abuse (23–26). One-fifth of women in a primary care population have reported some type of violence in their lifetime (14), but such data may be skewed because of restrictive research definitions (27). Information about abuse can be difficult to elicit, and questions must occur in a safe, patient-centered atmosphere of trust and compassion (24). All patients are potential recipients or perpetrators, and the extent of abuse may vary from frequent and severe to infrequent and mild. Women, children, and the elderly are particularly susceptible. Such stories of abuse are quite common in those with both medical and psychological illnesses.

Because obtaining all HI items is a time-consuming task, clinicians and advanced clinical level students may not cover all of them at the first visit and instead complete them over time. Beginning clinical level students, however, are advised initially to obtain complete information in all areas as a way of learning the categories and of beginning to appreciate the rich diversity of patients.

Continuation of Vignette with Mrs. Jones

DOC: Let me ask you some other questions about what you do to stay healthy.

[A good open-ended start into health issues. Because of space constraints, I again simply summarize the findings about Mrs. Jones, some of which required a return to a patient-centered process of inquiry.]

She has done nothing about advance directives but does think that they are a good idea. Her church attendance has decreased since moving here because of her busy schedule. She has no functional limitations. The student knows about her work but she also learns that Mrs. Jones worries about being a "workaholic" and about not taking enough time for her painting, which she doesn't do every day. She and her husband socialize frequently. She is trying to be a good model for her "lax husband" and always uses her seat belt, exercises three times weekly in a 45-minute aerobics class, maintains her weight around 120 pounds, and eats a low-fat and low-salt diet. She wants to do more to relax better, but she isn't sure what to do. She has yearly Pap smears and performs a breast self-examination about a week after each menstrual period. She had her "baby shots" years ago and a tetanus shot 2 years ago when she punctured her hand with a nail. Except for an occasional cup of coffee and glass of wine, she has never used any addictive substances.

She has been satisfied with her sexual life until the last 3 months when she has had less interest in sexual intercourse (now reduced from three to four times weekly to once weekly), and her husband has had inconstant difficulties with impotence; she has no reason to suspect her husband is not monogamous. She thinks the sexual problem "will take care of itself" when her job problems are resolved. She is not interested in talking any further about it at this point. She has had only two other sexual partners, prior to marriage. She has no history of sexually transmitted disease or sexual abuse (or other types of abuse now or in the past), and she and her husband are heterosexual.

Past Medical History (Step 9)

The past medical history (PMH) elicits information about significant past medical events unrelated to the HPI/OCAP. Events from the past that are related to the HPI/OCAP are elicited as part of them. For instance, in a patient presenting with chest pain, the prior history of myocardial infarction usually is obtained in the HPI rather than the PMH. Similarly, because of the close association of diabetes and coronary artery disease, if this patient also is a diabetic of 20 years duration, those data are elicited in the HPI. On the other hand, if the same patient presents with diverticulitis or a hip fracture, the cardiovascular history is obtained in the PMH as long as it is not an active problem. **These distinctions are not always clear, and no rigid right or wrong mandates where the interviewer can place or when she or he should obtain historical data.** Of course, the clinician or student sometimes elicits data pertinent to the HPI while obtaining the PMH; this information is relocated to the HPI when being written-up or presented.

Similar approaches to those used with the doctor-centered process of the HPI/OCAP elicit the PMH. Each major area shown in Table 5.5 is addressed with a focused, open-ended screening question (e.g., "Tell me about any previous hospitalizations." [any other medical problems, or surgeries]). This is followed with enough closed-ended questions to get the necessary details for all items mentioned. Simple closed-ended inquiry suffices for obtaining much data within these categories (e.g., "Ever had any broken bones?").

TABLE 5.5. PAST MEDICAL HISTORY (STEP 9)

A. Discuss hospitalizations: surgical, nonsurgical, psychiatric, obstetric, rehabilitation, other.
B. Inquire about other medical, surgical, or psychological problems: injuries, accidents, illnesses, unexplained problems, procedures, tests, psychotherapy, other.
C. Screen for major diseases: rheumatic fever, diabetes mellitus, tuberculosis, venereal diseases, cancer, heart attack, and stroke; major treatments in the past (cortisone, blood transfusions, insulin, digitalis, anticoagulants); and visits to the doctor during the last year.
D. Cover medications and other treatments: prescribed, over the counter, alternative therapies and health care, and "nonmedications" (laxatives, tonics, hormones, birth control pills, vitamins).
E. Verify allergies and drug reactions: allergic diseases (e.g., asthma, hay fever), drugs, foods, environmental.
F. Review menstrual and obstetric history (for women): onset of menses, duration, cycle length, discomfort, number of pads daily, birth control pills and other hormonal preparations, pregnancies, abortions (spontaneous), abortions (induced), deliveries of living children, other deliveries, complications of pregnancy, menopause.

The interviewer should continue to support the patient and to ensure a patient-centered atmosphere. **As interviewers, we also inquire periodically about how the patient is responding to the interview itself.** We realize that it can be tiring, confusing, and even upsetting. Furthermore, we almost always reassure patients that certain questions do not reflect a suspected condition but, rather, are routinely asked of everyone (such as those regarding cancer, diabetes mellitus, or memory loss).

I will now expand on the outline in Table 5.5. When a problem with significance for the patient's health is found in any of the areas listed, the interviewer should review the symptoms and make her or his own diagnosis, which often requires outside records to be certain. She or he cannot accept as final a patient's understanding of diagnoses or her or his interpretations of treatments. The interviewer should follow the procedure already described—convert complaints to symptoms in the System Review, refine them with the seven descriptors, and then order relevant primary data (symptoms) and secondary data (doctors, hospitals, tests) into chronologic sequence.

For PMH problems with little significance to present health (appendectomy or tonsillectomy many years ago), little detail, other than getting the patient's version of the diagnosis and complications and her or his statement that no subsequent problems have occurred, is needed. **Indeed, time constraints and patients' comfort discourage acquiring unnecessary data.**

The interviewer identifies significant past problems by inquiring in the following areas.

Hospitalizations

Hospitalizations often identify the most serious problems patients have experienced: surgical, nonsurgical, psychiatric, obstetric, rehabilitation, and any other type. The more recent and serious a hospitalization is, the more data that are required, sometimes more extensively than the HPI. For example, in a patient who is admitted with a hip fracture as the primary problem but who had a history of three heart attacks, the interviewer would need to elicit extensive details of all primary and secondary cardiovascular data. Hospitalizations usually are obtained in chronological order.

Other Medical, Surgical, or Psychological Problems

Here, the interviewer seeks significant past problems by specific inquiry about childhood illnesses (e.g., measles, mumps, German measles, chickenpox), injuries, accidents, illnesses requiring several visits, unexplained problems, procedures, tests, and psychotherapy.

Screen for Major Diseases

To screen for problems that might not yet have been identified, the clinician or student should make specific inquiry about potentially serious conditions, including diabetes, tuberculosis, venereal diseases, rheumatic fever, heart attacks, strokes, or cancer. Similarly, she or he asks about prior treatment that suggests serious problems, such as with cortisone, insulin, blood transfusions, digitalis, and anticoagulants. Finally, she or he inquires about all health visits to the doctor or to others during the last year.

Medications and Other Treatments

Prescribed and other medications are listed with dose, duration of use, reason for use, and any adverse reactions. The interviewer should also obtain a listing of medications that were used during the last year but that are not presently being taken. Specific inquiry about agents that sometimes are not considered medications, such as laxatives, tonics, hormones, birth control pills, and vitamins, is necessary as well. Questioning about agents obtained over the counter, from alternative healers, or from other sources, such as a friend, should also be conducted. In all instances, the interviewer must identify the contents, which often entails either contacting the pharmacy or having the patient bring in the actual medications so that they can be definitively identified, particularly when all the patient knows is that "I'm taking a brown pill for my circulation." Sometimes consulting the *Physicians' Desk Reference,* which has color photographs of many commonly used brand name medications, also helps (28).

The clinician or student should also ask about nonpharmacologic forms of treatment, whether administered by self or others, including physical therapy, biofeedback, relaxation techniques, yoga, acupuncture, psychotherapy of any type (e.g., individual, group), diet, and exercise. She or he must specifically inquire about so-called alternative methods of treatment (e.g., homeopathy, herbal medicine, chiropractic) because the patient often does not mention these out of embarrassment or for fear of angering the physician (29).

Allergies and Drug Reactions

The clinician or student asks about asthma, hay fever, hives, and atopic eczema if these have not already been ascertained because they are common allergic disorders; asthma has nonallergic dimensions as well. These patients also may be more sensitive to certain medications (e.g., aspirin in asthmatics).

Drug reactions can be allergic (rash caused by penicillin) or nonallergic (candida vaginitis caused by an antibiotic). Patients seldom make this distinction, but the interviewer must because allergic reactions usually militate against subsequent use of the medication, whereas alterations in dosage and frequency sometimes allow later use if a drug reaction was nonallergic. The student or clinician lists all allergic or other drug reactions, dose and duration of use of the agent, specific symptoms (e.g., hives, anaphylaxis, rash), as well as secondary data (e.g., desensitization, skin tests, cortisone), recurrence, history of re-exposure, and final outcome.

Menstrual and Obstetric History

Obtaining information from women and girls about menses is essential; included should be the age at onset, duration, cycle length, discomfort, and number of pads daily. Use of birth control pills or other hormonal preparations also is sometimes elicited at this point. Obstetric histories include the number of pregnancies, spontaneous abortions, and induced abortions; deliveries of living children and their outcome; other deliveries and the reason for adverse outcome; and any complications of pregnancy. Additionally, menopausal problems can be elicited here. When genitourinary (GU) problems are the focus, the menstrual and obstetric history is often elicited in the HPI.

I now return to Mrs. Jones for demonstration of this.

Continuation of Vignette of Mrs. Jones

DOC: Tell me about any hospitalizations you've had, you know, other than that time for the colitis.

[Although this was not recounted in the doctor-centered HPI/OCAP or PMH for space reasons, the student already has addressed Mrs. Jones' colitis and cough; the results of this inquiry are given in the write-up in Appendix D.]

PT: I had my tonsils out as a kid.

DOC: Any other hospitalizations?

[She might have asked about any complications or subsequent problems.]

PT: Well, I did break my arm in high school and they had to set it.

DOC: How's that been since? Any problem?

[Knowing how it was broken should also be important.]

PT: No, it's just fine. I play tennis and have no trouble.

DOC/PT: Other hospitalizations (no), injuries (no), accidents (no), or sickness (no)? [These questions were asked and answered individually.]

DOC: Didn't you mention having kids?

PT: Oh, yeah. I forgot! They're 6 and 8. But I had no trouble delivering.

[At this point, they sound uncomplicated, and the interviewer will get the details of the menstrual and obstetric history at the end of the PMH, although she could do that just as easily now.]

DOC/PT: I'm going to give you some specific diseases now; just tell me if you've ever had them. These, by the way, are routine questions; I'm not asking because I suspect something: Rheumatic fever? (no) Scarlet fever? (no) Diabetes? (no) Tuberculosis? (no) Sexually transmitted diseases? (no) Cancer? (no) Stroke? (no) Heart attack? (no) Any other diseases? (no)

[In a series of questions like this is, each one is asked individually and the patient is allowed sufficient time for an answer; the patient should not feel pressured, nor should a whole string of questions be asked at once. Remaining sensitive throughout the patient's responses to all inquiries and responding to her or his questions are important. In particular, reassuring the patient that items being inquired about are routine and that the clinician has not noticed something to make her or him suspicious almost always helps.]

DOC/PT: Besides the cortisone for your colitis, I need more specifics now about major league treatments you might have had: blood transfusions? (no) Insulin? (no) Digitalis? (no) Anticoagulants? (no)

[This is an additional way to screen for any major problems that have not yet been mentioned.]

DOC: Any visits to your doctor during the last year or so for anything we haven't covered?

PT: Well, I did have a bladder infection once and got some medicine for it.

DOC: What were your symptoms?

[The student is not taking her word for the diagnosis and, correctly, wants to know the symptoms; she will also want to know any secondary data.]

PT: One morning when I woke up I had to go all the time—it burned—and I'd have to go all of a sudden, but I felt ok.

DOC: When was this?

PT: Last July, just before the Fourth.

DOC: How long did it last?

PT: Oh, with the medicine it was gone in about 2 days, but I took the medicine for a week.

DOC: Did the pain, the burning, move any place like up into the bladder or back?

PT: No.

DOC: How many times a day would you go?

PT: Oh, that first day it must have been every hour.

DOC: Anything help it?

PT: Just the medications.

DOC/PT: Did any of these symptoms go with it: Fever? (no) Chills? (no) Blood in the urine? (no) Back pain? (no) Pass anything in the urine? (no) Getting up at night? (a couple times when it started) Unable to pass urine? (no) Unable to control your bladder? (no)

[Again, these are addressed individually; these particular questions provide information about other symptoms in the GU system.]

DOC: Any tests done, like looking up in your bladder or cultures of the urine?

PT: No, he just gave me some medicine, a sulfa drug of some kind.

DOC: Ever had this before?

PT: Nope, it didn't amount to much.

[The student has a good profile of pertinent symptoms from the urinary system, knows the attendant secondary data, and has established the chronology of what sounds like an uncomplicated lower urinary tract infection. This is a very simple and straightforward problem, but the student must evaluate each significant (to present health) PMH problem in a similar fashion.]

DOC: Any other problems you've seen your doctor or anyone else for?

PT: No.

DOC: If there's nothing else, I'd like to shift and find out about medications and some other things.

[A good open-ended start into this new area. Because of space constraints, I'll simply summarize the student's findings about Mrs. Jones. Except for the birth control pill and aspirin (detailed doses and other data obtained) with the headaches, she is taking no medications or other treatments from either prescribed or other sources. The history of prednisone use is reviewed. She has no allergic diseases and no history of adverse reactions to any drugs or other substances. Her menstrual and obstetric history are recounted in Appendix D.]

Social History (Step 10)

The social history (SH), also called the psychosocial history or the patient profile, provides two types of data: (a) the details, if any, of current personal or psychological problems not obtained in the HPI/OCAP and (b) routine personal data about noncurrent issues.

The SH completes, if necessary, the personal profile that was begun during the patient-centered process and is guided by the "Current Personal Situation" category of Table 5.6. Although, many times, much of the information in Table 5.6 has already been obtained, the guidelines given often provide additional specific details that sometimes must be addressed, as the following vignette illustrates.

As in the HI and PMH, the interviewer obtains the SH by screening open-ended questions (requests) followed by closed-ended questions for details. Also like the HI and PMH, although this does not intend a return to the patient-centered process, she or he does so if significant issues or emotions de-

TABLE 5.6. SOCIAL HISTORY (STEP 10)

A. Ask about current personal situation.
   1. Demographic: age, sex, race, current work and living situation.
   2. Impact (meaning) of illness on self or others.
   3. Beliefs or explanations about illness.
   4. Relationships and support system.
   5. Practical issues.
   6. Stress.
   7. Financial situation.
B. Inquire about other personal factors.
   1. Early developmental outline: birth and early development, early family setting and other caretakers, relationship with parents and siblings, others' relationships in family, early schooling and progress, places of residence, major losses and other adverse events, medical–surgical problems, happy events, later education and progress, social life and relationships, dating, adolescence, military or other service, getting away from home.
   2. Marriage/other relationships and outcome: significant relationships (origin, course, outcome), children.
   3. Work history and outcome: jobs and duration, satisfaction, toxic or other dangerous exposure (fumes, radiation, noise, dusts, chemicals).
   4. Recreational history.
   5. Retirement.
   6. Aging.
   7. Life satisfaction.
   8. Cultural and ethnic background.

velop or if a previously reticent patient begins to open up. Going back and forth between patient-centered and doctor-centered processes many times is not uncommon.

Because the "Other Personal Factors" category potentially is very extensive, as Table 5.6 demonstrates, the experienced clinician focuses on the "Current Personal Situation" data so that the SH is obtained in a timely way; she or he often only completes the entire SH over many visits, if ever. The bottom line is an attempt to understand the patient better and to fill in any necessary gaps. Beginning clinical level students, however, initially should obtain answers to all items. Doing so is essential for learning the questions and for understanding the many dimensions of human beings.

Continuation of Vignette of Mrs. Jones

DOC: We need to shift gears again and get some more details about your personal situation.

[A nice transition]

PT: Seems like I've told you everything.

DOC: Well, I need to get a few more details. First, though, how are you doing with all this questioning?

[Always attending primarily to the patient's needs, the student takes time to inquire about the process of the interview itself.]

PT: No problem. I like how thorough you are.

[She is doing well and makes a positive comment about the student, indicating that a good relationship exists.]

DOC: Thanks. Sometimes it feels like pressure to get so many questions. I appreciate your patience. Now, I need to get some more information. How old are you?

[The student is beginning to get some basic demographic data. Age is sometimes asked much earlier for basic orientation.]

PT: 38. I just had a birthday.

DOC: And your family has been here for how long?

[The student is not clear on how long the patient has actually been in the city.]

PT: About 4 months.

DOC: I think I know the answer to this but I'll ask anyway. How have these headaches affected you and your family's lives?

[Open-ended inquiry about impact of the headaches on her and others' lives. Although the patient has not raised the issue of impact, the interviewer introduces it in the SH. The doctor-centered process allows the student to take the lead like this to obtain necessary details about personal data.]

PT: It's been very disruptive. We were always quite happy and enjoyed things together. I told you about our sex life, and now the kids seem to get on my nerves all the time too. Things need to get settled down. The job, not just the headaches. I'm not sure I'll stay in this job if things don't change.

DOC: It's been a difficult time. I do think we can help with the headaches, but I don't know about your boss.

[Interspersing a patient-centered intervention—in this instance with naming and supporting statements—continues to be important.]

PT: He's supposed to retire in 6 months. If the headache comes around, I can make it that long.

DOC: I know you think the headaches are from your boss, but any other ideas why you might be getting them?

[She is leading and is shifting away from the boss and is probing for any other beliefs about why she is ill.]

PT: Only punishment! I was raised with that always there.

[Depending on the amount of time available, the interviewer could return to the patient-centered process and could explore this, allowing Mrs. Jones' ideas to lead. On the other hand, this issue is not current and she is exhibiting no distress so it can also be comfortably left until another time, as the student does here.]

DOC: That's a hard time for you. If it's ok to change, though, I'd like to ask you something else. (She nods approval.) You mentioned your husband earlier. Anybody else around that you can talk with?

PT: There's another new person there with the same problem and we commiserate all the time. He's taking over in another area but has the same boss. We get along great and seem to help each other. And, a couple other guys there know what's going on and have been very helpful—and had some good advice: Stay away from him.

[As with the rest of this dialogue, nothing urgent has arisen, so the student, recalling the need to be timely, simply obtains the information and does not pursue these issues in any depth.]

DOC: Is it possible to avoid him?

[A closed-ended question addresses a practical, personal issue that has therapeutic implications and that once again shows how inextricable is the link between disease and the personal dimension.]

PT: Actually, it is. I have to do a lot of traveling and can schedule it around him and things are much better then. I figured it out and I can miss him for at least half the time in the next 6 months!

[If it weren't possible to avoid him and to treat the headaches, the student and Mrs. Jones would have a bigger problem on their hands. In that event, this could be further addressed now or, more likely, at a subsequent visit that might be set up specifically for developing a strategy.]

DOC: You've sure had a lot of stress. Are financial issues a problem, you know like medical insurance or anything?

[Changing the subject to another important potential problem that must be raised by closed-ended means.]

PT: No! That was one of the benefits here. They cover everything with their insurance plan. I only pay a few dollars for everything, even medicines.

DOC: Let me change a little and ask now about some of your childhood.

[The student has now explored salient SH areas for Current Personal Situation issues, as noted in Table 5.6, and is beginning to obtain some of the more routine information that do not relate to current personal issues. Mrs. Jones' situation admittedly is very straightforward, and she is a bright, resourceful patient. The circumstances and details, however, don't always fall together so easily, so this inquiry can take much longer. Because of space constraints, I will not recount the remainder of the SH; rather, the reader should know that the student inquired about each remaining item in Table 5.6 that had not already been covered. This information can be found in the written report of Mrs. Jones in Appendix D.]

Family History (Step 11)

The family history (FH) is another rich source for completing the personal database where necessary. With families, the complexity of multiple interactions comes to the forefront (30). The interviewer most wants to know who is who, who is available to the patient, and in what way that person is available. In general, the interviewer should obtain information for at least two generations preceding the patient, as well as for any subsequent generations, and should include parents, siblings, and children for each generation. This should include spouses, adoptees, and other significant members of the family outside the bloodline even though they are not significant for familial or heritable disorders.

Once again, the interviewer uses open-to-closed coning inquiry to obtain the material in Table 5.7. After a screening open-ended question (e.g., "Tell me about any illnesses or other problems running in your family."), specific diseases are mentioned, including tuberculosis, diabetes, cancer, heart disease, bleeding problems, kidney failure or dialysis, alcoholism, tobacco use, weight problems, asthma, and mental illness (depression, schizophrenia, multiple somatic complaints, suicide, violence).

The student or clinician constructs a genogram to organize these data (30–32). Genograms can improve the amount of information in the FH and can help identify dysfunctional family patterns (31) and high medical utilization (32). As Mrs. Jones' genogram in Appendix D notes, this graphic form depicts myriad features in the family. Ages, gender, state of mental and physical health, and current status are obtained for each; when an individual is de-

TABLE 5.7. FAMILY HISTORY (STEP 11)

A. Make a general inquiry.
B. Inquire about specific diseases or problems: tuberculosis, diabetes, cancer, heart disease, bleeding problems, kidney failure or dialysis, alcoholism, tobacco use, weight problems, asthma, and mental illness (depression, suicide, schizophrenia, multiple somatic complaints).
C. Develop a genogram.
  1. Two generations preceding the patient and all subsequent should be included if they involve parents, siblings, children, and significant members outside the bloodline for each generation.
  2. Age, sex, mental and physical health, and current status are noted for each; note age at death and cause.
  3. Note interactions among family members for psychological and physical or disease problems.
    a. Psychological
      • dominant members and style (e.g., love, anger, alcoholism)
      • major interaction patterns (e.g., competition, abuse, open, distant, caring, manipulative, codependent)
      • family gestalt (e.g., happy, successful, dysfunctional)
    b. Physical or disease
      • patterns of disease (e.g., dominant, recessive, sex-linked, no pattern)
      • patterns of physical symptoms without disease (e.g., bowel trouble, uncoordinated, flighty)
      • inquire about others with similar symptoms (e.g., infection, toxic, anxiety)

ceased, the age and cause of death are noted. Depending on the length of time available, data can profitably be extended to include education, work, psychological style, and a host of other features for each member.

The interviewer learns also about dominant and nondominant family members and their specific styles (e.g., controlling, passive, caring). In addition to individual psychological profiles, the interactions among family members (e.g., direct, indirect, conflicted, close) are equally important. She or he also ascertains the gestalt of the family and its unique persona (e.g., the patient came from a successful family or a fighting family).

The classic use of the FH has been to obtain data about organic diseases by providing information about contagious (pinworms, varicella), toxic (carbon monoxide, lead), familial (breast cancer, coronary artery disease), and heritable (hemophilia, sickle cell anemia) diseases. In screening for these, the student or clinician asks if anyone in the family has similar physical problems to the patient's or if anyone at home has been ill lately with similar complaints.

Many patients, however, report illnesses in the family that do not refer to the same disorder (e.g., the statement "My father had a heart attack and I've got a murmur." likely refers to different problems) or even to any disease at all (e.g., "We all have bowel trouble."). Finally, especially following the death of a relative, patients worry that they are at increased risk because of familial connections (e.g., a healthy 21-year-old presents with chest pain and worries about having a heart attack 10 days after her grandfather died suddenly of a myocardial infarction). Most of these symptoms relate to the patient's concern, which is understandable. Although this is not the intent of the FH, the interviewer should become supportive and should address emotional material if it arises (e.g., in discussing the dates of death of his parents, the patient becomes sad and tearful). As was mentioned before, returning to the patient-centered process is essential.

With the large amount of potential data, the FH focuses on family data relevant to current problems. Beginning students, however, are again urged to obtain all FH data during initial interviews in order to learn the categories themselves and the richness and variability of the FH in different people. Busy clinicians often must acquire these data over many visits and are often guided by questionnaires that patients complete.

Continuation of Vignette with Mrs. Jones

DOC: Well, that's a lot of information. You've sure had a lot going on (referring to the SH). We've still got a little more information to gather and need to switch now to your family.

[The interviewer continues to weave a patient-centered, respectful atmosphere into her comments to Mrs. Jones and makes yet another transition, now into the FH.]

PT: That's fine.

DOC: Are there any medical problems in your family, you know, illnesses or any problems?

[Focused, open-ended beginning.]

PT: Nothing really. You made me think earlier about that one aunt who had some kind of headaches.

DOC: Even besides headaches, is there anything running in the family?

[The student makes sure Mrs. Jones knows that any familial problem is being inquired about.]

PT: Well, my grandmother had diabetes; is that what you mean?

DOC/PT: Yeah, that's it. Any other diabetes in the family? (no). Let me give you some things and tell me if anyone in the family has it when I mention it: Tuberculosis? (no) Kidney failure? (no) Bleeding problems? (no) Heart attacks? (no) Alcoholism? (no) Cholesterol? (no) Tobacco use? (no) Mental problems? (no)

[This helps the patient understand what the interviewer is requesting; the student screens for a number of diseases of possible familial origin, asking each individually.]

DOC: I need now to get some information on your immediate family, and then we'll go to your parents' and grandparents' families. Can you start by giving me the ages of your kids and your husband.

[The student began by getting a listing of each family member for this and the preceding two generations. This includes their ages, sex, mental and physical health, and current status. I do not recount the interview here because of space constraints, but Mrs. Jones' genogram is presented in Appendix D. Note the interactions among many members.]

DOC: Well, we're just about done. Before we go on, though, how are you doing?

PT: A little weary but I'm fine.

DOC: You've been very helpful. Anything I can do for you before we go on?

[Once again, the student returns to the patient-centered process and attends to the patient's needs.]

System Review (Review of Systems) (Step 12)

The Review of Systems (ROS) is less important than are other parts of the history (33); I already have discussed the System Review in another context (a resource that lists most symptoms) in Chapter 4, where a detailed list is seen in Table 4.2. Indeed, by this point, the interviewer ordinarily knows everything of significance. **The ROS is not used to obtain pertinent HPI/OCAP, HI, or PMH data; rather, it serves only as a final screening (33).** Indeed, the reader should recall that HPI and OCAP data often are discovered after repeated inquiries of "What else?" during agenda-setting (Step 2), meaning that little, if any, new, important, or current data should arise here. Nonetheless, relevant data are sometimes acquired (34); the interviewer then fits them into the HPI/OCAP, HI, or PMH during the write-up or presentation.

The ROS concerns primary and secondary data from systems that have not yet been considered. The interviewer returns to the System Review and inquires about still unaddressed symptoms and any secondary data, including specific diseases, such as psoriasis or cataracts.

The student or clinician often learns about many minor problems. For example, when screening for nasal symptoms, the patient may relate each cold and upper respiratory illness he or she has had over the last 20 years. Rather than obtaining details, interviewers want to know only if the problem has been out of the ordinary, if it has caused any disability, if it represents a significant change, or if it has not completely cleared. Refocusing patients, with comments such as, "I don't need all the details, but I do want to know if there have been any major problems." helps. As before, unnecessary data are not collected so that the interview is timely and does not overtax the patient. In like fashion, the interviewer should not probe for or encourage symptoms except in pediatrics (see Chapter 6). Most frustrating is the patient who answers positively to most questions, exhibiting a "positive system review." If this persists following clarification, it suggests still unrecognized diseases or a psychological disorder known as somatization in which patients present with multiple physical complaints that have no disease explanation.

The ROS proceeds almost entirely by rapidly paced, brief closed-ended questioning after an initial, orienting statement like "I need to ask you now about any other important or current problems or symptoms you might have had, so we don't miss something." For example, if the gastrointestinal system has not yet been addressed, the interviewer might begin open-endedly with "Any trouble with your digestion or bowels?" and may then inquire, "Have you ever had trouble with your appetite?" (no); "weight loss?" (no); "weight gain?" (no); "difficulty swallowing?" (no); "nausea?" (no); and so on until all of this system has been explored. Of course, questions are asked and answered individually. **When the more advanced clinical student has memorized all symptoms on the System Review list, she or he is urged to obtain ROS material when performing the physical examination to save time as experienced clinicians do.** For example, while she or he examines the nose, she or he would ask questions about nasal symptoms; while examining the eyes, about eye symptoms; and so on. The interviewer must always remain attentive to the patient's responses and needs and must tell her or him that questions are "routine" and that the clinician or student has not noticed something to make her or him suspicious.

When the ROS is concluded, the student or clinician summarizes briefly, asks if the patient has anything to add, and usually indicates that the physical examination will follow. A patient-centered atmosphere of courtesy, respect, and support should continue throughout.

Final Vignette of Mrs. Jones

DOC: I need to ask you now about some symptoms we haven't yet talked about, you know, to be sure we haven't missed something so far.

[An effective open-ended introduction to the ROS.]

PT: Fine, but I don't think there's much more.

DOC: We haven't talked yet about any skin problems; any problems there?

[An open-ended introduction to the integument system.]

PT: I thought I had some infection in my elbow once in 1980, but it turned out I'd used too strong a soap. It cleared long ago.

DOC/PT: Any problems since? (no) Or other skin problems like sores? (no) Itching? (no) Rashes? (no) Changes in moles? (no) Abnormal hair growth? (no) Or nail problems? (no)

[The student is getting an idea of how significant this is to Mrs. Jones' current health and then completes the ROS for the integumentary system.]

DOC:

[The student now proceeds to other systems that have not yet been addressed and inquires about all possible symptoms in each, as Table 4.2 of Chapter 4 outlines (e.g., hemopoietic, endocrine, breasts, genital). At its conclusion, she or he concludes the interview as follows.]

DOC: Well, you've done a nice job telling me a lot about the problems with headaches and your boss and about the colitis. I think I have a very good picture of what's going on. Is there anything else you'd like to add?

[A brief summary conveying understanding and support for her performance, and a patient-centered invitation for any final words.]

PT: No, I don't think so.

DOC: In that case, I'll step out now so you can get undressed and I'll be back in a few minutes for the physical examination. If you'd like to use the bathroom or get a drink of water, that's ok.

[Further material about the transition to the physical examination in a respecting, patient-centered way.]

SUMMARY

In the doctor-centered HPI/OCAP, the interviewer converts complaints to one of the symptoms in the System Review and then refines them with the seven descriptors. She or he then orders primary and secondary data into chronological sequence, progressively learning to test disease hypotheses as she or he proceeds. The HI inquiry concerns ethical-social-spiritual issues, functional status, health-promoting and health-maintenance activities, and various health hazards. The PMH mainly recounts important but not current problems. The SH and FH complete the personal and, to a lesser extent, the primary and secondary database. The ROS screens for still undetected primary and secondary data.

The interviewer better understands previous personal and symptom data from the patient-centered process and, in addition, acquires other essential parts of the database to complete the interview by the repeated coning-down process of brief open-ended screening followed by closed-ended acquisition of necessary details. Although the patient-centered process is not now as prominent, the student or clinician returns to it frequently by making supportive comments and by inquiring about how the patient is doing; and she or he returns to more extensive patient-centered, open-ended inquiry when the patient becomes emotional or presents important, new personal data.

The student or clinician now has completed the medical interview, summarized in Fig 5.1, and can make a full biopsychosocial description of the patient using integrated patient-centered and doctor-centered interviewing processes. That is, she or he now can be most scientific because she or he fully appreciates the patient's disease problems and the personal and emotional context in which they occur.

LEARNING EXERCISES

1. Describe the primary function of doctor-centered interviewing.
2. Why is hypothesis testing important?*
3. Distinguish an inductive approach from a deductive approach.
4. As you develop experience and want to become more efficient, which symptoms in the ROS might you want to emphasize? List five in each body system.
5. After you have learned all of the questions in Steps 8 to 12 in the doctor-centered interview, why is it important to truncate many of them?*
6. What do you use as a guide to determine whether you will spend more or less time in a given area of the doctor-centered interview?
7. List several guidelines to minimize bias from closed-ended questioning.*
8. List concerns patients may experience during a lengthy doctor-centered inquiry.*
9. Where would you include a family history of diabetes in a patient presenting with chest pain? Could there be more than one location, depending on the nature of the pain? Explain.
10. Give two functions of the System Review. How valuable is it in making diagnoses?
11. Draw your own genogram.*

*Good test questions.

PRACTICE QUESTIONS

(These would likely be spread over several sessions.)

Note: All **the following exercises are preceded by 3 to 5 minutes of** *patient-centered interviewing* **with a smooth transition into Step 6.** This emphasizes the *integration* of the two processes, which should not be practiced in isolation from each other.

1. Conduct Steps 6 and 7 multiple times in role-play, taking 5 to 15 minutes. Initially, use very straightforward disease problems, much as with Ms. Jones, over 5 minutes or so. As you become comfortable with developing the chronological description of symptoms (Step 7), the role-play 'patient' can begin to have more complicated problems, such as angina pectoris of 3 years duration but worsening over 3 weeks in conjunction with cigarette smoking and a family history of high cholesterol. See the vignette of Ms. Jones and the videotape demonstration for examples.

2. When comfortable in role-play, begin the same exercise with real or simulated patients.

3. Try to do some hypothesis testing with each exercise. When doing role-plays, have the 'patient' tell you in advance what problem she or he will depict so you can read up on it beforehand and therefore have some hypotheses and relevant questions in mind.

4. Each student should perform a complete history, including Steps 8 to 12, on a family member or fellow student. Ask all questions in each substep of Steps 8 to 12. I recommend that you use the book or a 'crib sheet' as a reminder of the many questions.

References

1. Smith RC. Videotape of Evidence-Based Interviewing: (1) Patient-Centered Interviewing and (2) Doctor-Centered Interviewing. Marketing Division, Instructional Media Center, Michigan State University. Contact information: PO Box 710, East Lansing, MI 48824; 517-353-9229 (tel); 517-432-2650 (fax); http://www.msu-vmall.msu.edu/imc.

2. Elstein AS. Psychological research on diagnostic reasoning. In: Lipkin M, Putnam SM, Lazare A, eds. *The medical interview.* New York: Springer-Verlag, 1995: 504–510.

3. Norman G. The epistemology of clinical reasoning: perspectives from philosophy, psychology, and neuroscience. *Acad Med* 2000;75:s127–s133.

4. Barrows HS, Pickell GC. *Developing clinical problem-solving skills. A guide to more effective diagnosis and treatment.* New York: WW Norton Medical Books, 1991.

5. Humes HD, DuPont HL, Gardner LB, et al, eds. *Kelley's textbook of internal medicine,* 4th ed. Philadelphia: Lippincott Williams & Wilkins, 2000.

6. Elstein AS, Kagan N, Shulman LS, et al. Methods and theory in the study of medical inquiry. *J Med Educ* 1972;47:85–92.

7. Fletcher RH, Fletcher SW, Wagner EH. *Clinical epidemiology. The essentials,* 3rd ed. Philadelphia: Lippincott Williams & Wilkins, 1996.

8. Sackett DL, Haynes RB, Tugwell P. *Clinical epidemiology: a basic science for clinical medicine.* Boston: Little, Brown & Company, 1985.

9. Griner PF, Panzer RJ, Greenland P. *Clinical diagnosis and the laboratory: logical strategies for common medical problems.* Chicago: Year Book, 1986.

10. Sox HC. *Common diagnostic tests: use and interpretation.* Philadelphia: American College of Physicians, 1987.

11. Platt FW. *Conversation repair: case studies in doctor-patient communication.* Boston: Little, Brown & Company, 1995.

12. Kuhn CC. A spiritual inventory of the medically ill patient. *Psychiatric Med* 1988; 6:87–100.

13. Ware JJE. Conceptualizing and measuring generic health outcomes. *Cancer* 1991; 67(suppl):774–779.

14. Garr DR, Lackland DT, Wilson DB. Prevention education and evaluation in US medical schools: a status report. *Acad Med* 2000;75(7 suppl):s14–s21.

15. Rivara FP, Grossman DC, Cummings P. Injury prevention. *N Engl J Med* 1997; 337:613–618.

16. Sox JHC. Preventive health services in adults. *N Engl J Med* 1994;330: 1589–1595.

17. McBride JL, Arthur G, Brooks R, et al. The relationship between a patient's spirituality and health experiences. *Fam Med* 1998;30:122–126.

18. Tierney WM, Dexter PR, Gramelspacher GP, et al. The effect of discussions about advance directives on patients' satisfaction with primary care. *J Gen Int Med* 2001;16:32–40.

19. Roter DL, Larson S, Fischer GS, et al. Experts practice what they preach—a descriptive study of best and normative practices in end-of-life discussions. *Arch Intern Med* 2000;160:3477–3485.

20. Tanner BL. *The open door.* Orange City, FL: RL Kruse Publishing, 2001.

21. Clark W. Effective interviewing and intervention for alcohol problems. In: Lipkin M, Putnam SM, Lazare A, eds. *The medical interview.* New York: Springer-Verlag, 1995:284–293.

22. Williams S. The sexual history. In: Lipkin M, Putnam SM, Lazare A, eds. *The medical interview.* New York: Springer-Verlag, 1995:235–250.

23. Eisenstat SA, Bancroft L. Domestic violence. *N Engl J Med* 1999;341:886–892.

24. Gebert B, Caspers N, Bronstone A, et al. A qualitative analysis of how physicians with expertise in domestic violence approach the identification of victims. *Ann Int Med* 1999;131:578–584.

25. McCauley J, Kern DE, Kolodner K, et al. The "battering syndrome": prevalence and clinical characteristics of domestic violence in primary care internal medicine practices. *Ann Int Med* 1995;123:737–746.

26. Bauer HM, Rodriguez MA, Perez-Stable EJ. Prevalence and determinants of intimate partner abuse among public hospital primary care patients. *J Gen Int Med* 2000;15:811–817.

27. Wagner PJ, Mongan PF. Validating the concept of abuse—women's perceptions of defining behaviors and the effects of emotional abuse on health indicators. *Arch Fam Med* 1998;7:25–29.
28. *Physicians' desk reference,* 55th ed. Montvale, NJ: Medical Economics, 2001.
29. Eisenberg DM, Kessler RC, Foster C, et al. Unconventional medicine in the United States: prevalence, costs, and patterns of use. *N Engl J Med* 1993;328:246–252.
30. Mullins HC, Christie-Seely J. Collecting and recording family data: the genogram. In: Christie-Seely J, ed. *Working with the family in primary care: a systems approach to health and illness.* New York: Praeger, 1984:179–191.
31. Hahn SR, Feiner JS, Bellin EH. The doctor-patient-family relationship: a compensatory alliance. *Ann Int Med* 1988;109:884–889.
32. Greenwald JL, Grant WD, Kamps CA, et al. The genogram scale as a predictor of high utilization in a family practice. *Families, Systems Health* 1998;16:375–392.
33. Hoffbrand BI. Away with the system review: a plea for parsimony. *Br Med J* 1989;298:817–818.
34. Mitchell TL, Tornelli JL, Fisher TD, et al. Yield of the screening review of systems: a study on a general medicine service. *J Gen Intern Med* 1992;7:393–397.

6 Advanced Interviewing
Adapting the Interview to Different Situations and Other Practical Issues

In multiple areas the student must adapt the interview to different clinical situations. Such fine-tuning occurs primarily during Steps 1 to 5 (setting the stage, agenda setting, opening the history of the present illness [HPI], continuing the HPI, and transition). In this chapter, I focus only on interviewing processes and do not consider details of the specific clinical situations. For the details that must be incorporated into many of the interviewing processes discussed here, I refer readers to clinical texts.

Balancing Patient-Centered and Doctor-Centered Processes

Even though the student or clinician knows how much time she or he can spend with the patient, no fixed rule mandates how to distribute the time between the patient-centered and doctor-centered processes. Based on the patient's needs, the interviewer determines the initial balance during Steps 1 to 5. I might average 10% of my time in the initial patient-centered process for most patients, but this allocation of time can vary from 2% (e.g., a patient who needs a medication refill and has no personal issues) to more than 50% (e.g., a patient with severe marital problems) depending on the severity and urgency of the patient's personal issues. Of course, returning again and again to a patient-centered approach even late in the interview may be necessary.

The interviewer's main block of controllable time lies in Step 4, continuing the HPI, during the patient-centered process. Steps 1 to 3 and 5 usually take little time and are similar from patient to patient. Consider the following examples.

New Patient Without Urgent or Complex Personal Problems

First consider a prototypic new patient, like Mrs. Jones, who comes to the doctor without urgent (i.e., immediate action is required) or complex personal problems. Physical symptom complaints often predominate, and I usually devote about 5% to 10% of my time to the initial patient-centered process of the interview. This is the student's or clinician's experience with most new patients, whether outpatient or inpatient, in a medical setting. Such patients, like Mrs. Jones, have definite personal issues, but they are not urgent or overwhelming. For example, a patient with known cancer is admitted to the hospital for chemotherapy, but he is more worried about his wife being alone and having the flu; or an outpatient presents with a weight loss of 5 pounds—she is somewhat concerned about possible cancer and wants "to be sure."

New Patient with Urgent or Complex Personal Problems

However, some new medical inpatients and outpatients do have more urgent and complex personal problems. For example, as clinicians or students you might see the following situations: acute marital discord led to sleeplessness, depression, headaches, and diarrhea for an outpatient who requested a "check-up;" a recent unexpected business set-back immediately preceded the hospital admission of an extremely angry man with chest pain; or a patient who was admitted for pneumonia is overwhelmed and crying after being informed of her AIDS diagnosis. In these instances, you give more time to personal issues by increasing time in Step 4 and, very likely, you also spend time during the doctor-centered process (Steps 6 and 7) to understand the details of what could be a serious psychological problem, such as depression, better (Chapter 5). If, for example, Mrs. Jones had shown evidence of depression or inability to function at work, the patient-centered process would have taken longer, and many relevant details would be revisited during doctor-centered interviewing.

Follow-Up Patient Without Urgent or Complex Personal Problems

Just as with new patients, most follow-up patients do not have urgent or complex personal problems, but their visits differ because they have much less time with the student or clinician. In a 5- to 15-minute follow-up visit, either inpatient or outpatient, for predominantly physical complaints, the interviewer quickly proceeds through Steps 1 to 4 and ascertains that few pressing personal issues need to be addressed in this brief visit. She or he will then shorten Step 4 and will make a transition (Step 5) into the doctor-centered process (Steps 6 and 7) where the agenda that was just determined with regard to the patient's physical symptoms is addressed (e.g., worsening or new symptoms after treating the patient's strep throat one week ago or any change from the preceding day in an inpatient's chest pain). In both instances, the clinician or student listens for new personal contextual material (e.g., wants to get back to work, wants to go home) and responds; but most personal data already are known, and the patient's symptoms are the primary focus. The personal issues of follow-up patients often concern the treatment and disposition. Because the database is more complete, as interviewers, we can more easily investigate treatment issues during the patient-centered process than with new patients.

Vignette of Mr. Gomez

(Setting: Ward rounds on a patient with primarily physical symptoms on his second day of hospitalization with no more than 15 minutes available at this time)

DOC: (Observes patient for comfort, helps with pillow, and sits down) Anything new you'd like me to look at today before I do some of my things (pointing to stethoscope)?

[The student sets the stage by attending to the patient's comfort, gives his own agenda (stethoscope), and asks about the patient's agenda so that both Steps 1 and 2 are addressed in no more than a few seconds.]

PT: Nothing new.

DOC: How you doing?

[An open-ended question to start Step 3]

PT: The pain is better. Can I go home?

[The patient gives both symptom and personal data.]

DOC: Go home?

PT: Yeah, my job. Remember, we talked about it?

DOC: Sure, anything new?

PT: No, but they still need me and my wife's in a fix.

DOC: Well, I sure understand you're anxious about your job and that's a tough situation for your wife to be in, but there's a little more. Our (pointing to the patient and himself) biggest concern now is to be certain that you are okay and that you don't have an appendicitis. We aren't sure yet.

[Note that, in a brief visit, the student addresses the personal issue to start Step 4, but does not re-explore what she or he already knows except to ascertain that there is no change. The student also incorporates naming, understanding, and support into his response. The response was supportive both verbally and nonverbally—it involved the patient by pointing and by using the terms `our' and `we.']

PT: You still think tomorrow?

DOC: Well, if the blood count and x-ray turn out ok and the pain clears up, it's possible. But don't count on it yet. Our main need now is your health and getting you back to your job in good shape. Sounds really difficult for you, though.

[The student continues addressing personal issues in Step 4 by staying focused on the question raised by the patient and again makes a supportive statement about wanting to help the patient and indicates respect.]

PT: Yeah, thanks.

[The patient seems satisfied.]

DOC: Let me shift now and have you tell me more about the pain.

[This is Step 5, the transition, and the beginning of Step 6 of the doctor-centered process still using open-ended requests. Note that the student effectively conducted the patient-centered process in about 1 minute and will now address the patient's medical condition in Steps 6 and 7.]

PT: Well, the pain yesterday was more around the belly-button but now it's down here on the right (right lower quadrant). It hurts to push on it but isn't bad otherwise.

DOC: Any bowel movement yet? . . .

[The student spends the next several minutes determining symptom descriptors and changes in symptoms from yesterday and searching out and defining any new symptoms. He then examines the patient, reviews the laboratory data, and makes further plans in conjunction with the resident and supervising physician. Steps 8 to 12 of the doctor-centered process are unnecessary because the student obtained these data when the patient was admitted to the hospital the previous day. The student also informs the patient that he will be back when the results of the lab tests and x-ray are available. Note how closely the patient's personal issues revolve around the symptom.]

Such a predominantly doctor-centered follow-up interaction can also concern personal data. When the interviewer wants to address a specific issue that the patient has not raised, such as sexual habits or cessation of cigarette use, this also requires that a majority of the time be spent in the doctor-centered process.

Follow-Up Patient with Urgent or Complex Personal Problems

On the other hand, the interviewer may have a follow-up patient who presents with urgent or complex personal issues that often, but not always, have few physical complaints. The interviewer quickly determines this during Steps 1 to 4, and then takes more time in Step 4 to develop the personal issues better, which results in a predominantly patient-centered interview. Even with no physical complaint from the patient, the student or clinician should make a transition to the doctor-centered process and should briefly inquire about the patient's physical health (e.g., "No more problems with the heartburn or constipation?"). In other words, she or he must always integrate the personal and symptom data.

Vignette of Mrs. Wong

(An outpatient who has been seen previously for other problems now presents with a predominantly personal problem in a 15-minute appointment slot.)

DOC: Hi, Mrs. Wong. Hadn't seen you for a while. Is that comfortable sitting there? (She nods.) Anything you need before we get started?
[Step 1]

PT: No, unless you can fix my son. He is getting a divorce. And that means the grandchildren will have to leave town. And then . . .
[The patient is introducing tension-laden personal material already.]

DOC: That sounds pretty heavy. We're going to need to get back to this in a minute but before we get started, could you tell me if there was anything else you wanted to look at today, you know, other problems?
[The clinician determines that, as is usually the case, to interrupt briefly in order to get the agenda is appropriate.]
[Step 2]

PT: Well, I came because of my back. It's a little worse, and you did all those tests a year ago that were ok. I think it's the stress.

DOC: Anything else to look at today?
[He is being certain that the entire agenda is elicited.]

PT: No, that's enough!

DOC: So, tell me more about your son. Sounds like a tough time for you.
[When the patient has already begun with strongly felt personal data, returning directly to the material that was raised to start Step 3 is appropriate.]

PT: Well, they've been married for nearly 15 years and everything always seemed ok. I think they thought so too. And now this. She's just furious at him.

DOC: (Silence)

[He is in the nonfocusing Step 3 and is simply letting the patient lead.]

PT: He's always been a bit of a lady's man and, well, that's caused problems before too.

DOC: Sounds like a tough time for you. How're you doing with all this?

[Beginning to grasp the problem and recalling the need to be timely, the clinician introduces Step 4 by changing the focus to her emotions. While following the steps in sequence, he no longer needs to address all substeps such as, in this example, addressing physical symptoms before proceeding to emotion. The details of the son's problem are less important also and can be developed later, if necessary.]

PT: (Starting to cry) I'm mad at him for being so stupid. And I can't stand having to be away from the little kids. She'll get them and they'll move back to her home. (More crying)

[The clinician would now develop this in much the same way Mrs. Jones' story was. That is, he would use active open-ended, emotion-seeking, and emotion-handling skills over and over in a cyclic way. In so doing, he obtained more details and learned that Mrs. Wong is depressed, as she was once before following her husband's death. I pick the interview back up at this point to show the transition to the doctor-centered process.]

DOC: You've sure been through a lot and I'm glad you've told me about it. Do you feel okay to change gears now so I can ask a few more questions?

[He is in Step 5 and is checking to see if the patient is finished talking about this difficult problem.]

PT: Sure, and thanks again for listening. I feel better.

DOC: I wanted to ask about your sleep. How's that going?

PT: Not very good.

DOC: Do you have trouble getting to sleep?

[Because he has learned that Mrs. Wong is depressed, he is starting to inquire about physical (vegetative) symptoms that often accompany depression. In addition to sleep disturbances, he learns that Mrs. Wong has a poor appetite and that she no longer enjoys previously enjoyable activities (anhedonia), further supporting the diagnosis of depression, which is an urgent problem that requires treatment. He then ascertains, continuing to use predominantly closed-ended inquiry, that Mrs. Wong is not suicidal. I pick up the conversation again where the student is addressing the back pain that brought the patient in.]

DOC: Well, that's been a hard time for you. Could you now say more about the backache?

[The clinician or student should still address physical symptoms, no matter how insignificant they may seem or how much the patient downplays them. Note again how closely the symptoms and personal problems often are related.]

PT: It's the same place. And it never did go down the leg after that one time 4 years ago. I don't think it's anything . . .

[During the next few minutes the student reviews the symptom descriptors and then examines her. When the patient has dressed, the clinician makes recommendations about the depression and back pain.]

Disease-Prevention Visit

Patients often come without a particular problem to focus on and want, rather, to address how they might prevent health problems in the future in what is frequently called a "regular or routine physical exam." As a clinician or student, you should proceed in the same stepwise fashion. In Step 2, the patient often has a large number of issues he or she wants to discuss (e.g., flu shot, exercise program, diet, mammograms, and Pap smear). Because the patient has no particular complaint and may have many agenda items, to keep asking, "Anything else?" until all her or his concerns have been elicited is essential. In Steps 3 and 4, you often focus on why the patient has come in at this particular time; you should not be surprised to learn that some health problems have occurred in her or his family or friends or that she or he has noted some alteration in body function and, therefore, that the patient wants to be sure that she or he does not have something wrong, such as cancer, high cholesterol, or osteoporosis. On eliciting this story open-endedly, you use the emotion-seeking skills to explore the attendant worry and anxiety. Then, you can use NURS, especially to praise them for coming in and for working to achieve maximum health status.

However, many patients simply come in for routine visits without a specific reason. In these instances, the patient-centered process may be no more than 1 to 2 minutes of largely agenda-setting, praising, and supporting the patient for coming in. In all disease prevention visits, a lot of time is spent in the doctor-centered process pinning down details of the patient's health-related activities: (a) present exercise pattern, how many minutes, how vigorous, and any related injuries and (b) specific daily diet, understanding of caloric and fat content, interest in making major changes, and prior attempts to diet. Chapter 9 provides the details of how you can inform and motivate patients to change when it is necessary (e.g., cigarette cessation). In addition, even though a patient may not have routine health prevention on his or her agenda, you should determine her or his interest in pursuing routine recommendations for their age (e.g., colonoscopy, mammograms). During such visits, you should address all pertinent (to the patient's age, gender, and status) aspects of health issues in Chapter 5: ethical-social-spiritual practices, functional status, health-promoting and health-maintenance activities, and health hazards.

Of course, as clinician and students, you will see a spectrum of patients between the urgent and less urgent personal categories, and no method currently exists for predicting how many physical symptoms will be present in either category. What should you do in a difficult situation where both personal and symptom data are plentiful, urgent, and complex? Careful agenda setting (Step 2) should be used to define what seems most important to both you as the doctor and the patient. Even so, some issues may have to be deferred to a later appointment.

How Common Interviewing Situations Are Addressed

Even after an interviewer knows how to distribute time between the initial patient-centered and doctor-centered processes, some patient styles and situations still influence interviewing and affect how time will be spent in the process (e.g., a loquacious patient can require more time, more interrupting, and less encouragement to talk than a reticent one with the same story would). I now consider some variations on our theme. As before, most decisions about how to proceed will be made during Steps 1 to 5.

The Reticent Patient

As clinicians and students, we must get reticent patients talking about anything, no matter what it takes. Typically, the agenda (Step 2) is limited and is about physical symptoms, and the patient gives little response to our initial open-ended inquiry (Step 3). The nonfocusing open-ended skills (silence, nonverbal encouragement, neutral utterances) may be ineffective, and, in Step 4, we must rely on the focusing open-ended skills (echoing, requests, summary) and emotion-seeking skills (direct, indirect). Among the latter skills, self-disclosure can be particularly effective (e.g., "I once had chest pain and was very concerned—how about you?"). Even though the patient may express no emotion, we should direct emotion-handling skills toward what we do know about the patient (e.g., "It sounds like some difficult problems you've had; you were right to come in so we could help out [naming, praising, supporting].") This often facilitates obtaining additional information about his or her story.

To get some conversation going, we can talk about a patient's symptoms using closed-ended questions in Step 4 (e.g., "What brings you in?" "Where is the back pain?" "Does it go down your leg?"). Once we begin to hear the symptoms, we elicit their immediate personal dimensions, and the broader personal context will follow. We look for any thread of personal data to facilitate this flow of information, such as if the patient mentions the family dog (e.g., "I can't walk the dog anymore."). When we find it, we then focus on it to get some more personal conversation going.

Ordinarily, these patients will talk, and we can elicit satisfactory stories, although they will be briefer and less complete than those of other patients. Symptom data are easier to obtain in the doctor-centered process because we have more control of the conversation. Sometimes, these patients, seemingly warmed up by what has preceded, offer personal data during the doctor-centered process (e.g., while giving the Family History (FH), the patient begins to talk about personal issues). We then, of course, alter our style to become patient-centered and to develop these personal data further.

The Overly Talkative Patient

As a clinician or student, we try to establish a personal and emotional focus in a timely way with overly talkative patients, especially by focusing too detailed or diffuse conversation. These patients may begin without us saying anything. Developing the agenda (Step 2) typically is difficult. Nevertheless, we can develop a list of complaints, often by respectfully interrupting and by refocusing frequently. We seldom need to use an open-ended beginning question because patients already are giving a lot of data. Indeed, silence alone often suffices as patients talk on in Step 3. However, after no more than 1 minute with a new patient (sooner with follow-up patients), we should get involved actively to prevent our becoming nonparticipatory.

Some patients need to recount every detail. That sort of verbal output interferes with our ability to get personal and emotional data. In this situation, we respectfully and tactfully interrupt and redirect, sometimes repeatedly. Other patients discuss issues that do not relate to themselves directly, such as other people and politics. Still others focus on remote past events with no apparent relevance to their present situation. In all these instances, we actively refocus the patient (Step 4) on herself or himself in the here and now (e.g., "I understand your concern about the President's health policy, but how does it apply to you, you know, personally?"), and in particular, on her or his emotional reactions by using emotion-seeking skills (e.g., "Those are important details, but how did that affect you emotionally?"). Also, we can use the NURS tetrad as a means for achieving a modicum of control of the interview (e.g., "That's been a long spell for you. I can sure understand how upsetting it might be. Thanks for giving me that background. Let's move on now to what happened yesterday."). On the other hand, if patients are talking about themselves in the present and are giving emotional data, we should stay with and should facilitate this focus. Once such a focus is established, our difficulty then is to complete Step 4 in a timely way. We can use a firm, clear transition statement to change the focus effectively to the doctor-centered process. For example, after summarizing and using the NURS tetrad, we can say, "We need now to change so I can learn more about your constipation if that's ok."

Talkative patients produce plentiful personal data, and the interviewer may easily obtain a long story. Because of time constraints, she or he should avoid a prolonged return to such personal data if the patient reintroduces them later in the doctor-centered process. The most important data usually will already have arisen. Nonetheless, if emotion is expressed, the interviewer must address it. Listening for a brief amount of time and using emotion-handling skills usually suffices.

These patients can seem "easy" to the interviewer who is inclined to passivity and "irritating" to those who like to take control. The clinician or student should be aware of his or her own characteristics to maximize his or her effectiveness. Chapter 7 details further strategies for addressing her or his personal responses and for managing these patients.

The Patient Who Persists in Symptoms and Secondary Data During the Patient-Centered Process

I now focus on a difficult, though uncommon, problem. When, after developing a good personal description of symptoms during the patient-centered process, the patient persists in communicating physical symptoms and secondary data, our strategy as interviewers must change.

Open-ended skills are sometimes not enough to encourage expanding the information to the patient's general personal and contextual data; we may have to direct the patient actively with emotion-seeking skills. The symptoms pointing to medical disease in these patients may be prominent and may frighten the patient. We first summarize this information and then immediately follow the summary with emotion-seeking skills. Direct and indirect emotion-seeking inquiry typically establishes a personal focus. In addition, the respectful use of interrupting often facilitates the transition. As with the reticent patient, the patient's personal stories often are more truncated and less complex.

These patients are very frustrating because conducting the interview is difficult and they are hard to get to know personally.

Vignette of Mr. Swenson

PT: (The patient gave limited personal descriptions of arm pain, headache, loose stools, and nausea from medication in Steps 3 and 4 without expression of concern, emotion, or anything more personal. The patient also tells the interviewer of a negative CT scan and Dr. Johnson's diagnosis of arteritis.)

[The student knows that she is going to have to work harder than usual to draw out the broader personal context of these symptoms.]

DOC: (She first summarizes the physical problems and then immediately follows with this entry.) Boy, you've sure had a lot of things going on. How does that make you feel, you know, personally?

[She summarizes the symptoms and secondary data but then directs patient toward the personal context by a direct emotion-seeking question.]

PT: I don't know. This pain keeps going right over here. And I've also been coughing. That started last . . . (student interrupts)

[The patient is staying with the symptoms and is not responding, as hoped for, with more general personal contextual information; the student interrupts quickly to try again to establish a more personal focus; otherwise, the symptom focus will continue.]

DOC: What I'm asking about are other things, like what do you think is going on. Why is all this happening?

[She tries indirect emotion-seeking to probe the patient's beliefs instead of repeating the direct inquiry about feelings.]

PT: Dr. Johnson says it's arteritis. It's a blood vessel disease . . . (student interrupts)

[The student continues to look for personal clues, but she has found none yet; she will keep trying.]

DOC: But why you? Why did you get it?

[She persists in the probe for beliefs; most patients usually have some opinion about this, which will lead eventually to personal data.]

PT: I don't know.

[The patient isn't saying much; the student needs to use another indirect inquiry or to return to direct inquiry about feelings.]

DOC: With so much going on, how has it affected your life?

[This is usually a more productive indirect emotion-seeking inquiry because it forces some personal data; the patient can hardly say that he doesn't know.]

PT: Not much. I retired and wasn't doing anything anyway, until all this stuff came. That pain is right in . . . (student interrupts)

[At last, she has some personal data; she now actively focuses on this.]

DOC: Tell me more about that—retiring and not doing much.

[Combined open-ended summary and request; now that personal data have appeared, she uses focusing open-ended skills repeatedly to maintain the focus and to develop the personal story, as already described. Earlier, rather than using indirect inquiry about beliefs and personal impact, she could also have used self-disclosure or she could have asked about the impact of illness on others' lives. If the patient lapsed back into symptom data, she would now use these.]

In many of the common interviewing situations, patients often frustrate and disappoint interviewers, either because the they are reticent or because they don't have inherently complex stories. Students especially sometimes lament that they "didn't get much." Nevertheless, the patient still feels understood, and a good doctor–patient relationship develops. **The amount of material obtained, especially emotional, is not a marker of a successful in-**

terview. Rather than measuring a good interview by getting the patient to cry, successful deployment of the steps determines success.

When Necessary Personal Data Are Not Forthcoming During the Patient-Centered Process

So far, I have assumed in this text that the personal data that we have obtained during the patient-centered process are the most important personal data. Indeed, generally this is so, but such data are not always complete, especially with topics about which patients are embarrassed or afraid that others will perceive them as abnormal (e.g., sexual practices, substance use, suicidal intent, and abuse).

When proceeding through Steps 1 to 5, the interviewer often first suspects an occult problem. For example, a story of severe depression may raise the question of suicidal intent or a story of frequent fractures may broach the issue of alcoholism. Sometimes, however, awareness does not arise until later (e.g., a story of recurrent pneumonia and diarrhea during the past medical history [PMH] raises the question of AIDS and, thereby, of homosexual activity or drug abuse; or the clinician observes unusual bruises during the physical exam, which leads to thoughts of physical abuse).

Doctor-centered inquiry allows us as interviewers, usually at the start of the doctor-centered process (Steps 6 and 7), to obtain the necessary information, although we sometimes might not elicit it until later on (e.g., health issues [HI], PMH, and social history [SH]). In one of these situations, we begin with a focused open-ended question (e.g., "I want to focus now on your use of alcohol") and follow up with progressively more closed-ended inquiry until all significant information is obtained. The HI section of Chapter 5 (Step 8) shows the key data that must be elicited about sexual activity and addictive behaviors.

As interviewers, we perform this inquiry with sensitivity and respect. We remind patients of how important these data are to help them medically, and we reassure them of doctor-patient confidentiality. Often, the patient has strong feelings that we must elicit with emotion-seeking skills and then address using emotion-handling skills.

I recommend using the doctor-centered approach in this way whenever we do not obtain pertinent personal data during patient-centered interviewing. For example, if the patient does not seem to be following our treatment recommendations, we might start the doctor-centered process (Steps 6 and 7) open-endedly with a question like, "Let's talk about how you're taking each of your medicines each day;" we may then follow up with more narrowly focused inquiry until we achieve clarity (e.g., "Let's count how many pills you have left in the container to be sure you're taking them like I think you are."). Thus, we often must use doctor-centered inquiry that is predominantly closed-ended to supplement the personal database.

Students usually find addressing issues that the patient is avoiding and has strong feelings about to be difficult. The student may personally experience fear, concern, abhorrence, or voyeuristic curiosity. An interviewer who is self-aware can keep these responses from interfering with her or his patient interaction, as we discuss in more detail in Chapter 7.

When More Than One Person Is Present

Although the family interview (1) is beyond the scope of this text, other situations exist where the student or clinician faces more than one person for the interview. The interviewer might decide to consult a relative or friend of the patient, hoping that she or he can provide unique information (e.g., a parent reporting on her or his child, to investigate what happened while the patient was unconscious, or to refresh what the patient has forgotten or denied). A properly conducted interview with a relative or other third person provides information that is otherwise unavailable, including how the patient interacts in this relationship (e.g., domineeringly, passively, distantly, angrily, or lovingly). Many hours of interviewing the individual patient would be needed to provide this much "hard data" about the patient's interactional style. For instance, an interviewer might obtain a story of great personal independence and achievement only to see the patient behave in a very dependent way when her or his spouse arrives, or she or he might find that a person who appeared very sensitive and considerate during the interview becomes hostile and sharp with a family member.

During Step 1, the clinician or student must first learn who the third party is and then must discover if both the parties (i.e., the patient and the third party) want the third party to be present. Next, the interviewer should ask whether the third party has special information that she or he would like to convey. If this seems pressing for the individual, then she or he hears it out. The patient interview then takes place as described. The interviewer tries to monitor how the third party is doing, how she or he interacts with the patient, and what effect she or he has on learning about the patient. She or he should weigh whether more or less data are being obtained because of the third party's presence. Problems arise when the third party interrupts or nonproductively lengthens the interaction. This potential has led many interviewers to dismiss all third parties reflexively without ever attempting to include them. If they are interfering, the interviewer should focus on them, should obtain any other data they might have, and then should respectfully excuse and thank them. Ensuring privacy while discussing sensitive issues and during the physical examination are other reasons for excusing some third parties. However, relatives and friends typically remain quiet. The interviewer may involve them for points requiring clarification or at the end of a successful interview to see how they view the problem (e.g. a spouse may see the patient as at great risk for cancer although the patient denies this, or a spouse may have practical questions the patient did not raise).

The pressure of a group of relatives and others, often with an acutely ill or dying patient, provides the clinician with another complex interaction. If conducting an interview with the patient is possible, the earlier guidelines apply. The less responsive the patient is, the more important her or his relatives are, and the more important identifying who knows the most about the patient is. Once the interviewer has attended to the patient's needs, she or he must consider her or his obligation to the relatives. They also need to be heard and understood. She or he should listen to their concerns and emotions, use emotion-handling skills, answer their questions, and help them find solutions.

Involving third parties usually takes little time and produces data that otherwise would not be available. Nevertheless, the additional time required, the need to incorporate data from new sources, and having to focus on the needs of third parties do increase the demand on the clinician or student. Understanding personal feelings of frustration (e.g., loss of control, the aggravation of an already inefficient approach, strict time orientation) can help the interviewer avoid adverse, often reflexive responses, such as impatience, dismissal of third parties, or avoidance of relatives.

Working With an Interpreter

Non–English-speaking patients are very common; these patients report more problems and less satisfaction with care (2–4). With these patients, we as clinicians are often less patient-centered (4). Therefore, I now consider the interview mediated by an interpreter (5).

When the third party is an interpreter (translating a foreign language or sign language or for a dysarthric patient), the interaction may take considerably longer, although recent data indicate that physicians spend no more time with non–English-speaking patients. However, the quality of the interactions was not evaluated (6). At the outset, learning how much the interpreter already knows about the patient, what her or his relationship to the patient is, how well she or he understands the patient, and vice versa can help. Many interpreters are family members or friends, and confidentiality is an issue; in this case, the interviewer must understand their relationship. Professional interpreters independent of the patient are best, but they are seldom available. Nonprofessional translators should be advised of the requirements of their position. For example, the interviewer might say, "I'm going to speak to your mother and she to me. I need you to translate exactly what I say and exactly what she says back. I know you'll be tempted to add or to subtract because of what you know already but, for now, I need a precise translation only. Can you do that for me?" If necessary, the clinician or student should ask the interpreter to identify which remarks are her or his own. The clinician or student then conducts the interview using the interpreter as the mediator, but she or he should address the patient directly, making eye contact and keeping her or him involved and central. The interviewer must be more direct and should avoid jargon, technical terms, and abstractions. She or he should also periodically check with the interpreter on the patient's nonverbal reactions, her or his understanding, and for culturally sensitive issues. Even with such an effort, the interviewer may find that establishing the usual relationship is difficult. The experience can be frustrating for patient and doctor alike. Indeed, acknowledging this (e.g., "It may be harder for us to get to know each other, but I want you to know I'm going to work on it.") can be helpful (7). **Having the history written in advance** by the patient or a knowledgeable relative so that the interviewer can focus on the doctor–patient relationship and on major problems can also facilitate the interview. For the patient to find a doctor who speaks the same language, especially for complicated or long-term care, may be the best solution (7). A new approach puts doctors and their patients in touch with skilled interpreters at remote sites and shows promise for enhancing the care of millions of non–English-speaking patients (8).

Patients with Communication Challenges

Developing a patient-centered focus requires special attention when communication problems exist. The patient's handicap and the measures required to address it can distract the student or clinician from a patient-centered approach. As interviewers, we try not to overlook special needs, such as allowing a deaf patient to see our lips clearly; to omit usual needs, such as touching the patient; or to overcompensate for perceived but nonexistent needs, such as speaking loudly and simply to a blind patient.

The relationship requires special attention. Nonverbal means can be especially effective; these can include touching the patient, a well-timed smile or friendly gesture, and an accepting demeanor (9). Because of these patients' impairments, many have been relatively isolated and are leery, particularly of insincere interactions, so genuinely felt expressions that lead to a relationship that develops more slowly are most effective (9). Some who have speech or hearing impairments may seem cognitively impaired to the unwary interviewer who then oversimplifies ideas and speech, often presenting material as though to a child (9).

Having the written history in advance often helps. This allows a more relaxed atmosphere and more focus on the relationship and key events. The following section presents additional measures that can enhance data-gathering and the relationship; it often focuses on setting the stage for a successful interview and on attending to comfort (Step 1).

Deaf or Hard of Hearing

Hearing impairment, which is most common with older patients, can cause great difficulty (10); it is associated with higher than normal mortality because of lower health status (11). If the patient has a hearing aid, encourage the patient to use it. Inquire specifically about what can be most helpful with an attitude of mutual decision making (12). Patients appreciate the invitation and attention to their special needs, in which they are experts as they have much experience in how best to communicate. Determine if the patient lipreads (speech reads) and, if so, ensure that she or he can see the interviewer's face adequately. Reducing background noise, pointing, and using gestures also helps. Because the patient has learned to read lips of normally speaking people, the interviewer should not slow down, shout, or overarticulate her or his speech. The student or clinician should speak at a moderate rate, pitch, and volume; pause at the end of sentences; use complete sentences; and inform patients of changes in topics being discussed. When necessary, repeat statements using different words and write out certain words or ideas.

Mute

Writing is essential for a signing patient if a translator is not available and the interviewer is not versed in sign language. With planning and instructions, the time that is required can be shortened by having others available who can provide information and by having the patient or others record the history before the visit.

Blind

Blind people, although they communicate verbally in normal ways, lack many cues that sighted people routinely and unconsciously experience. Blind patients use auditory compensatory mechanisms to understand mood, style, friendliness, and other features of the interviewer. Such nonvisual cues are not necessarily in accord with what others would perceive; therefore, paying special attention to their perceptions is important (9). The interviewer might ask, "Things are going ok for me, but I wanted to check with you on how I'm coming across and how our interaction is going."

As before, inquiring if the blind patient has special ways of proceeding, if she or he needs assistance from the interviewer, and if she or he has any particular requests relating to her or his blindness can be useful; the interviewer should give the patient freedom to refuse unwanted help. This allows her or him to take the lead and to know that the interviewer is available and open to her or his needs and that she or he respects the patient's self-sufficiency (9). Verbal orientation to furniture and doors, others in the room, and the interviewer's movement during the history and physical examination are helpful. The interviewer's speech quality, intensity, and pace should remain normal and should not be "adjusted" for the blind patient.

Cognitively Impaired

Cognitive disturbances present a different problem. Even though these patients perceive and speak, they do not intellectually process the information in a normal way; therefore, data are less reliable and meaningful, especially when the cognitive loss is severe.

Cognitive dysfunction is a vast topic that is dealt with during clinical rotations in medicine, pediatrics, surgery, psychiatry, and neurology. Such dysfunction is common, it can be acute or chronic, and it may have many causes (e.g., congenital, head injury, dementia, brain tumor, alcohol withdrawal, drug abuse, meningitis, medications, anemia, uremia, sepsis, hypoxia, poisoning, postoperative state). In addition, psychiatric disorders of mood, altered thinking, and abnormal mental experiences can present with cognitive changes as part of their presentation (e.g., schizophrenia, depression) (13,14).

To this point, I have assumed that the patient is a reliable authority for primary and secondary data. Cognitively impaired patients often vary considerably with each telling in reporting symptoms, and the chronology typically is unreliable. Similarly, emotions and other personal issues often are quite variable and nonreproducible. In general, **these data often are incomplete and cannot be definitively relied on.** Therefore, the student or clinician needs to **obtain external corroboration.** Nonetheless, while gathering these data from the family and others, the interviewer must attend to the patient's needs and to the relationship.

The interviewer begins in the usual way. With severe cognitive dysfunction, she or he easily recognizes the problem during Steps 1 and 2 as patients do not know where they are, that they are in a medical setting, or who is with them. They make little sense, and their stories are grossly inconsistent. Additional psychiatric symptoms (e.g., hallucinations) may be present if the cognitive changes are part of a psychiatric problem. Mildly affected patients who remain aware that they are losing their cognitive capacities often compensate by keeping detailed notes of events and appointments to assist their failing memory and carefully guard against showing evidence of cognitive dysfunction. Nevertheless, such loss of thinking capacity can be suspected during Steps 1 to 5 by the patient's vagaries, inconsistencies, undue focus on familiar areas, and deft circumvention of areas where her or his memory has failed. The patient may use humor to mask her or his confusion and failing memory. With this patient, unlike the more severe forms, the interviewer usually needs systematic mental status evaluation to be certain. Once the interviewer suspects these problems, she or he shifts to the doctor-centered process (Steps 6 and 7) and conducts systematic testing.

The formal Mental Status Evaluation (MSE) is presented in Appendix E and is summarized in Table 6.1. Where inquiry rather than simple observation is needed, the investigation is conducted in the usual doctor-centered way, beginning with a general open-ended statement in relevant categories and then pinning down details using closed-ended inquiry. The interviewer might say, "Tell me about your memory." (No problems.) He or she would follow with, "Good, I need to ask you some specific questions so we can get the details." The interviewer then asks specific questions about important dates and well-known facts (e.g., "Who is the President?" "What is today's date?"). Full MSE requires knowledge of the various psychiatric, neurologic, and medical conditions that cause abnormalities of mental status. As standard clinical textbooks outline in greater detail (13–16), the interviewer makes observations or inquiry in the areas shown in Appendix E and summarized in Table 6.1.

With most patients, the clinician's or student's usual interaction and observation constitute sufficient mental status evaluation and can confirm intact

TABLE 6.1. MENTAL STATUS EVALUATION

A. Appearance: age, physical stigmata, dress, depression, general health, cleanliness, neatness
B. Attitude: cooperative, angry, guarded, suspicious, attentive, seductive, playful, obsequious
C. Activity: increased (hyperactivity, agitation), decreased, catatonic; abnormal movements (tics, tremors); visual–motor integrity
D. Mood (sustained objective emotional feeling): sad, happy, anxious, angry, depressed, detached, irritable
E. Affect (transitory, immediate emotional expression): full, flat, blunted, inappropriate, anhedonic, labile
F. Speech: normal, slowed, reduced, increased, pressured, mute; dysarthria, puns, rhymes
G. Language: bizarre, distracting, colorful, word salad, circumstantial, tangential; loosening of associations; neologisms
H. Thought content: logical, incoherent, derailed, content-poor, obsessive, delusional, paranoid
I. Perceptions: illusions, hallucinations (visual, auditory, olfactory, tactile), depersonalization, derealization
J. Judgment and insight: realistic, unrealistic; la belle indifference
K. Neuropsychiatric evaluation
   1. Level of consciousness: comatose, stuporous, drowsy, alert, hyperalert
   2. Attention and concentration: repeating digits, serial 7s, spelling backward, immediate memory
   3. Language function: fluency, comprehension, naming, repetition, reading, writing
   4. Memory: recent (orientation to time, place, and person; recall three unrelated objects); remote (past events); amnesia (retrograde, anterograde)
   5. Other higher functions: abstraction (proverbs), calculation, intelligence

Andreason NC, Black DW. *Introductory textbook of psychiatry*. Washington, D.C.: American Psychiatric Press, 1991:37–40.
Leon RL, Bowden CL, Faber RA. The psychiatric interview, history, and mental status examination. In: Kaplan HI, Sadock BJ, eds. *Comprehensive textbook of psychiatry*, 5th ed. Vol. 1. Baltimore: Williams & Wilkins, 1989: 449–462.

cognitive function. As clinicians, we routinely obtain full MSE in its entirety when we suspect dysfunction (of behavior, thought, or emotion) and in most new psychiatric and neurologic patients. I advise medical students in beginning clinical clerkships to complete the full MSE in all new patient evaluations, again as a way of becoming familiar with it in both normal and abnormal circumstances. Written reports of the patient should include comments on MSE in conjunction with the physical examination of the neurologic system. The MSE is part of the "physical examination" of the brain and its functional integrity although it is mostly obtained earlier during the doctor–patient interaction.

A screening MSE may quickly detect cognitive dysfunction, and it is useful when cognitive impairment is suspected (17). This testing can be performed in 5 to 10 minutes and can help both diagnosis of and follow-up for the course of cognitive dysfunction.

Pediatric Patients

Integrated interviewing applies with children and adolescents as well as adults (18). As clinicians, we still hope to establish a relationship and to obtain adequate personal and symptom data, but we also emphasize growth, development, and family interactions (19,20). Relationship issues necessarily extend to parents and other family. The younger the child is, the more age-related issues that are involved, including decreased ability to communicate, shorter attention span, less physical and mental development, and increased dependency on parents (19).

The usual conduct of Steps 1 to 5 has to be modified with many pediatric patients and even some adolescents. **Children often lack the psychologic and physical maturity to participate fully at this level of independence and self-directedness, and the interviewer sometimes relies more on a doctor-centered process.** Nevertheless, the child's concerns are always sought and the interviewer must recognize that children become increasingly autonomous as they grow older. Research has shown that direct involvement of younger patients in treatment discussions and decisions is important for their comfort and understanding (18). **The interviewer should also use a patient-centered approach with a major focus on the child's problems in interacting with the parent.**

The student or clinician should continue to attend to the various steps of the interview, while modifying the approach to the age and initiative of the patient. In Step 1, age-appropriate opportunities and facilities should be made available (e.g., toys, chairs, and games; appropriate place for teens who frequently do not want to sit with children or in childlike circumstances) (19,20). Older children and adolescents can often provide their own agenda, but parents usually formulate the issues for younger children (18).

The age of the child determines how Steps 3 and 4 are best carried out. The interview involves the parent more when the patient is a younger child. Even then, the interviewer should address the child first in an open-ended style, and the child should remain the focus of the inquiry (18,19). The interviewer should directly interview children who can speak, irrespective of age, and must recall their unfamiliarity with many medical terms and other words (18). The younger the patient is, the more concrete, simple, and brief the questions must be. The clinician or student should always try to use an open-ended approach, which can sometimes be productive even in the very young (19). In fact, as interviewers, we often underestimate how much information we can get from little children (e.g., "Mommy says Daddy needs to get a better job."). Nevertheless, initiating conversation is sometimes aided by giving the child age-appropriate "menus" of topics to choose from (20); for example, the interviewer may open-endedly inquire about recent birthdays, siblings, athletic events, school, social events, friends, and so on. Her or his task is to get the child talking about whatever interests she or he has. In addition, the interviewer wants to see the child interact with the parent and others and may even observe them in the waiting room (19). The interviewer and child should also try to interact, even briefly, without the parent present. The clinician or student then observes the child's behavior, as well as her or his communication skills.

In Steps 6 and 7 (HPI), the student or clinician obtains information from the child, parent, or both in the fashion already described in Chapter 5. Steps 8 (HI) and 9 (PMH) require an additional emphasis. Because growth and development are critical, the younger the child is, the more detail that is required about the mother's pregnancy, delivery, newborn and infancy periods, and subsequent developmental landmarks (e.g., feeding, growth, walking, talking, toilet training, progress in school, social development). Personal habits, immunization status, usual childhood illnesses, hospitalizations, poisonings, accidents, and injuries are biomedical data that merit special attention. As the child ages, the approach more closely resembles that of the adult HI and PMH.

Steps 10 (SH) and 11 (FH) also have unique foci. The SH contains information about the pertinent social aspects of the family (e.g., father's job), as well as the patient (e.g., less fighting at school and improved reading). The interviewer inquires about salient family interactions as well (e.g., ignoring a new brother, parents getting along better since the strike was settled). Speaking with a child's teacher to understand the SH better can also be helpful, especially if the child is having problems.

The FH and genogram (Step 11) include the health histories of grandparents, parents, and siblings. Because genetic disorders and precursors of adult diseases frequently begin in childhood, the interviewer must obtain a careful family pedigree. The mother's health, with attention to menses, contraception, marriages, pregnancies and outcomes, subsequent progress of children, and plans for more pregnancies, is especially important. The interviewer must also ascertain her feelings about her pregnancy with the patient and should learn about her physical and psychologic health. Her own rearing (e.g., punishment practices, abuse) and expectations of what being and raising a child are like are germane. The student or clinician assesses what kind of mother she will be and looks for areas where an intervention may be helpful; she may need support for her own competence. As mothers increasingly support families, their work situation is important as well. As fathers become more central to rearing children, many of the preceding considerations apply to them also. Indeed, fathers frequently are ignored and often feel left out at all levels of their child's care. The clinician must actively include and involve them.

The student or clinician accords Step 12 (review of systems [ROS]) more importance than she or he does with adults (20). Because children have much shorter histories and because obtaining pertinent symptoms during the HPI can be more difficult, detailed inquiry in all systems should be made prior to physical examination; more attention should be paid to transient or "minor" complaints (e.g., increased urinary frequency off and on again can signify severe disease).

Adolescence is a tumultuous period both physically and psychologically. An interviewer must take this into account. Some adolescents are perfectly comfortable with the standard patient-centered approach to an adult, whereas this can make others uncomfortable and anxious; they may benefit from a more structured, doctor-centered approach. Prominent issues and themes that can emerge are dependency on parents, feeling that he or she was forced to come to the doctor, conflict with the parents and others, confidentiality, desire to see an "adult doctor," obliviousness of health risks, hypochondriasis, mood changes, and rebelliousness (20). Ordinarily, the interviewer begins with the patient-centered approach, but she or he should be prepared to change to a more doctor-centered approach if the adolescent seems anxious or uncomfortable. Providing support and comfort may be more important than obtaining open-ended information, particularly at the beginning of the relationship. Seeing the adolescent alone is often more effective than seeing him or her with a parent and can lead to a better relationship.

Elderly Patients

With geriatric patients, although we as clinicians continue to focus on the relationship and gathering data, we must address their unique issues (10,21,22). These are occasioned by multiple medical problems, which are combined with greater functional, social, psychologic, and economic impairments (10). To understand and to integrate this multiplicity of biopsychosocial problems, the student often must involve other professionals, such as a nurse, a social worker, and therapists.

Setting the stage and ensuring comfort in Step 1 requires special attention. We should consider our patients' comfort and pride (e.g., dentures available, full dress) and their ease of hearing and seeing, and we should show proper respect (e.g., use surname). During the interview, many will tire if the pace is too fast and they do not have time to formulate their responses. Therefore, we must check frequently. In addition, friends and relatives may make the patient more comfortable and may provide additional information; confidentiality issues, of course, must be clarified.

Agenda setting in Step 2 can be difficult if many problems are present. Both the doctor's and the patient's time, as well as the patient's fatigue, may necessitate the deferral of less pressing problems to a later visit; obtaining a full history may sometimes take two or three visits. Completion of a previsit history questionnaire form (and sometimes other forms assessing functional status, mental status, and psychosocial status) can be useful adjuncts that provide necessary information without overtaxing the patient (10).

Steps 3 and 4 usually are conducted as I have already described. The following can sometimes greatly facilitate the interaction: touching the patient sensitively and caringly, showing interest and patience, and addressing the older person's priority items (10). Because many patients are familiar with the medical system and know "what it wants," getting older patients to talk on their own, rather than to respond to questions, can sometimes be difficult. Moving them from physical symptoms to personal issues may also be hard. Nevertheless, most respond to a patient-centered approach if the interviewer persists in its use.

Some older patients tend to recite long stories about the past, which can pose a difficulty for the interviewer. Patients often tell "old war stories" to impress the student or clinician that they were, and therefore still are, people of value and dignity (10). To shift the conversation, we as interviewers must acknowledge what the patient is trying to tell us. For example, to a patient relating his successes with a job in 1949, we might say, "That's quite an accomplishment; you sure did a lot. Thanks for telling me. We'll get back to that if we can, but let me shift gears and get you to say how things are going for you now."

The HPI and other current active problems [OCAP] take longer in most elderly patients because they usually have more than one problem, their multiple problems interact, and many problems are chronic with long histories. The interviewer should focus primarily on currently active problems. Falls, painful feet and toes, incontinence, sexual dysfunction, waning memory, depression, insomnia, and decreased hearing and vision are common. Similarly, functional difficulties, such as dressing, bathing, feeding, using the toilet, transferring, using a telephone, shopping, cooking, cleaning, driving, taking medications, and managing finances, are increasingly common as people age.

Multiple losses (of spouses, siblings, and friends) and loneliness are prominent. The patient may have more concerns about death and disability, as well as about living circumstances and remaining independent.

Health issues (Step 9) are essential. Interviewers should not overlook, for example, the fact that elderly patients have active sexual interests and a high alcohol abuse rate. Health maintenance activities are important but are frequently ignored; making a nutritional assessment, not only for caloric excesses but also for deficiencies, is particularly important. The student or clinician should make sure that the patient has the opportunity to discuss advance directives and end-of-life issues. The past medical history (Step 9) also can be quite extensive. Once again, the interviewer should focus on problems relevant to the patient's health.

If the social history is not ascertained in the HPI/OCAP, it is covered in Step 10; it determines the patient's social situation and her or his support structure. As patients age, they may lose capacity in what was previously routine (e.g., bathing, cooking). Therefore, learning specifically what their support structure is and how it is affecting their health (e.g., senior citizens' center, church groups, Meals on Wheels) is essential.

The family history (Step 11) can become quite complex, so only information that is still important to the patient's health should be obtained (e.g., a family history of elevated blood pressure or diabetes in an 80-year-old is of little value); however, asking about family members who are available to help is a critical question. Similarly, the review of systems (Step 12) should address only issues that are salient to the patient's health.

Unique Issues for the Student

How Much Time to Spend with Patients

Students at the *start of the third year* obtain complete histories from new patients, often those who are inpatients. Beginning clinical students can ignore the need for efficiency. As experience accumulates, efficiency follows. Initially, the student takes at least 30 minutes with the patient-centered process of the HPI/OCAP (Steps 1 to 5) and 2 or more hours in the remainder of the HPI/OCAP, HI, PMH, SH, FH, and ROS. Physical examination takes another hour or more at the outset; students must carefully attend to the patient's comfort and sometimes may have to return at a later time to complete the evaluation if the patient tires. This is only the beginning. The student reads, discusses, synthesizes data, obtains data from other sources, plans and analyzes diagnostic interventions, participates in treatment decisions, and then again interviews the patient.

By graduation, most students can conduct a full interview in 60 to 90 minutes and by completion of their residency, in 30 to 60 minutes. New patients typically receive 40- to 60-minute appointments in residents' and advanced students' clinics. Follow-up visits with both inpatients (ward rounds) and outpatients (clinic visits) involve patients known to the doctor or student; these ordinarily range from 5 to 30 minutes.

Audiotape Recording of Interviews

During initial instruction in patient-centered interviewing (Steps 1 to 5), teachers often introduce students to audiotaping or videotaping; they will have learned how to critique interviews. **Because the interview is a core skill, clinical students are urged to continue taping interviews on their own, much as a musician or an athlete hones his or her most important skills on a daily basis.** Self-critique and input from other students or faculty leads to continuing improvement.

Inexpensive audiotape recorders can be used with minimal inconvenience and great benefit. Students should inform patients that taping is confidential and that the tape will be erased when its use is completed; patients of course should know if others will listen to the tape and who they are. In getting permission to tape, the student benefits from the usual willingness of patients to help. He or she may say, "Before we get started talking, I'd like to ask your help. I'm interested in improving my communication skills and would like to tape record our interaction. I (and my instructor—or my group) will listen to it afterward to see how I could have communicated better. Nobody else will hear it. Then we'll erase it. It's nothing you have to do, but it would be a big favor to me." Patients rarely refuse. Critiquing Steps 1 to 5—one's patient-centered skills and transition into the doctor-centered process—is especially important.

Taking and Using Notes

During Steps 1 to 5 (patient-centered process), the student can unobtrusively jot down a few pertinent words or dates. This helps when the patient is giving the chronology of her or his physical problem and can preclude the student asking about it again during the doctor-centered process. Nevertheless, she or he should avoid any excessive break in eye contact, disruption of information flow, or other hitch in the relationship. During the doctor-centered process, the student almost always takes notes, which are sometimes quite extensive, but she or he should still keep the primary focus on the patient.

Students frequently need to use notes themselves as reminders to recall all components of the HI, PMH, SH, FH, and ROS. Reminder notes, however, should be minimal during the patient-centered process.

The interviewer can explain her or his notetaking and should ask the patient to give feedback if it interferes. For example, the student might say at the outset, "I'll be making an occasional note early on, and later I'll be taking more notes and using some of my own notes to refer to. This helps me get all the information about you and to keep it in order. If that becomes disruptive for you, please let me know."

Clinical Conduct

Many of my students and residents have debated the appropriateness of certain behaviors and attitudes and, in many discussions, generated the guidelines presented here. These suggestions are not comprehensive, however, and the student can add more.

The consensus has been that the *following behaviors are the most important:* unconditional positive regard, empathy, acting as the patient's ally, acting in the patient's interest, respect, self-confidence tempered with humility, encouraging patient autonomy without forcing it, recognizing at least one patient strength or unique attribute, awareness of the role of spirituality, and honesty balanced by hope; informing the patient about the student's role in her or his care and the student's reason for seeing her or him; introducing oneself and all others present; arranging a mutually satisfactory time to interact; attending to the patient's physical comfort before interviewing; anticipating issues that could disturb the patient; openly addressing confidentiality; providing service beyond the usual; and meeting specific requests from the patient.

My students and residents believed the *following behaviors were seldom, if ever, appropriate when one was with the patient:* smoking, drinking anything, or eating; chewing gum or a toothpick; swearing; behaving seductively or making sexual remarks or jokes; poor personal hygiene; uncomfortable joking or teasing; stating personal opinions about others; going beyond appropriate self-disclosure to discuss one's own problems; and making value judgments about the patient or others.

These discussions raised other difficult issues. Although we certainly wanted to avoid seductive behavior, we struggled with the role of touching the patient outside of the physical examination. The students and residents generally agreed that this was appropriate, but only if the student or resident felt comfortable with it, if it was motivated out of genuine personal concern, and if it would appear professional. Although hugging or putting one's arm around a well-known patient can be appropriate and professional, they preferred more limited touching, such as a pat on the back or arm.

We also puzzled over the conversations that one conducts during the physical examination, especially during the more tension-laden portions (e.g., pelvic, breast, or rectal examination). All agreed that calm, confident discussion of what one is doing and why is appropriate, while, of course, attending to the patient's experience and comfort. Inquiry about symptoms and problems in the areas being examined also defuses tension. In addition, the interviewer can explain self-examination and other preventive techniques (e.g., during breast examination, the student could instruct a woman in self-examination).

Treatment

As has already been noted, the intention of this book is not to outline specific treatments for various medical conditions. Nevertheless, I must comment on the fact that the student now has two powerful therapeutic tools at his or her command. **Using NURS and being present with the patient in times of difficulty, whether medical or psychologic, are highly therapeutic in and of themselves (23,24).** They are the active ingredients of the drug "doctor" that Balint referred to and are the key determinants of the provider–patient relationship (25).

Caretakers often believe that they have nothing to offer patients who are beyond hope medically and surgically (e.g., terminal cancer) or for whom no disease explanation has been found for their physical symptoms (somatization), but from research we know that being with patients in a supportive way and using NURS are highly effective treatments, not only from a humanistic standpoint but also from a scientific respect (23,26–33). Further, for the many patients with diseases that are responsive to biomedical treatments, we also know that we contribute tremendously to their health outcomes and satisfaction by using these skills (34–41)(see Rationale section of Chapter 1). We have now come full circle—these are the benefits that accrue from being patient-centered, and the student now knows how to achieve them!

SUMMARY

In the clinic or at the bedside, the advanced interviewer makes key practical decisions during Steps 1 to 5. These have many nuances. They guide fine-tuning of the interview that is required for balancing the patient-centered and doctor-centered processes; for dealing with patients who are reticent, talkative, focused on biomedical material, or in for a routine exam; for situations when all necessary personal data do not arise during the patient-centered process and when more than one person is present; for coping with communication problems (deaf, mute, blind, cognitively impaired); and for interacting with pediatric and geriatric patients. Interviewing issues unique to the student include taking sufficient time for the interview, conducting self-critiques using audiotapes, using notes strategically at the bedside, and following recommendations for appropriate clinical behavior. Finally, by one's simple supportive presence with the patient and by using NURS, one now has a powerful treatment tool readily available to all patients.

LEARNING EXERCISES

1. Estimate how much time you would be likely to spend in the patient-centered process in the following situations if you have a total of 45 minutes available for new patients and 15 minutes for follow-up patients:
    a. Routine physical with no problems (new)
    b. Severe medical problem with difficult to control diabetes mellitus and worsening depression (follow-up)
    c. Severe anxiety (follow-up)
    d. Acute emergency with periodic loss of consciousness and severe chest pain (new)
    e. Average patient (new)
    f. Average patient who requires an interpreter (new)
2. Describe how you can be therapeutic in all of the above situations.*
3. How do you know if the patient-centered process has been effective?* (There can be several good answers.)
4. Describe circumstances in nonacute patients where you might not want to spend as much time in the patient-centered process as is usual.*

*Good test questions.

PRACTICE EXERCISES

1. To get the feel for short patient-centered interactions, practice (in role play) using all 5 steps in 2 to 3 minutes. Touch all five bases but don't worry about each substep, except in Step 4—be sure that you always start with the physical, switch to personal, and end up with emotional and NURS.
2. When you are comfortable with question #1, try omitting some of the substeps.
   a. Ignore physical symptoms in an emotion-laden situation; ignore personal data in the same situation; in each case, proceed directly to NURS and rely upon that as your sole patient-centered activity.
   b. In a low-key emotional situation that has many serious medical problems, use just NURS even though the patient has little or no emotion.
3. When you have mastered questions #2 and #3 in role-play, do the same with real or simulated patients.
4. Perform an in-depth, patient-centered interview, lasting 15 to 20 minutes, with a patient who has significant personal issues. The key here is in Step 4 where you keep using the cycle of skills to develop chapter after chapter of the patient's story.
5. In role play or with patients, practice Steps 1 to 5 in the following circumstances: reticent patient, talkative patient, deaf patient, using an interpreter, blind patient, pediatric patient, geriatric patient, terminal patient, with a relative present, with a demented patient.

References

1. Campbell TL, McDaniel SH. Conducting a family interview. In: Lipkin M, Putnam SM, Lazare A, eds. *The medical interview.* New York: Springer-Verlag, 1995:178–186.
2. Hornberger JC, Gibson Jr CD, Wood W, et al. Eliminating language barriers for non–English-speaking patients. *Med Care* 1996;34:845–856.
3. Carrasquillo O, Orav EJ, Brennan TA. Impact of language barriers on patient satisfaction in an emergency department. *J Gen Int Med* 1999;14:82–87.
4. Rivadeneyra R, Elderkin-Thompson V, Silver RC, et al. Patient centeredness in medical encounters requiring an interpreter. *Am J Med* 2000;108:470–474.
5. Hardt EJ. The bilingual interview and medical interpretation. In: Lipkin M, Putnam SM, Lazare A, eds. *The medical interview.* New York: Springer-Verlag, 1995:172–177.
6. Tocher TM, Larson EB. Do physicians spend more time with non–English-speaking patients? *J Gen Int Med* 1999;14:303–309.
7. Billings AJ, Stoeckle JD. *The clinical encounter—A guide to the medical interview and case presentation.* Chicago: Year Book, 1989.

8. Lotke M. She won't look at me. *Ann Int Med* 1995;123:54–57.
9. Enelow AJ, Swisher SN. *Interviewing and patient care.* New York: Oxford University Press, 1986.
10. Mader SL, Ford AB. The geriatric interview. In: Lipkin M, Putnam SM, Lazare A, eds. *The medical interview.* New York: Springer-Verlag, 1995:221–234.
11. Barnett S, Franks P. Deafness and mortality: analyses of linked data from the National Health Interview Survey and National Death Index. *Public Health Reports* 1999;114:330–336.
12. Barnett S. Clinical and cultural issues in caring for deaf people. *Fam Med* 1999; 31:17–22.
13. Leon RL, Bowden CL, Faber RA. The psychiatric interview, history, and mental status examination. In: Kaplan HI, Sadock BJ, eds. *Comprehensive textbook of psychiatry,* 5th ed. Vol. 1. Baltimore: Williams & Wilkins, 1989:449–462.
14. Andreason NC, Black DW. *Introductory textbook of psychiatry.* Washington, D.C.: American Psychiatric Press, 1991.
15. Humes HD, DuPont HL, Gardner LB, eds. *Kelley's textbook of internal medicine,* 4th ed. Philadelphia: Lippincott Williams & Wilkins, 2000.
16. Strain JJ, Putnam SM, Goldberg R. The mental status examination. In: Lipkin M, Putnam SM, Lazare A, eds. *The medical interview.* New York: Springer-Verlag, 1995:83–103.
17. Folstein MF, Folstein SE, McHugh PR. "Mini-mental state": a practical method for grading the cognitive state of patients for the clinician. *J Psychiatric Res* 1975; 12:189–198.
18. Lewis C, Pantell B. Interviewing pediatric patients. In: Lipkin M, Putnam SM, Lazare A, eds. *The medical interview.* New York: Springer-Verlag, 1995: 209–220.
19. Greenspan SI, Greenspan NT. *The clinical interview of the child,* 2nd ed. Washington, D.C.: American Psychiatric Press, 1991.
20. Enzer NB. Interviewing children and parents. In: Enelow AJ, Swisher SN, eds. *Interviewing and patient care,* 3rd ed. New York: Oxford University Press, 1986: 122–147.
21. Blazer D. Techniques for communicating with your elderly patient. *Geriatrics* 1978;33:79–84.
22. Fletcher CR. How not to interview an elderly clinic patient: a case illustration and the interviewer's explanation. *Gerontologist* 1972;12:398–402.
23. Frank AW. Just listening: narrative and deep illness. *Families Systems Health* 1998;16:197—212.
24. Stuart MR, Lieberman III JA. *The fifteen minute hour.* London: Praeger, 1993.
25. Balint M. *The doctor, his patient, and the illness,* rev ed. New York: International Universities Press, 1957.
26. Smith GR Jr, Monson RA, Ray DC. Psychiatric consultation in somatization disorder. *N Engl J Med* 1986;314:1407–1413.
27. Smith RC. Somatization disorder: defining its role in clinical medicine. *J Gen Intern Med* 1991;6:168–175.
28. Smith GR Jr, Rost K, Kashner TM. A trial of the effect of a standardized psychiatric consultation on health outcomes and costs in somatizing patients. *Arch Gen Psychiatry* 1995;52:238–243.

29. Rost K, Kashner TM, Smith GR Jr. Effectiveness of psychiatric intervention with somatization disorder patients: improved outcomes at reduced costs. *Gen Hosp Psychiatry* 1994;16:381–387.
30. Spiegel D, Bloom JR, Yalom I. Group support for patients with metastatic cancer. *Arch Gen Psychiatry* 1981;38:527–533.
31. Spiegel D, Bloom JR, Kraemer HC, et al. Effect of psychosocial treatments on survival of patients with metastatic breast cancer. *Lancet* 1989;2:888–891.
32. Fawzy IF, Fawzy NW, Arndt LA, et al. Critical review of psychosocial interventions in cancer care. *Arch Gen Psychiatry* 1995;52:100–113.
33. Fawzy IF, Fawzy NW, Hyun CS, et al. Malignant melanoma—effects of an early structured psychiatric intervention, coping, and affective state on recurrence and survival 6 years later. *Arch Gen Psychiatry* 1993;50:681–689.
34. Kaplan SH, Greenfield S, Ware JE. Impact of the doctor-patient relationship on the outcomes of chronic disease. In: Stewart M, Roter D, eds. *Communicating with medical patients*. London: Sage, 1989:228–245.
35. Shear CL, Gipe BT, Mattheis JK, et al. Provider continuity and quality of medical care—a retrospective analysis of prenatal and perinatal outcome. *Med Care* 1983; 21:1204–1210.
36. Egbert LD, Battit GE, Welch CE, et al. Reduction of postoperative pain by encouragement and instruction of patients—a study of doctor-patient rapport. *N Engl J Med* 1964;270:825–827.
37. de Groot KI. The influence of psychological variables on postoperative anxiety and physical complaints in patients undergoing lumbar surgery. *Pain* 1997;69: 19–25.
38. Kiecolt-Glaser JK, Page GG. Psychological influences on surgical recovery: perspectives from psychoneuroimmunology. *Am Psychol* 1998;53:1209–1218.
39. Williams GC, Frankel RM, Campbell TL, et al. Research on relationship-centered care and healthcare outcomes from the Rochester Biopsychosocial Program: a self-determination theory integration. *Families Systems Health* 2000;18:79–90.
40. Stewart MA. Effective physician-patient communication and health outcomes: a review. *Can Med Assoc J* 1995;152:1423–1433.
41. Williams S, Weinman J, Dale J. Doctor-patient communication and patient satisfaction: a review. *Fam Pract Res J* 1998;15:480–492.

7

Advanced Interviewing
The Provider–Patient Relationship

Interviewing elicits information about the patient. In addition to the informational dimension, a second determinant of a successful interview exists—the doctor–patient relationship (DPR). Integrated interviewing incorporates additional measures (beyond the relationship-building skills we already have addressed with NURS [naming, understanding, respecting, and supporting]) to foster the DPR. This chapter addresses these determinants of the dyadic aspect of the DPR, but it does not consider more general determinants (e.g., the sociocultural matrix, patients' and doctors' roles, and subcultures). Nor do we address relationships in medicine that are outside the dyad, a wider area often called relationship-centered care (1–4) (e.g., relationships among nurses, administrators, doctors, educators, and community representatives within a hospital).

The DPR is a fundamental dimension of care, and, as clinicians, we *monitor our relationship* with the patient as closely and continuously as we do his or her temperature, blood pressure, and pulse rate. First, we inquire how things are going between ourselves and the patient, both overall (e.g., "You've been in the hospital several days now and I wanted to check how we're doing") and in the immediate interaction ("That's a difficult problem—what is it like talking about it with me?"). This provides direct feedback on the relationship and, in turn, allows us to make necessary changes. Doing so also validates the patient by showing that her or his reactions are important. In addition, we always observe the patient's body language, behavior, what he or she says and how it is said, her or his emotional comfort, and the ability to interact and negotiate. For example, a comfortable, safe, and otherwise healthy DPR is suggested when the patient's arms are not folded defensively across her or his chest, appropriate (intermittent) eye contact is made, and the patient arrives on time and follows the negotiated agreements and when she or he openly expresses personal concerns, including negative aspects of care, is comfortable expressing emotions, and is able to negotiate care solutions. Of course, many variations do exist. When the relationship is effective, the patient and physician alike experience respect, trust, and an effective interchange of data. Both feel comfortable and note rapport, satisfaction, compliance, confidence, and openness to negotiation. The opposite features characterize an ineffective relationship.

To understand the dyadic aspects of the DPR, consider **the doctor's and the patient's personalities as two interacting gears.** The gears must engage to establish the relationship; otherwise, as clinicians we find ourselves in an uninvolved, distant interaction, in which, perhaps, the doctor and the patient address different agendas. On the other hand, if the gears engage too deeply, the mechanism itself can be destroyed, resulting in overinvolvement of doctor and patient (e.g., a sexual relationship). Therefore, we must understand both the patient's personality and our own. This understanding allows us to **adjust our behavior so as to mesh better with our patient.**

Unrecognized Responses Affect the Relationship with the Patient

The student or clinician often must change to maximize the effectiveness of the relationship because the patient cannot be expected to change. Interviewers frequently exhibit personal responses that are counterproductive (5); therefore, changing them improves the DPR. Most problems occur during Steps 1 to 5 (patient-centered process) because the relationship is just beginning, and here the patient expresses most of the personal material that can be stressful to the interviewer. Nevertheless, her or his personal responses affect the DPR throughout.

I define a "personal response" as an individual's emotional reaction and its behavioral result. For example, one student became afraid of an authoritarian patient who reminded him of his father. This led him, in turn, to allow the patient to take over the interview, even though he knew better. Another interviewer became anxious and felt out of control when a patient began talking about death. This led her, in turn, to take excessive control of the interview by switching prematurely to the doctor-centered process. In both instances, the emotions (fear and anxiety) led to a nonproductive interviewing behavior.

Any aspect of a patient (e.g., personality, job, illness, family, or odor) can trigger our adverse emotions and behaviors. Some doctors feel negatively about people with AIDS, perhaps owing to unwarranted fears of catching it (6); some, about patients who abuse alcohol, which often reflects negative feelings about the patient's seeming unwillingness to take responsibility for her or his actions; and some, about patients with no definable disease, often from frustration at their own inability to make a disease diagnosis (7). Negative feelings produce negative behaviors, such as avoidance, criticism, or superficiality.

Deleterious responses also can feel positive, as in the example already given of sexual attraction to patients. Similarly, "liking" a patient because that patient reminds the interviewer of a positive person in her or his life can be harmful if, as a result, the student or clinician treats the patient as though she or he were that other person. That ignores the patient's real self and needs; for example, an interviewer might avoid a discussion of cancer in an elderly woman because she reminds the interviewer of her or his own much-loved grandmother.

The Problem

My research with medical students, house staff, and fellows demonstrates that interviewers' responses to patients almost universally have negative components and deleterious potential. Thirteen of 15 sophomore medical students (8) and 16 of 19 residents and fellows (9) exhibited potentially harmful responses when *each* were observed in a *single interview*. Table 7.1 lists the potentially deleterious feelings and their resulting behaviors. Common fears of losing control, addressing psychological material, or appearing unpleasant generate interviewing behaviors that are, respectively, overly controlling, avoiding, and superficial. The reader can imagine their potential for harm. Consider, for example, the life-threatening impact of avoiding data about suicidal intent, noncompliance, and specific symptoms—in addition to the effects of these behaviors on data gathering and the relationship itself!

A study of board certified physicians with an average age of 50 showed that experienced doctors continued to exhibit potentially deleterious responses, particularly when threats to their integrity or self-esteem occurred (10). Although these seasoned practitioners reacted adversely to fewer patient circumstances than students, residents, and fellows did, their reactions did not diminish with age or experience. Once a pattern has been established, it remains. This suggests that experience alone does not change potentially harmful behaviors unless instructors attempt specific educational interventions.

TABLE 7.1. UNRECOGNIZED FEELINGS AND RESULTING BEHAVIORS IN STUDENTS, RESIDENTS, AND FELLOWS DURING ONE INTERVIEW*

I. Unrecognized feelings elicited immediately after a patient interview
  A. Common
    1. Fears of losing control, addressing psychological material, appearing unpleasant, harming the patient
    2. Unique personal issues (e.g., reminds one of own difficult divorce, fear of cancer in self)
    3. Performance anxiety
  B. Uncommon
    1. Sexual feelings, attitude favoring biomedical data, anger, fear of involvement, intimidation by patient, inadequacy, disdain
    2. Identification with the patient
  C. Not found—severe anxiety, depression
II. Unrecognized behaviors observed during a patient interview
  A. Common
    1. Overcontrol of the patient and interview (e.g., inappropriate interrupting or changing subject)
    2. Avoidance of psychological material (e.g., death, loneliness, disability)
    3. Superficial behavior (e.g., overly reassuring, overly social, cocktail party atmosphere)
    4. Passivity (e.g., no control or direction, inactive, detached)
  B. Uncommon
    1. Seductiveness
    2. Critical, intimidating, passive–aggressive
    3. Lack of respect and sensitivity
    4. Withdrawal, distancing
    5. Awkward interactions

---

*These data were obtained by the author during and following training interviews. The author personally observed the learner–patient interview and noted untoward behaviors that were potentially unrecognized behaviors. The teaching critique followed immediately and always was begun with open-ended inquiry. This produced data about the learner's emotional response to the patient and also provided data showing whether the interviewer was fully aware of the behaviors observed by the author. When the interviewer previously was fully aware of the emotions or behaviors observed by the author, they were not included (i.e., only incompletely recognized emotions and behaviors are recorded here).
Smith RC. Teaching interviewing skills to medical students: the issue of 'countertransference.' *J Med Educ* 1984;59:582–588.
Smith RC. Unrecognized responses by physicians during the interview. *J Med Educ* 1986;61:982–984.

My team recently studied residents who were learning interviewing and associated psychosocial skills (11). Fifty of the 53 had negative reactions that interfered with learning interviewing and that were harmful to patients. Fortunately, with teaching, 44 out of 50 changed these negative reactions and improved their communication and relationship skills.

Because these personal responses are universal and understandable and because they are viewed as part of the human condition, *we as humans consider them normal* (8,9,11). Nonetheless, unrecognized responses have harmful potential; therefore, to maximize the DPR, I like to address them. Why?

Unlike most disciplines, where the relationship is not as central to the outcome, the relationship in medicine is key for effective medical care; and these quite human reactions can interfere with learning, as well as with care. Troublesome, unrecognized responses often interfere with or override new learning. Patient-centered practices entail relinquishing some control and addressing patients' emotional material, but, because of understandable personal responses, many interviewers act as if they wish to seize control and to avoid emotions. Even though the student or resident may demonstrate an ability with newly learned patient-centered skills, long-ingrained emotions can interfere with her or his use of those very skills.

What the Interviewer Can Do About Unrecognized Responses

Unfortunately, most people do not fully recognize most of their interfering responses. Although effective coaching by a teacher or mentor (12) best helps an interviewer become aware of her or his previously unrecognized responses, she or he can nevertheless make significant progress even working alone or just with colleagues (13).

Diagnosing the Problem

As clinicians, to diagnose difficulties with our personal responses, we must make our emotional responses more conscious and recognizable. As an interviewer, you can reexperience emotions by recalling negative or otherwise difficult experiences with patients, clinical situations, peers, and family. By thinking individually or talking freely with peers, you can become more aware and can begin to understand your personal responses. First, identify the emotion. Then, link the emotion to a specific behavioral outcome (e.g., you were angry about a slight and then ignored the provocateur). By considering many difficult situations, you can usually find a common pattern (e.g., one individual realized that perceived slights provoked anger and withdrawal from nurses, friends, his spouse, and a teacher).

Another exercise for better recognizing your interfering emotions relates specifically to the interview. A good first question you can ask yourself following any interaction is, "What was my emotional reaction to the patient, and how did it affect my interviewing behavior?" You should look for one positive and one negative emotion with each patient and then identify your behavioral responses. You should consider imagined, as well as actual, behaviors (e.g., "I wanted to shake a patient abusing alcohol 'for being so stupid'."). Reviewing a video or audiotaped interaction can allow you to re-experience your emotional reactions and to observe any untoward responses, such as unnecessarily changing directions or avoiding certain topics. If, as a student, you are not yet seeing patients, you can increase emotional awareness by considering other medical encounters: working on cadavers, operating on animals, having blood drawn, drawing blood, watching an uncomfortable procedure, reading about awful diseases, experiencing difficult contacts with teachers or peers, and the general educational atmosphere. You should identify the emotion and any behavioral consequence (e.g., while observing a pelvic examination, one student became fearful that it was causing pain, which led her to skip the next demonstration on pelvic exams).

Other routes may increase your awareness of emotions. You can read stories of patients' courage in the face of severe suffering (14–18). Also, reading emotion-laden material, watching emotional movies, recalling personal emotional events, revisiting music and art, working with emotional people, or considering likely emotional events in the future (births, deaths) can help. You should seek positive, as well as negative, emotions. Other self-help or centering measures can be valuable to hard-working students and physicians. Increased calmness and poise usually help, as do regular exercise, relaxation (19), meditation (20), taking personal time, nonintellectual pursuits, hobbies, creative endeavors, meeting different people, altruistic activities, and renewing your spiritual dimension.

Successful self-analysis and honesty go hand in hand (13). Realizing that **"negative" feelings are normal and universal** helps (8,9). As humans, we often make things worse by ignoring them. Surprise awaits you if you believe emotions can be suppressed; a consequence always exists for doing so. For example, feeling angry at a patient or a peer always has some behavioral expression, such as being distant, overly friendly, or aggressive. Following an honest diagnosis of yourself, you must determine if your observed responses are taking you where you want to be in relationships. Once you are aware, you can choose to change that response.

Treating the Previously Unrecognized Behavior and Emotion

Repeatedly acknowledging the problem sometimes leads to improvement; for example, a student or clinician might remind herself or himself before each interview that "discussing death and other painful issues is difficult and I need to be on the lookout." Often, though, the interviewer must select a specific healthier behavior, but not the ultimate, perfect behavior, as a replacement. Progressing a step at a time works better; for example, learning to make a few comments is a good start for someone who has trouble talking in the presence of a professor. You should rehearse the desired new behavior in your mind and then in role-play. You take your own role and then switch to the other person's (or patient's) role in the problematic situation in a role-play with a peer. You then perform both roles again using the planned new behavior. Doing this provides important reinforcement and insight about the old pattern and promotes satisfactory change toward the new one.

Changing the emotion is more difficult. Sometimes, self-supportive statements help (e.g., a student might think that "He just reminds me of my father. I have important things I want to begin saying.") Using emotion-handling skills with yourself also helps. You should consciously recognize that the work is uncomfortable, that you are working hard and trying new behaviors, and that progress, although slow, is occurring. You can reinforce your self-esteem with positive self-talk and recall that this work will make you a better doctor (21).

In general, students and clinicians can make remarkable changes as they get to know themselves better, take some risks, and stretch personally. Interviewers' innate capacity for adult growth and maturation uncovers unexpected strengths and capabilities that can then lead to more effective relationships with patients and others (22,23).

Attempting these changes with a few colleagues produces the best results. Others provide support, accurate feedback, and insightful suggestions for new behaviors. Within such groups, the following useful guidelines can aid progress (24,25). (a) Meet regularly for the sole purpose of self-awareness work. (b) Observe strict confidentiality. (c) Urge people to speak only for themselves and to participate only when they are ready and to the extent that they are comfortable. (d) Direct feedback to focus on behaviors rather than on the person; be sure the feedback is descriptive and nonevaluative, contains a balance of positive and negative, and provides only a manageable amount of information for the next step (26). (e) Focus on emotions and here and now events; intellectual discussions are appropriate but they should not dominate the session. (f) Ask members not only to work with their own problems but also to try to be supportive and empathic to colleagues. (g) Give a nonjudgmental attitude and unconditional positive regard for each member; this keeps the setting safe and comfortable for the sharing that makes the process work. (h) Use predominantly open-ended questioning and remain person-centered. (i) Facilitate problem solving and provide support. These are more valuable than advice, analysis, trying to change others, and "the hard truth."

(j) Foster patience, understanding, and recognition that each person's behavior is what works best for her or him right now; this offsets frustration with slow or inapparent progress. Many people often do not understand or even recognize some very obvious aspects of themselves. The same issue often surfaces repeatedly and requires additional exploration even after it has been addressed. (k) Encourage others toward self-disclosure and responding to their own emotions by doing it yourself. (l) Recognize that respectfully and supportively discussing personal issues cannot harm another and that others can take care of themselves; this assists when the group is working with "painful" material. (m) Address feelings about other members of the group, especially when conflict occurs. (n) Always link personal issues and professional issues. (o) Expect to find that healthy, positive feelings often are among the most guarded and suppressed in many individuals. (p) Realize that support leads to hope. (q) Use appropriate touching, which does help, to the level of each member's comfort. (r) Enhance the group's work with a facilitator where appropriate. Seek help if problems or conflicts arise that interfere with the group work.

This process works even better if you, as the learner, carefully analyze your emotions and behaviors by keeping a journal (25). You can synthesize self-awareness work and can identify specific issues and behaviors to address in the future. Some items that benefit from recording include the following: most memorable events, most important learning experiences, applying new knowledge, emotions (and resulting behaviors), how behaviors and emotions have changed, specific new learning goals (including the immediate next step), successes as well as problems, and whether the personal and group work are meeting expectations and why or why not.

A little anxiety and tension can help you with this process, but you should not experience depression, marked anxiety, disruption of work or relationships, or other evidence of psychologic disturbance. These outcomes require help from a mental health professional. The reader should note that self-awareness work does not "cause" problems but, rather, sometimes provides the venue for them to surface and, in turn, allows early identification.

Dimensions of the Patient That Affect the Relationship: The Patient's Personality Style

Most people have several of the features of basic personality characteristics noted next, and I encourage the reader to look for these features in herself or himself. Many people in medicine, however, have been described as having predominantly obsessive and authoritarian features. These are very useful characteristics for ensuring our success as clinicians, but they also can have adverse consequences for us personally and for the provider–patient relationship (27), which I note in discussing each of the following personality types.

The patient's personality is far more difficult to change, and we should not try to do so. Nevertheless, if we understand the patient's personality style, we can improve the relationship by adjusting our behaviors to the patient's unique style. *Personality style* is defined as that group of enduring personal characteristics that describe how a person thinks, feels, behaves, and interacts in relationship to others and the environment (28–33). Personality partially determines how people respond to the various stresses in life, including illness. It determines how the patient recognizes and presents her or his illness, relates to the doctor and nurses, responds to treatments and procedures, and deals with discomfort and disability and how she or he will return to health and activity. Knowledge of a patient's personality alerts us to circumstances likely to be stressful that can be avoided or ameliorated. Designations of personality styles apply to ourselves, as well as to patients. We can identify and name these styles, but we must be careful to not use the terms pejoratively as in name-calling or blaming.

Most personalities are within the range of normal, and readers will recognize parts of themselves in most styles described (28–33). Moreover, multiple styles usually are combined; many people have both dramatic and organized styles. Personality characteristics form the bedrock of psychological structure, and they are the basis for success as people make their way in the world; for example, a dramatic flair can be essential for a good performer or politician, whereas an organized style is essential for an effective professional or a good homemaker.

A personality is abnormal only when it is maladaptive and when it then interferes with successful functioning; this is called a *personality disorder* (32). For example, overconcern about appearance can lead a patient to mutilative procedures (numerous tattoos, unnecessary facial or breast reconstruction), or another patient might obsessively count ceiling tiles and wash her or his hands the entire day. Maladaptive patterns can be precipitated by or exacerbated in response to a medical illness. These patterns then may puzzle and obstruct physicians and may lead us to label these patients as "problem," "hateful," or "difficult" patients (34,35).

The interviewer can assess a patient's personality style during Steps 1 to 5 of the interview and then can use the appropriate skills based on his or her assessment. She or he can further diagnose the style in Step 4 by focusing on corroborating features and by considering whether the style is adaptive or maladaptive. The sooner she or he accomodates the patient's style, the smoother the interaction will be.

This section describes how to enhance the relationship by using knowledge of the patient's personality style, which is comprehended from a constellation of features rather than from any one or two of them. **After identifying a personality style, the interviewer meets the needs of its predominant feature to maximize the relationship.** With normal, well-adapted patients, this process is simply woven into each visit and the doctor proceeds as usual. **Normal patients present no unique problems in the medical setting.** Establishing the initial relationship with maladaptive patients, however, is just the start. **Maladaptive patients usually require ongoing care by a mental health professional, whose goal is to develop more adaptive traits and to wean patients gradually from their maladaptive features,** a topic that is beyond the scope of this text and that is addressed in psychiatry. The interviewer will note that each personality style has unique features that dictate different and sometimes opposite behaviors by her or him.

I only present summaries of some major personalities and how they affect the DPR (28–33). *For illustrative purposes, I emphasize the maladaptive patterns (personality disorders), but the reader must remember that normal patients exhibit minor variations of these as I also summarize.* Further, although this review presents each type singly, the reader should consider how different patterns might be combined. Most of us have features of several different personality styles.

Dependent Style

Basic Problem. The basic problem in *maladaptive* dependent patients is a wish for boundless interest, attention, and care. Such attention represents love to these patients and assuages their fears of abandonment, starvation, and helplessness that were learned very early.

Clinical Presentation. Maladaptive patients, with naive expectations for endless love, reach out quickly and impulsively to doctors. They demand urgent, special attention, and behave as though no one else exists. The simplest instructions often require repetition and assistance (e.g., how to get to the lab for a test). Losses and separations from loved ones are particularly stressful; they can lead to illness and psychological deterioration. Because illness leads to caretaking, relinquishing its nurturing aspects when health is regained may be difficult.

The student or clinician observes the following in *better-adapted* patients: normal and greater degrees of requests for advice, a need for detailed directions, checking plans in order to do things "right," "superindependent" behaviors wherein the patient delights in single-handedly performing many activities, living in the parental home as adults, deferring to a spouse for answers and decisions, using the collective "we" to indicate another's close involvement in their activities (e.g., "We took the medicine and then we did the physical therapy."), repeated stories of how others help and support them, and problematic oral habits (eating, smoking, drinking, addictions).

Maladaptive patients can pose difficult problems in medical settings; they can become angry and frustrated when their needs are not met. Incessant demands make the doctor feel "sucked dry." Doctors who are mothers have likened the situation to having a child constantly tugging at their breast. Passivity, helplessness, and a sense of entitlement often preclude following directions, paying bills, and performing other responsible acts.

Response of the Interviewer. We, as interviewers, can meet dependency needs during our initial contacts by incorporating much support into our conversation and actions; by evincing a positive outlook and showing interest in patients independent of disease; by giving guidance, advice, more detailed instructions, and special favors; and by arranging for more frequent visits.

Problems for the Interviewer. The common authoritarian interviewer typically interacts nicely with dependent patients at the outset (i.e., these doctors like to take charge and these patients like to be taken care of). Because maladaptive patients keep trying to get more and more attention, however, the clinician or student faces two possible relationship problems. First, she or he may try to meet the endless dependency needs so that the relationship becomes overinvolved, enmeshed, terribly time-consuming, and unproductive. She or he then becomes frustrated from trying hard and failing, and the patient becomes upset by not getting enough. Second, the doctor may reject it and may distance herself or himself from the patient so that the relationship dies.

Obsessive-Compulsive Style

Basic Problem. The basic problem with *maladaptive* obsessive-compulsive patients is their need to maintain control, especially of emotional expression. Control assuages unconscious fears of the following: emotion, dirtiness, disorderliness, impulsive aggression, and pleasurable indulgences—it is often the result of excessive childhood punishment.

Clinical Presentation. Maladaptive patients use knowledge as a tool for controlling these fears. Thinking substitutes for emotion in them. Ritualistic behaviors and obsessive thinking replace action, and their rationalizations are elaborate. Patients may bring extensive written notes for reference and may give detailed, boring accounts of routine body functions and symptoms. Although they may ask many questions, they do not listen and instead obsessively focus on selected details as a way to control anxiety (rather than to satisfy intellectual need). They typically try to take control of medical interactions, and they often succeed because illness bespeaks loss of control. Obsessive patients guard against emotions. When they are asked how they feel or what their emotional reaction is, they characteristically respond with what they think.

The student observes the following in *better-adapted* patients: normal and greater degrees of orderliness, precise speech, detailed information, self-discipline, tidiness, punctuality, conscientiousness, a well-organized approach, responsibility, conservatism, and a concern with right and wrong.

Maladaptive patients in medical settings demand a great deal of time, have many questions, and present detailed expositions of symptoms. Anger, depression, and anxiety may supervene when their control falters. Self-doubt, indecisiveness, and vacillation can pose problems when medical decisions (especially urgent ones) have to be made.

Response of the Interviewer. Meeting an obsessive patient's needs means giving information with an appropriate level of detail, which can include written materials and which often must address specific plans for diagnosis and treatment. Repeated requests for information, however, can indicate an underlying anxiety that must be explored rather than simply supplying that patient with information. Involving the patient actively and giving her or him a sense of control in decision making (e.g., which consultant to see) and in determining the details of daily conduct (e.g., when blood is drawn, how bath will be given) can help. The student or the clinician puts the patient in charge, as long as the patient is comfortable and it is consistent with good care. Also, prominently complimenting such patients on their knowledge, reasoning, self-sufficiency, and high standards can prove helpful.

Problems for the Interviewer. The common authoritarian interviewer can have trouble interacting with these patients—who are often very similar—if a battle for control ensues. This will result in an unengaged relationship, and patients may become unhappy and may go elsewhere. If an authoritarian doctor yields the appropriate level of control and gives information, the doctor's remaining obsessive features, such as thoroughness, precision, and clear reasoning, will impress the patient.

Histrionic Style

Basic Problem. The basic problem with *maladaptive* histrionic patients is the need to merge with others emotionally, especially with those of the opposite sex. Interacting in an emotionally intensive way, regardless of the pain and discomfort it produces, gratifies them.

Clinical Presentation. Maladaptive histrionic patients communicate through emotions, feeling, and performing rather than through thinking and doing. They are overly dramatic, flamboyant, teasing, inviting, flighty, and impulsive. Concern about appearance and bodily integrity is paramount. Although histrionic patients can be quite personable, engaging, and entertaining at the outset, the interviewer soon notes a pervasive superficiality and lack of depth. These patients often are seductive in dress, style, and language. Women may present in a defenseless, vulnerable way or with sexual promiscuity. Histrionic men emphasize their manliness and courage before women; plentiful tattoos, sexually revealing dress, and "macho" remarks are characteristic. Alternatively, these men may present as effeminate, weak, and fragile. In the intellectual domain, maladaptive histrionics impress the interviewer as vague, imprecise, inconsistent, circumstantial, contradictory, and exaggerating. Such patients may have short attention spans, decreased ability to concentrate, and erratic handling of factual data.

The student or clinician observes the following in *better-adapted* patients: normal and greater degrees of charm, colorfulness, liveliness, attractiveness, sexual appeal, gregariousness, romanticism, sentimentality, artistic interest, and creativity. Many exhibit a zest for life and pleasure, have a rich fantasy life, and arouse the envy and admiration of others for these qualities.

Maladaptive patients in medical settings can become angry, depressed, and jealous if they are not noticed as attractive and outstanding. Dissatisfaction in the relationship can lead them, as in their personal lives, to leave precipitously for another caretaker. Their impulsivity and inexperience with sound reasoning lead to difficulties with drugs, medications, ill-advised surgery, and other decisions about care. Minor problems, especially perceived bodily defects, create ongoing anxiety. These patients can be particularly vulnerable when deforming disease (e.g., breast surgery, facial laceration) occurs.

Response of the Interviewer. Meeting a histrionic patient's needs includes giving brief compliments on the patient's appearance in a useful, tasteful, and nonsuggestive way. However, showing and expressing interest in such a patient as a person rather than as just an object of attention is essential. The interviewer should behave calmly and firmly when the patient behaves seductively. She or he should allow the patient to ventilate fears and concerns but should not foment or encourage them. Reassurance works better than intellectual explanations do. The interviewer should try to involve these patients in decision making, but she or he often must assist in the thinking process and should not be reluctant to provide guidance, advice, and support.

Problems for the Interviewer. These patients can prove disastrous depending on the extent to which the interviewer is susceptible to seduction or is seductive herself or himself. Sexual encounters between caretaker and patient can be a harmful outcome of such interactions. Similarly, fears of such involvement can lead to the opposite outcome—a distancing interaction. Most interviewers working with histrionic patients are troubled less by sexual issues, however, than by the patient's lack of sound cognitive skills, which can be a source of frustration to a more cerebral caretaker. This, perhaps, is a factor in the observation that physicians seem to discount the reality of histrionic patients' problems. For example, with the same clinical presentation of coronary artery disease depicted on videotape, physicians investigated only about half as many presentations with histrionic patients as they did with obsessive patients (36).

Self-Defeating (Masochistic) Style

Basic Problem. A need to suffer is the underlying problem with *maladaptive* self-defeating patients, a category of patients whose existence as an entity has been questioned (32,37). This results from a severely repressive upbringing (physical, sexual, and emotional abuse) that, nonetheless, symbolized love and attention to the child. She or he, therefore, felt loved only when suffering or when the parent showed remorse following punishment.

Clinical Presentation. Maladaptive patients repeatedly fail. They are typified by experiences of suffering, bad luck, and disappointments and by a general hard-time impression. They present as the helpless victim and believe that they do not deserve success and that, if success occurs, something bad will follow to offset it—often, a self-fulfilling prophecy. Such patients may precipitate their own misfortune, and they are often incapable of learning from prior mistakes, even when they are made aware of their repetitious patterns; for example, the spouse of an alcoholic may repeatedly return to the marriage, or she or he may leave but then find another alcoholic.

The student or clinician observes the following in *better-adapted* patients: normal and greater degrees of guilt and need to atone for misdeeds, complaints about their troubles, self-effacement and submission, expectations of adverse outcomes, feelings of unworthiness of success, an image of themselves as victims without recourse, and the desire to meet others' needs without a concern for their own.

In the medical setting, maladaptive patients complain bitterly about many problems. Moreover, when one problem is resolved, they are not happy but instead present additional difficulties. Reassurance typically leads to more complaints. Resistance to encouragement, denial of improvement, accentuation of yet unimproved aspects of health, and a spurning of efforts to help are common. Patients frequently reject advice that would improve their situations; for example, when a patient is told to quit riding a motorcycle that has caused five injuries, he does not. They often request painful procedures or surgery and sometimes even seek them out against advice.

Response of the Interviewer. In meeting these patients' needs, the student or clinician should avoid reassurance, suggestions of improvement, or promises of a cure. Instead, she or he should simply acknowledge and respect their plights. Emotion-handling skills work nicely for this. Certainly, the interviewer must never be abusive to the patient, but she or he can frame tests or treatment as yet another burden to discourage the patient. When patients exhibit a prominent martyr component, the interviewer can structure interventions in terms of another's need. For example, the interviewer might say, "You've been through a lot, but I've got another difficult task for you with this test. I also know that it will make your wife less worried about you."

Problems for the Interviewer. These patients create a situation with great potential for an unwitting, but nevertheless harmful interaction. They elicit much sympathy, and clinicians and students respond by wanting to help, reassure, and cure them. These responses are, however, counterproductive with self-defeating patients; they create dissonance and eventually lead to loss of both the relationship and patient. Rather, the interviewer must restrain her or his usual more positive approach, acknowledge the patient's plight, and provide a less hopeful, more austere atmosphere.

Narcissistic Style

Basic Problem. The basic problem with *maladaptive* narcissistic patients is low self-esteem and a lack of confidence in maintaining their personal identities. Intimacy with or accepting anything from others means, for this type of patient, merging with them and losing one's own individuality. Narcissistic patients overcompensate by attempts to be superior and unique. This offsets low self-esteem.

Clinical Presentation. Maladaptive patients present as all-powerful and all-important with an exaggerated self-confidence; they often appear to be smug, vain, arrogant, supercilious, disdainful of others' opinions, and grandiose and seem as if they possess mysterious knowledge. With others, they may be patronizingly superior, overbearing, callous, or aloof. Not surprisingly, they do not have close relationships, do have difficulty establishing new ones, and are not described by others as friendly or warm. They often irritate doctors, particularly by discoursing in prolonged monologues.

The interviewer observes normal and greater degrees of expressing their opinions and feelings when working with those narcissistic patients who are *better-adapted*. The distinction between well adapted and less well adapted is determined by whether this pattern represents a healthy self-respect and respect of others' needs and opinions or rather represents an attempt to salve one's own self-esteem.

In the medical setting, maladaptive narcissistic responses increase with illness; this is characteristically manifested by an attitude of superiority to physicians, by always trying to "one-up" them, by being content only with the "best" doctor (typically the Chief of Service), and by exhibiting disdain for or patronizing other physicians. These patients lose confidence as they dwell on the doctor's faults, incessantly search for weakness in their physicians, and thereby exacerbate both their stress and narcissistic behaviors.

Response of the Interviewer. The interviewer meets the patient's needs by acknowledging her or him as a person of unique achievement, but, at the same time, she or he must be careful to show expertise in a nonthreatening fashion, so that the patient does not lose confidence. Engaging the patient at medical levels by discussing recent journal articles and by sharing ideas with him or her as one might with a colleague can help. The patient benefits most from an attitude of respect and concern rather than from one of warmth and caring.

Problems for the Interviewer. These patients often challenge or threaten interviewers, especially those who are authoritarian, by their superior behaviors, lack of confidence, a search for other consultants, and refusals to follow advice. She or he may enjoy working with such a patient more if she or he can develop patience and can avoid feeling threatened.

Paranoid Style
Basic Problem

The basic problem with *maladaptive* paranoid patients is a fear of their own faults, weaknesses, impulses (which are often retaliatory), and infringement by others. These patients, who were often severely criticized as children, distrust others and displace their negative impulses by projecting them onto other people (e.g., they see their own aggressive impulses in others). Their suspicion is rigid and intense; it is characterized by a hyperalertness to anything that is out of the ordinary.

Clinical Presentation. Maladaptive paranoid patients are guarded, vigilant, quarrelsome, suspicious, and fearful. They complain bitterly of mistreatment and neglect, and they blame others for their problems. Oversensitivity to slights and alertness to the negative feelings of others are typical. They often feel persecuted and then respond with self-righteous counterattacks that are out of proportion to the magnitude of the perceived criticism.

The student observes the following in *better-adapted* patients: normal and greater degrees of suspiciousness, good critical evaluation skills, alertness to things that are out of order, cynicism, complaining, a tendency to plan ahead to avoid dangerous circumstances, self-righteous statements, rigid limit-setting, predisposition to ruminate on negative problems, and a constant anticipation of problems.

In medical settings, a maladaptive patient's querulous approach to demand more attention, better food, less noise, faster nurses, and better clinic personnel is disrupting and time-consuming. Such patients frighten and irritate clinicians and students by threatening legal action and blaming others. Anger and aggressive control of medical personnel engender an unhappy milieu. Depression and anxiety bespeak a deterioration in the patient.

Response of the Clinician. Meeting these patients' needs requires giving full information about plans and treatment with the expectation that one will have to be more detailed than usual and will be subjected to greater scrutiny. The interviewer should prevent inadvertent slights, including those by other staff members. A friendly, courteous approach that avoids closeness works best.

Attempts at more usual, closer relationships are met with great suspicion for what is perceived, by the patient, as an infringement. The interviewer should not reinforce, dispute, or ignore patients' paranoid assertions. Rather, she or he must create a sense of safety and should acknowledge how difficult the problems are for a sensitive person like the patient to have to tolerate during an illness; she or he can also praise the patient's grasp of facts, self-control, and sense of autonomy. This, of course, is done using emotion-handling skills. The interviewer should recognize feelings without either disputing or reinforcing them. The patient is then ready for an appeal for more tolerance.

Problems for the Interviewer. A paranoid patient creates considerable difficulty for interviewers, especially for those who are authoritarian, if they battle or ignore the patient. Even when these understandable tendencies are controlled, management proves difficult and is received without gratitude.

Schizoid Style

Basic Problem. The basic problem with *maladaptive* schizoid patients is a fear of disappointment when relating to others. These patients may have experienced repeated early emotional deprivation and the absence of long-term ties (e.g., absent caretaker, erratic caretaking, multiple foster homes, institutional rearing) or the influence of schizoid or otherwise distant parents, which makes them uninvolved, detached, and remote. They have never learned how to love or be loved. Aloofness is a protective denial in response to the many painful relationships gone awry.

Clinical Presentation. Maladaptive schizoid patients isolate themselves. They are unsociable and out of touch, relate poorly to others, and have solitary interests. Although they may appear to be independent and not easily impressed, they often are oversensitive, fragile, and lacking in resilience. They frequently have low socioeconomic status and draw on public support. Although they are usually uninterested, some patients have eccentric ideas and behaviors with regard to foods, health measures, religious movements, social betterment schemes, and dress.

The student observes the following in *better-adapted* patients: normal and greater degrees of distance in relationships and comfort in being alone. Healthy people have relationships of varying degrees of closeness and involvement.

With maladaptive schizoid patients, illness threatens their seclusiveness and can occasion denial and minimization of severe or even dangerous proportions. They may appear surprisingly undisturbed despite having very significant problems. Typically, well-meaning relatives or neighbors bring in these patients. Solitary drinking is common, but it may go unrecognized. Patients are extremely poor on follow-up; therefore, whatever needs to be done must be done at the initial visit. Compliance is poor.

Response of the Interviewer. Meeting schizoid needs means accepting the patient's unsociability and not threatening her or him with closeness or demands for relating; however, the student or clinician should not permit withdrawal. This difficult task entails maintaining a considerate interest that is quiet and reassuring and that does not demand reciprocation. The interviewer hopes to engage such patients to the degree that they can tolerate, although the relationships frequently remain distant and refractory to her or his best efforts.

Problems for the Interviewer. Many physicians find these patients unappealing because of their inability to relate. However, recalling their long-term deprivation can help the interviewer maintain steady but reserved interest.

Summary and Implications

The interviewer should conduct Steps 1 to 5 according to the guidelines outlined in the preceding chapters. In addition, during Steps 1 to 5, she or he should identify the personality style of the patient and should then meets its unique needs by matching her or his approach to the dominant patient style identified. This matching enhances the DPR by meeting the psychological (i.e., personality) needs of the patient. This process works with normal patients; however, maladaptive patients require much more work in consultation with a psychotherapist to develop healthier patterns.

Nonverbal Dimensions of the Relationship

Nearly all the material presented so far concerns the verbal aspects of interviewing. I now branch out to the nonverbal dimension and explore its powerful impact on the DPR (38,39). Prior to language acquisition, as humans, we all responded to stimulation solely by nonverbal (bodily, somatic) means (e.g., crying to express hunger or pain, smiling to express contentment) (40–43). We acquired a new route for expressing emotion with language acquisition (e.g., "I don't like you, Mommy.") (43); however, the original capacity to experience and to express emotions at a nonverbal level remains. Although normal growth and development requires that we integrate verbal and nonverbal expressions (41,44), much nonverbal material remains unintegrated (45,46). These nonverbal expressions may remain incompletely recognized. This dissociation leads to the classic "mixed message" (38), such as the patient who answers 'yes' to a request to stop smoking while she shakes her head in a negative way. The savvy interviewer knows this represents the patient's ambivalence.

Nonverbal responses give us, as interviewers, a picture that goes "beyond words" (seductive, angry, depressed). We get a better picture of the whole person by integrating nonverbal and verbal information during the interview. In this way, we can most fully understand the patient and her or his suffering and can make the most meaningful connection that is possible.

I have discussed some nonverbal expression of emotions when presenting relationship-building skills (e.g., addressing crying with emotion-handling skills); however, most people who are crying are aware of the associated emotion. This section helps the interviewer become aware of less apparent nonverbal expressions and of how to facilitate them.

Ensure Conducive Spatial Arrangements

An interviewer ensures that the spatial arrangement of the interview room promotes the relationship by paying attention to its geography. For example, she or he should not sit or stand higher than the patient (45). When dealing with a very ill patient who is lying supine or with a child, the interviewer can sometimes reduce the disparity by sitting down. She or he should empower rather than overpower (45). The interviewer should also try to avoid barriers, such as a desk, between the patient and herself and himself and should also try not to work either too close to the patient nor too far away.

TABLE 7.2. CATEGORIES OF NONVERBAL COMMUNICATION

A. Kinesics (body language): body position (angulation, tension), gestures, posture, gait, facial appearance, eyes (e.g., leaning forward tensely with chin projected, making a fist, tip-toeing walk, depressed facies, tearing of the eyes)
B. Touching: handshake; other touching, including during the physical examination (e.g., weak handshake, overpowering handshake, seductive pat on the arm)
C. Paralanguage (everything but content of language): rate and rhythm of speech, voice pitch, inflection, volume, sighs and grunts, tone of voice, pauses (e.g., rapid and jerky voice, low-pitched voice, peculiar inflection, very loud and frequent sighing, fearful tone, no pauses)
D. Spatial: vertical and horizontal distance to another, angles of facing each other, physical barriers in the space (e.g., doctor standing over a supine patient, far removed interaction, desk between two people)

Levinson D. *A guide to the clinical interview.* Philadelphia: WB Saunders, 1987:135–145.
Carson C. Nonverbal communication in the clinical setting. *Cortlandt Consultant*, February, 1990:129–134.

Observe Systematically for Nonverbal Cues

To observe the patient's nonverbal expressions, consciously tuning out verbal material briefly, as though watching a muted TV, and systematically looking for nonverbal data may help. Nonverbal cues, which are outlined in Table 7.2 (46,47), interact to give life to many of the emotions listed in Appendix C. The interviewer might consider what nonverbal cues characterize each emotion on the list; in other words, what unique somatic or nonverbal features typify anxiety, grief, despair, joy, love, devotion, or determination? Or, approaching this from another direction, what possible emotional meanings can be interpreted from the following commonly observed nonverbal responses: leaning away from the interviewer; frequent patting or stroking of the interviewer's hand, arm, or knee; quivering lower lip; arms tightly crossed over chest; frown; slumped shoulders; furrowed brow; standing to talk; glistening of eyes (tearing); or smiling? As Chapter 3 reviews, the interviewer also should integrate other nonverbal data concerning physical characteristics (emaciated), autonomic changes (sweaty palms), accouterments (tattered clothing), and the environment (no greeting cards).

As interviewers, we begin our conscious observation of the patient's emotional responses as early as the initial conversation of Step 1. This gives us an idea of the patient's associated nonverbal response pattern and allows us to recognize the responses more easily later on (45).

Up to this point in the book, I have discussed how we observe and interpret nonverbal behaviors but I have covered little about them. Now I will begin working with nonverbal material.

Pacing and Matching

Pacing is a neurolinguistic programming concept wherein the interviewer subtly matches a patient's nonverbal expressions to establish an unconscious rapport (45,48,49). The student or clinician mirrors the patient slowly to avoid distracting or alarming her or him; for example, observing that a patient has her head tipped to one side, the interviewer slowly adopts a similar position. While interacting with a patient who gestures a lot with his hands, the interviewer slowly begins to use similar hand gestures; or while talking to a patient who frequently purses her lips, the interviewer might emulate this unobtrusively. Pacing applies to a vast range of behaviors, especially to those in the kinesics and paralanguage categories of Table 7.2. Pacing need not be complex—it can be as simple as mirroring the way the patient crosses his legs, folds her arms, or rubs his chin.

Leading

When a good relationship is present, people in nonverbal synchrony with others may want to stay there. In such situations, a leading behavior by one member induces a reciprocal act by the other, as long as the behavior is introduced slowly and subtly (45,48,49). This provides the following two opportunities for the interviewer (45,46): (a) it confirms nonverbal connectedness if the patient follows a lead and (b) it leads the patient away from nonproductive behaviors (e.g., after matching a patient's persistent frown, the interviewer might gradually introduce a slight smile in the hope that the patient will follow the gesture and will feel better).

Addressing Nonverbal Behaviors

The interviewer addresses overt nonverbal expressions of emotion with emotion-handling skills (NURS) as discussed earlier; for example, she or he might say to a crying patient, "That is really sad for you and I can understand because . . ." With less overt nonverbal messages, the clinician or student must rely on emotion-seeking and focused open-ended queries, and she or he must concentrate on the nonverbal behavior (e.g., "You look a little down, how do you feel about that?" or "You seem kind of tense." or "You look like the cat who swallowed the canary.") This deepens the story and the DPR. Sometimes, she or he just notes, but does not address, the nonverbal behavior if she or he suspects that addressing the behavior would be poorly timed or offensive. In general, the interviewer should not address the fact that the patient's arms are tightly folded across the chest in a defensive way.

Mixed messages represent conflict, perhaps with the doctor, which must be explicated if communication and the relationship are to be maximized. The following steps can be helpful (45,46). (a) Indirectly acknowledge the disparity; to a patient who says that work is great but who, at the same time, is shaking his head negatively, the interviewer can say, "I hear what you say but I still get the feeling that things aren't going too well at work." If this prompts appropriate, congruent discussion, nothing else is necessary. She or he also might frame the incongruity in terms of a third person (e.g., "I know some people in your work situation where difficulties arose and they were concerned about their jobs."). (b) Address the incongruity directly, although the student or clinician usually has to know the patient well enough to be sure that her or his action will not be perceived as mocking. For example, she or he might say, "I notice you saying 'all is well' but shaking your head 'no.' What is that about?" Interviewers themselves often send mixed messages too. They might say, "I'd like to hear more about that" while they are standing up to leave.

SUMMARY

Facility with the informational aspects of integrated interviewing, which was presented in Chapters 1 to 6, goes only part way. Maximal flexibility and adaptability require the use of more advanced skills with the interactional aspects of interviewing. Conducting the interview and experiencing patients as human beings often creates untoward responses that can then produce harmful effects on the relationship and communication if they are not properly handled. The interviewer improves the DPR by vigorously pursuing self-awareness and by changing her or his own undesirable responses. In addition, patients' presentations and responses vary as a result of their unique personalities. The effective interviewer must recognize these styles and must interact with each patient according to her or his personality's unique dictates. Finally, the interviewer enhances communication and the DPR by recognizing patients' nonverbal emotional expressions and by responding to nonverbal, as well as verbal, cues. The interview takes little additional time because the student incorporates relational skills within a structure that is already present.

LEARNING EXERCISES

Doctor–Patient Relationship

1. Define the DPR and its dyadic components. What are nondyadic influences on the DPR?
2. Why and how does the student monitor the DPR? What characterizes a good DPR?
3. Discuss the obsessive-compulsive features of many physicians (27), why they occur, what is useful about them, what is potentially harmful, and what they can do to decrease their negative impact on the patient.*
4. What is an unrecognized response? Are students and doctors with unrecognized responses abnormal? Why is a focus on the interviewer the best way to improve the DPR?
5. Distinguish between the interviewer's unrecognized feelings and her or his unrecognized behaviors. Do these unrecognized responses feel good or bad to the interviewer?
6. What problems do unrecognized responses cause? How common are unrecognized responses toward patients? Do interviewers outgrow these responses as they gain experience? List the common unrecognized emotions and unrecognized behaviors.*
7. List several ways the interviewer can conduct "self-analysis" to increase personal awareness of emotions.
8. Why do interviewers not easily recognize these potentially harmful problems about themselves and, once recognized, why are they not easily changed? Is it possible for interviewers to prevent their emotions from becoming manifest to the patient?*
9. Why is it valuable to develop self-awareness of unrecognized personal responses concerning other people as well as patients?
10. If one chooses to change, should her or his focus be the behavior, the emotion, or both? Explain your answer. List several techniques that the interviewer can use to assist the patient in changing.
11. What principles are followed when working on self-awareness with colleagues?

Personality

1. Define personality style and contrast it to personality disorder. Why is the patient's personality important to the interviewer? When and how does the interviewer "read" the patient's personality?
2. For each personality that was described (dependent, obsessive-compulsive, histrionic, self-defeating, narcissistic, paranoid, and schizoid), answer the following questions.*
   a. Why does the personality occur?
   b. What are its general features in maladaptive and better-adapted patients?
   c. How do maladaptive and better-adapted patients present in the medical setting?

d. What unique problems do they pose?

e. What unique therapeutic measures are employed with each to enhance the DPR?

f. What problems might these patients pose for interviewers, especially those who are authoritarian?

g. Also, describe how control, intellectuality, emotionality, and ability to engage in a relationship vary from one personality to another.

3. Is it possible to change the patient or her or his behavior in order to enhance the DPR? If so, how?

4. What does "going with the flow" of the predominant personality feature mean for responding to the patient's personality?

5. Examine your own personality. What would your interactions be like with patients having maladaptive, as well as adaptive, personalities of each type? Would the interaction "feel" good or bad to you? Why?*

Nonverbal Behaviors

1. Why are nonverbal behaviors important? Are they more or less important than verbal behaviors in understanding the patient? What is meant by a "mixed message" or a mind–body split when verbal and nonverbal behaviors are compared?

2. What can the interviewer do to ensure that her or his own nonverbal behaviors do not create an adverse reaction?

3. Give the different categories of nonverbal behaviors as shown in Table 7.2 and list the different bodily or somatic (nonverbal) manifestations of at least 10 emotions (see Appendix C). What are likely meanings of the following nonverbal behaviors:
   - Leaning away from the interviewer?
   - Frequent patting or stroking of the interviewer's hand, arm, or knee?
   - Quivering lower lip?
   - Arms tightly crossed over chest?
   - Frown?
   - Slumped shoulders?
   - Furrowed brow?
   - Standing to talk?
   - Glistening of eyes (tearing)?
   - Smiling?

4. Define and describe pacing; include an example of how to perform it.

5. Define leading and describe it. Give an example of how to perform it. Why does it work and what is its potential utility?

6. How does the interviewer address nonverbal behaviors when emotion is overtly expressed, near the surface, or when a mixed message exists?*

*Good test questions.

PRACTICE EXERCISES

Doctor–Patient Relationship

1. In addition to your usual critique, identify one positive and one negative emotion that you experienced toward the patient you interviewed (e.g., like or dislike, warm or distant interaction).
2. Working with colleagues and mentors over time, identify one or more of your own responses to patients or others that could be harmful (e.g., overly controlling, overly 'nice,' avoidance of psychosocial issues, fear of discussing a specific issue such as death). Also, identify those responses that could be helpful (e.g., caring, respect, empathy, desire to help).
3. If you decide to change a previously unrecognized, potentially harmful response, develop a new one that is more conducive to a healthy DPR. Role-play the old response and the new response.
4. Maintain an active journal of experiences that demonstrate personal awareness.

Personality

1. Role-play the various personalities. The interviewer should practice Steps 1 to 5 with the additional assignment of identifying the "patient's" simulated personality. The simulation works best using the maladaptive patterns because the changes are easier to portray and to recognize. Have the person simulating the personality do it as an unknown so that everyone can make a diagnosis following the interview.
2. Role-play meeting the patient's predominant personality need (i.e., "going with the flow").

Nonverbal Behaviors

1. Watch the videotape of a student's interview with the sound turned off and identify nonverbal behaviors in both student and patient. Explain what they signify about the interaction and whether student and patient are synchronized or not.
2. Role-play different emotions using only nonverbal communication.
3. Watch any videotape in a foreign language and identify paralanguage (noncontent aspects) communication and tell what it means (e.g., voice pitch, rapidity).
4. Role-play the positive and negative impact of various common nonverbal behaviors (e.g., too close, too far, excessive eye contact, no eye contact, arms folded, supportive touching, appropriate smiling, eye level interaction).
5. Role-play appropriate and inappropriate nonverbal pacing.
6. Role-play appropriate and inappropriate nonverbal leading.
7. Role-play how the interviewer should address nonverbal behavior when emotion is overt (with emotion-handling skills), when it is not (with emotion-seeking or focused open-ended skills), and when a mixed message exists (with focused open-ended skills).
8. Role-play how the interviewer might convey right and wrong nonverbal messages.
9. Role-play a synchronous interaction and a nonsynchronous interaction.

References

1. Tresolini CP, Pew-Fetzer Task Force. *Health professions education and relationship-centered care.* San Francisco: Pew Health Professions Commission, 1994.
2. Inui TS. What are the sciences of relationship-centered primary care? *J Fam Pract* 1996;42:171–177.
3. Suchman AL, Botelho RJ, Hinton-Walker P, eds. *Partnerships in healthcare: transforming relational process.* Rochester, NY: University of Rochester Press, 1998.
4. Williams GC, Frankel RM, Campbell TL, et al. Research on relationship-centered care and healthcare outcomes from the Rochester Biopsychosocial Program: a self-determination theory integration. *Fam Systems Health* 2000;18:79–90.
5. Brody H. *The healer's power.* New Haven: Yale University Press, 1992.
6. Epstein RM, Christie M, Frankel R, et al. Understanding fear of contagion among physicians who care for HIV patients. *Fam Med* 1993;25:264–268.
7. Ford CV. *The somatizing disorders: illness as a way of life.* New York: Elsevier Biomedical, 1983.
8. Smith RC. Teaching interviewing skills to medical students: the issue of 'countertransference.' *J Med Educ* 1984;59:582–588.
9. Smith RC. Unrecognized responses by physicians during the interview. *J Med Educ* 1986;61:982–984.
10. Smith RC, Zimny G. Physicians' emotional reactions to patients. *Psychosomatics* 1988;29:392–397.
11. Smith RC, Dorsey AM, Lyles JS, et al. Teaching self-awareness enhances learning about patient-centered interviewing. *Acad Med* 1999;74:1242–1248.
12. Smith RC. Use and management of physicians' feelings during the interview. In: Lipkin M, Putnam SM, Lazare A, eds. *The medical interview.* New York: Springer-Verlag, 1995:104–109.
13. Reik T. *Listening with the third ear: the inner experience of a psychoanalyst.* New York: Farrar, Straus and Giroux, 1948.
14. Tanner BL. *The open door.* Orange City, FL: RL Kruse Publishing, 2001.
15. Nepo M. *Acre of light: living with cancer.* New York: Talman, 1994.
16. Nepo M. *The book of awakening—having the life you want by being present to the life you have.* Berkeley: Conari Press, 2000.
17. Young-Mason J, ed. *The patient's voice—experiences of illness.* Philadelphia: FA Davis, 1997.
18. Remen RN, ed. *Wounded healers.* Mill Valley, CA: Wounded Healer Press, 1994.
19. Benson H. *The relaxation response.* New York: William Morrow, 1975.
20. Kabat-Zinn J. *Wherever you go, there you are: mindfulness meditation in everyday life.* New York: Hyperion, 1994.
21. Wood JT. *The little blue book on power.* Winslow, WA: Zen 'n' ink, 1990.
22. Vaillant GE. *Adaptation to life.* Boston: Little, Brown & Company, 1977.
23. Erikson EH. *Childhood and society,* 2nd ed. New York: WW Norton, 1963.
24. Yalom ID. *The theory and practice of group psychotherapy,* 3rd ed. New York: Basic Books, 1985.

25. Lipkin M. *Standards Document: American Academy on Physician and Patient.* New York: NYU Medical Center.

26. Ende J. Feedback in clinical medical education. *JAMA* 1983;250:777–781.

27. Gabbard GO. The role of compulsiveness in the normal physician. *JAMA* 1985;254:2926–2929.

28. Shapiro D. *Neurotic styles.* New York: Basic Books, 1965.

29. Kahana RJ, Bibring GL. Personality types in medical management. In: Zaiberg NE, ed. *Psychiatry and medical practice in a general hospital.* New York: International University Press, 1964:108–123.

30. Lipkin M. The medical interview and related skills. In: Branch WT, ed. *Office practice of medicine.* Philadelphia: WB Saunders, 1987:1287–1306.

31. Andreasen NC, Black DW. Personality disorders. In: Andreasen NC, Black DW, eds. *Introductory textbook of psychiatry.* Washington, D.C.: American Psychiatric Press, 1991:333–354.

32. American Psychiatric Association. *Diagnostic and statistical manual of mental disorders,* 4th ed. Washington, D.C.: American Psychiatric Association, 1994.

33. Putnam SM, Lipkin M, Lazare A, et al. Personality styles. In: Lipkin M, Putnam SM, Lazare A, eds. *The medical interview.* New York: Springer-Verlag, 1995:251–274.

34. Smith RC. *The difficult patient* (CD-ROM, vol 9, no. 1); BD Rose, ed. *UpToDate.* In: Aronson MD, Fletcher SW, Fletcher RH, eds. *Primary care series.* Wellesley, MA: 2001.

35. Groves JE. Taking care of the hateful patient. *N Engl J Med* 1978;298:883–887.

36. Birdwell BG, Herbers JE, Kroenke K. Evaluating chest pain—the patient's presentation style alters the physician's diagnostic approach. *Arch Intern Med* 1993;153:1991–1995.

37. Skodol AE, Oldham JM, Gallaher PE, et al. Validity of self-defeating personality disorder. *Am J Psychiatry* 1994;151:560–567.

38. Feldman SS. *Mannerisms of speech and gestures in everyday life.* New York: International Universities Press, 1959.

39. Larsen KM, Smith CK. Assessment of nonverbal communication in the patient-physician relationship. *J Fam Pract* 1981;12:481–488.

40. Rodin G. Somatization and the self: psychotherapeutic issues. *Am J Psychother* 1984;38:257–263.

41. Barsky AJ, Klerman GL. Overview: hypochondriasis, bodily complaints, and somatic styles. *Am J Psychiatry* 1983;140:273–283.

42. Katon W, Kleinman A, Rosen G. Depression and somatization: a review (part 1). *Am J Med* 1983;72:127–135.

43. Stern DN. *Diary of a baby.* New York: Basic Books, 1990.

44. Engel GL. *Psychological development in health and disease.* Philadelphia: WB Saunders, 1962.

45. Carson CA. *The hidden language of medicine: nonverbal communication in clinical encounters.* Unpublished manuscript; Dept. of Medicine, The Genesee Hospital, Rochester, NY.

46. Carson CA. Nonverbal communication in the clinical setting. *Cortlandt Consultant* February, 1990:129–134.

47. Levinson D. *A guide to the clinical interview.* Philadelphia: WB Saunders, 1987.
48. Bandler R, Grinder J. *Frogs into princes: neuro linguistic programming.* Moab, UT: Real People Press, 1979.
49. Christensen JF, Levinson W, Grinder M. Applications of neurolinguistic programming to medicine. *J Gen Intern Med* 1990;5:522–527.

 Summarizing and Presenting the Patient's Story

The interviewer has generated a database of symptoms and personal issues, has translated it to a biopsychosocial story about a human being and her or his illness, and has worked to create an effective doctor–patient relationship. Now what? How does she or he now summarize and transmit this information to others?

Summarizing the Patient's Story

Even if the student or clinician has gathered a great deal of information and has synthesized it sensibly, the task of meaningfully summarizing it to reflect the essence of the patient and her or his biopsychosocial story, which includes disease diagnoses, still remains (1). Our proposed multidimensional scheme integrates mind (psychosocial) and body (biomedical) components to describe the whole person and her or his dynamically interacting parts.

Three components of the patient's biopsychosocial description are found: Relationship story, Personal story, and Disease story/diagnoses (recalled by the mnemonic RPD). These are outlined in Table 8.1 and are illustrated at the end of this chapter and at the end of Appendix D, where Mrs. Jones' story is summarized.

Relationship Story

The interviewer's experience during the entire interview allows her or him to synthesize a story of the doctor–patient relationship (2,3). Students often can be as successful as experienced practitioners in this domain because its cardinal skill seems to be using the emotion-handling skills (naming, understanding, respecting, and supporting [NURS]).

TABLE 8.1. THE COMPONENTS OF THE PATIENT'S BIOPSYCHOSOCIAL STORY*

A. **R**elationship story
   1. Interviewer's responses
   2. Patient's personality
   3. Doctor–patient interaction
B. **P**ersonal story
C. **D**isease story (diagnoses)
   1. Biomedical
   2. Psychiatric

*The mnemonic RPD aids in remembering these components (see bold and underscore).

The Interviewer's Responses

The interviewer first needs to sort out and to address consciously her or his personal feelings and any resulting behaviors toward the patient or the patient's circumstance that occurred at any time in the interview. For example, fear of harming the patient could lead to avoidance of the discussion of death; fear of catching AIDS could lead the interviewer to avoid touching the patient; or a feeling of sexual attraction to the patient could lead to excessive attention or avoidance. As the following examples note, the student or clinician protects her or his own confidentiality and publicly expresses (in a written report or verbal presentation) only material that he or she is comfortable having many others know. More personal material is neither written nor presented and is reserved for discussion with preceptors or mentors.

The Patient's Personality

The interviewer makes her or his observations throughout the interview and identifies the patient's dominant personality style as dependent, histrionic, obsessive, self-defeating, narcissistic, paranoid, or schizoid (or other types), as Chapter 7 outlines. For most people, this designation depicts the style of interacting with others. When personality style interferes with normal functioning, however, it is called a personality disorder and is identified as such in the summary (4).

The Doctor–Patient Interaction

Finally, the interviewer must consider the interactional process itself and note any difficulties. Did the interview feel strained? Did it have a nice give and take? Was the tone of the interview formal, collegial, parent–child, or charged?

Personal Story

Synthesis of the multiple bits of the personal data, which were gathered largely during the patient-centered process, produces a psychosocial story or theme. This ordinarily is quite straightforward. Students or clinicians should identify the major issues and then summarize them in two or three sentences. Although every patient is unique, the following themes occur frequently (5–7):

1. Fear of death, mutilation, and disability.

2. Dislike, distrust, and disbelief of the medical system.

3. Concern about loss of function, wholeness, role, status, and independence.

4. Denial of problems.

5. Separation, grief, and losses of many varieties.

6. Leaving home and becoming independent.

7. Retirement.

8. Marital or job problems.

9. Other unique personal problems of the patient.

10. Administrative issues relating to her or his disease diagnosis (e.g., requesting disability).

Disease Story

Similarly, the interviewer synthesizes multiple bits of primary and secondary data to make disease diagnoses or, at a minimum, high level designations of the disease problem. A list of problems or diagnoses represents the disease story. Such a list usually numbers three or four problems, but as many as 15 or 20 problems and diagnoses can be found in complex patients. Data for problems and diagnoses derive from the personal description of symptoms during the patient-centered process and their further clarification during the doctor-centered process and the physical examination. Of course, more knowledge of disease patterns makes identifying diagnoses easier for clinical students (e.g., angina or infectious hepatitis). Preclinical students, however, are not expected to make diagnoses; they simply describe and list the problems that were identified and characterize them as fully as possible (e.g., chest pain occurred with exercise and was relieved by rest; vomiting and jaundice of recent onset and one other family member who has the same problem).

Biomedical

The following are a few of the disease diagnoses common in adult nonpsychiatric settings, although they may not always be identified after just one interview and physical examination: hypertension, arteriosclerotic heart disease, diabetes mellitus, chronic bronchopulmonary disease, osteoarthritis, dermatitis, hypothyroidism, muscle strain and/or sprain, otitis media, upper respiratory infection, infectious sore throat and diarrhea, cataracts, glaucoma, acid peptic disease and gastritis, hemorrhoids, colonic polyps, urinary tract infection, cystitis, benign prostatic hypertrophy, prostatitis, sexually transmitted diseases, endometriosis, dysfunctional uterine bleeding, trichomoniasis, migraine, stroke, neuritis, radiculopathies, drug reactions, and health-maintenance problems (elevated cholesterol). For common psychiatric problems that present in nonpsychiatric settings, see below.

Even after thorough clinical and laboratory evaluation, many patients do not have a satisfactory disease explanation for their physical symptoms. Sometimes symptoms clear and we as clinicians may never know what caused them. Occasionally, symptoms persist and patients later are found to have a disease. The problems of many of these patients, though, are designated by the general term somatization, by which we mean the expression of emotional distress via physical symptoms that have no disease explanation.

Psychiatric

Twenty to thirty-five percent of medical patients have a psychiatric diagnosis, and over half of all psychiatric patients are seen only in a medical setting (8). These psychological diagnoses and problems include depression, anxiety, adjustment disorders, addicting behaviors (e.g., tobacco, caffeine, alcohol, drug), homelessness, and abuse (psychological, sexual, physical—primarily involving the elderly, children, and women).

The interviewer first needs to identify and then to update the RPD. By frequently returning to the RPD designation, the interviewer can decide which diagnostic area needs the most attention. She or he cannot put the story to rest as a fixed event or an unchanging "reality." The story changes as diagnoses are resolved, as treatment is implemented, as new personal responses occur, and as the relationship deepens. Indeed, the very act of telling the story leads the patient to new thoughts and emotions about herself or himself and, in turn, to new actions and attitudes so that a new, different story evolves as part of the narration process (9–12).

The Medical Record: The "Write-Up" of the Patient's Story

In the next step, the student or clinician records information in the medical record. This written description is usually called the "write-up." It follows the outline in Table 8.2. Appendix D contains a full write-up of Mrs. Jones' initial evaluation. See Chapter 5 for general guidelines for content and length.

As with most scientific endeavors, a well-organized, tightly knit written summary does not describe the discovery process itself. In fact, write-ups synthesize personal, primary, and secondary data from different parts of the interview. The order in which data are discovered sometimes has little bearing on just where these data will be displayed in the written version.

Many use the following format for recording the history, physical examination, initial diagnostic formulations and treatment interventions, assessment, and treatment and investigative plans. All but the history are outside the scope of this book, but I include the others to illustrate the integration of the interview with the other four basic components of a formal patient evaluation. These components are addressed extensively during clinical rotations.

Identifying Data

The student or clinician obtains identifying data (Table 8.2) from the admitting records and other data that accompany the patient by simple observation and inquiry.

Source and Reliability of Information

The source of data and their reliability reflect the quality of data obtained. The interviewer should note any concerns that she or he has.

TABLE 8.2. RECORDING THE NEW PATIENT EVALUATION: THE WRITE-UP

A. Identifying data: age, gender, job, race, marital status, immediate family status, address, telephone number of nearest relative in case of emergency, referral source (if any)

B. Source and reliability of information: patient, relative or translator (specify), outside records (indicate completeness), judgment of reliability of information from all sources

C. Chief complaint and agenda: the patient's most bothersome complaint and a summary (list) of all presenting complaint(s)

D. History of present illness and other current active problems
   1. Overview of symptoms and time of onset
   2. Complete description of the dimensions of each symptom (i.e., location, quality, quantification, chronology and timing, setting, moderating factors, and associated symptoms)
   3. Absence of pertinent symptoms
   4. Relevant positive and negative secondary data
   5. Personal contextual dimension of the preceding (e.g., story content, emotions, patient's beliefs and explanations, impact of illness on daily life, relationships, support systems, practical issues, and role of stress)

E. Health issues
   1. Ethical-social-spiritual issues: advance directives, living will, "do not resuscitate" wishes, power of attorney, whom to contact if the patient cannot speak for herself or himself, and spiritual practices
   2. Functional status: dressing, bathing, feeding, transferring, walking, shopping, using the toilet, using the telephone, cooking, cleaning, driving, taking medications, managing finances, and cognitive function; extent of interference with normal life
   3. Health-promoting and health-maintenance activities
      a. Health-promoting habits: diet, seat belts, use of a helmet when riding a bicycle or motorcycle, protection of self and others from poisonous substances (including medications) and dangerous circumstances at home and at work, exercise, relaxation, and recreation
      b. Health screening: periodic health exams, mammograms, Pap smear, sigmoidoscopy, stools for occult blood, cholesterol, blood sugar, serologic test for syphilis, tuberculosis skin testing, HIV testing, prostatic evaluation, dental check, audiograms, eye exam, tonometry; self-examination (breasts, genitals, and skin)
      c. Disease prophylaxis: diphtheria, pertussis, tetanus, polio, measles, German measles, hepatitis, influenza, and vaccines for pneumococcal pneumonia and for diseases in areas of foreign travel
   4. Health hazards
      a. Use of addicting substances: caffeine, tobacco, alcohol, street drugs, and prescription medications
      b. Sexual practices: activity, preferences, diseases, abuse, risky habits, contraception, and satisfaction
      c. Abuse: sexual, physical, verbal, psychological, or other

F. Past medical history
   1. Hospitalizations: surgical, nonsurgical, psychiatric, obstetric, rehabilitation, or other
   2. Other medical, surgical, or psychological problems: childhood illnesses (mumps, measles, German measles, chickenpox), injuries, accidents, illnesses, unexplained problems, procedures, tests, psychotherapy, or other
   3. Screening for major diseases: rheumatic fever, diabetes mellitus, tuberculosis, venereal diseases, cancer, heart attack, and stroke; major treatments in the past (cortisone, blood transfusions, insulin, digitalis, anticoagulants); and visits to the doctor during the last year
   4. Medications and other treatments: prescribed, over-the-counter, or alternative therapies and health care, and "nonmedications" (laxatives, tonics, hormones, birth control pills, vitamins)
   5. Allergies and drug reactions: allergic diseases (e.g., asthma, hay fever), drugs, foods, and environmental

(Table continued)

TABLE 8.2. *continued.*

6. Menstrual and obstetric history (for women): onset of menses, duration, cycle length, discomfort, number of pads daily, birth control pills and other hormonal preparations, pregnancies, abortions (spontaneous), abortions (induced), deliveries of living children, other deliveries, and complications of pregnancy

G. Social history

1. Current personal situation
   a. Demographic: age, sex, race, and current work and living situation
   b. Impact (meaning) of illness on self and others
   c. Beliefs and explanations about illness
   d. Relationships and support system
   e. Practical issues
   f. Stress
   g. Financial situation

2. Other personal factors
   a. Early developmental outline: birth and early development, early family setting and other caretakers, relationship with parents and siblings, others' interactions in family, early schooling and progress, places of residence, major losses and other adverse events, medical–surgical problems, happy events, later education and progress, social life and relationships, dating, adolescence, military or other service, and getting away from home
   b. Marriage and other relationships and outcome: significant relationships (origin, course, outcome) and children
   c. Work history and outcome: jobs and duration, satisfaction, and toxic or other dangerous exposure (fumes, radiation, noise, dusts, chemicals)
   d. Recreational history
   e. Retirement
   f. Aging
   g. Life satisfaction
   h. Cultural and ethnic background

H. The family history

1. General inquiry
2. Inquire about specific diseases or problems: tuberculosis, diabetes, cancer, heart disease, bleeding problems, kidney failure or dialysis, tobacco use, alcoholism, weight problems, asthma, and mental illness (depression, schizophrenia, multiple somatic complaints)
3. Develop a genogram
   a. Two generations preceding the patient and all subsequent; involves parents, siblings, children, and significant members outside the bloodline for each generation
   b. Age, sex, mental and physical health, and current status noted for each; include age at death and cause
   c. Note interactions among family members for psychological and physical problems
      • Psychological
        —dominant members and their style (e.g., loving, angry)
        —major interaction patterns (e.g., competition, abuse, open, distant, caring, manipulation, codependent)
        —family gestalt (e.g., happy, successful, dysfunctional)
      • Physical
        —patterns of disease (e.g., dominant, recessive, sex-linked, no pattern)
        —patterns of physical symptoms without organic disease (e.g., bowel trouble, uncoordinated, flighty)
        —inquire about others with similar symptoms (e.g., infection, toxic, anxiety, anniversary reaction)

(Table continued)

TABLE 8.2. *continued.*

I. System review items not already considered: review of systems*
1. General symptoms
   a. Poor appetite
   b. Excessive appetite
   c. Weight loss
   d. Weight gain
   e. Fever, chills, and sweats
   f. No enjoyment of life (anhedonia)
   g. Pain
   h. Fatigue and lack of energy
2. Integumentary symptoms
   a. Sores or skin ulcers
   b. Itching (pruritis)
   c. Rash
   d. Change in size or color of moles
   e. Abnormal hair growth
   f. Changes in nails
3. Hematopoietic symptoms
   a. Enlarged glands (lymphadenopathy)
   b. Lumps anywhere
   c. Urge to eat dirt (pica) or ice
   d. Abnormal bleeding or excessive bruising
   e. Frequent or unusual infections
4. Endocrine symptoms
   a. Heat intolerance
   b. Cold intolerance
   c. Decreased sexual drive
   d. Salt craving
   e. Enlarging glove and hat size
   f. Excessive thirst (polydipsia)
5. Musculoskeletal
   a. Frequent fractures
   b. Muscular weakness
   c. Painful muscles
   d. Joint pain and swelling
   e. Low back pain
   f. Paralysis
   g. Movement difficulty
   h. Pain in calf with walking (intermittent claudication)
   i. Swollen leg
6. Eyes, ears, nose, and throat
   a. Change in vision
   b. Bright flashes of light
   c. Image of light with jagged, shimmering appearance (scintillating scotomata)
   d. Spots in visual field
   e. Double vision (diplopia)

(Table continued)

TABLE 8.2. *continued.*

     f. Loss of hearing
     g. Ringing in the ears (tinnitus)
     h. Drainage from nose
     i. Decreased or altered sense of smell
     j. Bloody nose (epistaxis)
     k. Sore throat
     l. Impaired speech
    m. Painful tooth
     n. Hoarseness
  7. Head and neck
     a. Headache
     b. Dizzy (vertigo)
     c. Lightheadedness
     d. Loss of consciousness (syncope)
     e. Stiff neck
  8. Breasts
     a. Lump or mass
     b. Discharge
     c. Tenderness
  9. Cardiovascular and pulmonary
     a. Chest pain
     b. Shortness of breath (dyspnea)
     c. Shortness of breath when lying down and need to sit to breathe (orthopnea)
     d. Wakening at night with dyspnea (paroxysmal nocturnal dyspnea)
     e. Wheezing
     f. Cough
     g. Yellow or green sputum
     h. Clear sputum
     i. Bloody sputum (hemoptysis)
     j. Pounding sensation in chest (palpitations)
     k. Peripheral arterial and venous symptoms—see Integumentary
10. Gastrointestinal
     a. Appetite and weight changes—see General
     b. Sticking sensation in throat (globus hystericus)
     c. Difficulty swallowing (dysphagia)
     d. Heartburn
     e. Upper abdominal pain
     f. Mid-lower abdominal pain
     g. Nausea
     h. Nonbloody vomiting (emesis)
     i. Bloody emesis (hematemesis)
     j. Black stools (melfsena)
     k. Bloody stools (hematochezia)
     l. Difficult or infrequent bowel movemements (constipation)

(Table continued)

TABLE 8.2. *continued.*

     m. Loose or frequent bowel movements (diarrhea)
     n. Yellow discoloration of sclerae and skin (jaundice)
     o. Dark urine that is the color of tea or a cola drink
     p. Excessive upper (belching or eructation) or lower (flatus) bowel gas
     q. Rectal pain (proctalgia), discharge, mass, hemorrhoid, or itching (pruritis ani)
     p. Lump in groin or scrotum
11. Urinary
     a. Increased urinary frequency (polyuria)
     b. Burning with urination (dysuria)
     c. Getting up more than once during the night to void (nocturia)
     d. Need to urinate suddenly and urgently (urgency)
     e. Loss of urinary control (incontinence)
     f. Bloody urine (hematuria)
     g. Particulate matter in urine
     h. Slow to get urinary stream started (hesitancy)
12. Genital, male
     a. Urethral discharge
     b. Penile sores or growths
     c. Painful or swollen testicle
     d. Impotence
     e. Bloody ejaculation (hematospermia)
     f. Retrograde ejaculation into bladder
     g. Premature ejaculation
     h. Decreased sexual drive
13. Genital, female
     a. Vaginal discharge or itching
     b. Sores or lumps
     c. Painful menses (dysmenorrhea)
     d. Absence of menses (amenorrhea)
     e. Irregular, heavy menses (menometorrhagia)
     f. Hot flashes
     g. Decreased sexual drive
     h. Painful intercourse (dyspareunia)
     i. Nonorgasmic
14. Neuropsychiatric
     a. Cranial nerve symptoms—see Head and Neck and Eyes, Ears, Nose and Throat
     b. Motor symptoms—see Musculoskeletal
     c. Numb, tingling sensation in extremities (paresthesia)
     d. Decreased (hypesthesia) or absent (anesthesia) sensation
     e. Tremor
     f. Loss of balance
     g. Staggering gait (ataxia)
     h. Seizures
     i. Bizarre, unrealistic thoughts (intrusive thoughts)
     j. Bizarre, unrealistic perceptions (hallucinations)

(Table continued)

TABLE 8.2. *continued.*

      k. Depression
      l. Mania
     m. Poor judgment, orientation, memory, attention, and concentration
     n. Inability to get to sleep or stay asleep (insomnia)
     o. Hypersomnolence
     p. Nightmares
     q. Anhedonia
     r. Suicidal
     s. Anxiety, nervousness
     t. Symptoms without a disease explanation (somatization)
J. Physical examination†
K. Initial diagnostic formulations and treatment interventions (if any)†
L. Assessment: the biopsychosocial description—the patient's story**
  1. Relationship story
    a. Interviewer's responses
    b. Patient's responses
    c. Doctor–patient interaction
  2. Personal story
  3. Disease story and diagnosis
    a. Biomedical
    b. Psychiatric
M. Treatment and investigative plan†

*Many of these symptoms can occur in systems other than where listed.
†Not addressed in this book.
**Addressed in this book only to show the RPD designation.

Chief Complaint and Agenda

The Chief Complaint and the patient's agenda clarify the reason for the patient's visit and arise mostly from Step 2. While one should recall that the Chief Complaint, or the most bothersome symptom, may not have been presented first during the history, she or he should remember that it serves as a powerful tool for directing the focus of the written story. When possible, I advise citing the Chief Complaint in the patient's own words. Then, a list of the full agenda should be summarized.

History of Present Illness and Other Current Active Problems

Five specific aspects of the history of present illness (HPI) or other current active problems (OCAP) exist, as noted in Table 8.2 and the following:

1. An overview of pertinent symptoms (those that fit together to describe the underlying disease process best) and their time of onset.

2. Specific symptom descriptors.

3. The absence of pertinent symptoms.

4. Relevant secondary data.

5. The personal context of these data.

The student can convey a dynamic understanding of the patient's situation through these five aspects of the history and can thus prepare the reader to understand the full biopsychosocial description of the patient that is to be provided later. Putting each category in a separate paragraph may be helpful for beginning clinical students as the following outlines; as students gain experience, these categories can be condensed and interwoven considerably.

Paragraph 1. An overview of all relevant symptoms, reflecting the Chief Complaint and other current problems. It also identifies when each began. This information will most likely have arisen during the patient-centered process or during Step 6 (getting an overview).

Paragraph 2. Records all symptoms (primary data) relevant to the problem and expands on each with a full recording of the seven descriptors (location, quality, quantification, chronology and timing, setting, moderating factors, and associated symptoms). The descriptors can be recorded in this order, as the example for Mrs. Jones in Appendix D shows, and they must be clearly anchored in the chronology and timing dimension. **Rather than including all the descriptors, experienced clinicians often record only those of diagnostic significance.** Students and beginning clinicians are advised, however, to remain comprehensive until their skills develop more fully. As their skills and understanding of diseases increase, they recognize more and more symptoms that belong in this paragraph; in other words, their 'associated symptom' category of the descriptors increases. Most data in this paragraph will have arisen in Step 7 of the doctor-centered process.

Paragraph 3. The student or clinician next records the absence of pertinent symptoms. Thus, she or he will record the absence of symptoms from the same system of involvement as the chief complaint. As the student becomes more facile with hypothesis testing and develops a better understanding of disease, the absence of other pertinent symptoms also is included. For example, in a patient with chest pain, the preclinical and beginning clinical student would record the absence of hemoptysis and dyspnea in this paragraph, whereas the more advanced clinical student would also indicate the absence of joint pains and excessive sunburning if systemic lupus erythematosus was a diagnostic consideration (these can be useful diagnostic symptoms). Data for this paragraph usually come from Step 7 of the doctor-centered process.

Paragraph 4. Pertinent positive and negative nonsymptom (secondary) data are included in this paragraph. This includes data, for example, about previous doctors and health care facilities, diagnostic tests and results, treatments and results, specific habits, occupation, and other nonsymptom information important for understanding the patient's disease problem, especially its etiology (cause) and pathogenesis (mechanism) (e.g., a history of smoking in someone with possible lung cancer, a recent coronary angiogram that was normal in a patient with chest pain, the use of birth control pills in a patient with headaches, a family history of sickle cell anemia in an African-American boy with pain in his legs). These data often will have arisen in Step 7, but also may have occurred in Steps 8 to 12.

Paragraph 5. Although personal data are usually obtained first in the interview, mostly during the patient-centered process (primarily Step 4), they often are recorded last to enhance our understanding of how personal factors interact with the physical. The interviewer explicitly links symptoms and psychological and emotional dimensions. In this final paragraph, the mind–body link is established. Although it was notable in Mrs. Jones' situation, we as clinicians do not always find a clear causal relationship between personal factors and the disease problem. However, we can describe a personal context of the physical problem in all patients.

The HPI, the most important part of the history, synthesizes the patient's personal and physical dimensions. Preclinical students simply record the chronology of primary data (including symptom descriptors), secondary data, and their personal dimensions. As students understand more about disease patterns later in training, they begin to **record the patient's data in a way that will lead other students or physicians to the same diagnostic conclusion.** The clinical student learns to highlight selectively certain portions of the story, while still utilizing the preceding five dimensions, so that she or he provides data for and against the diagnosis she or he has made. She or he follows strict rules of clinical reasoning that proceed from a growing knowledge and skills base in clinical medicine. Accordingly, data both for and against the proposed diagnosis (hypothesis), as well as reasonable alternative diagnoses, are painstakingly and fairly recounted so that another professional (often a preceptor) can make an informed decision. Mrs. Jones' HPI in Appendix D illustrates this diagnostic process.

The student includes only primary and secondary data in the HPI. Discussion and interpretation of the patient's problem can be found in the Assessment section. Interpretative comments, however, can be made when the clarity of data is in question (e.g., "The patient says she or he underwent some type of heart surgery when hospitalized in 1983 but doesn't know what it was. We have no records of it yet.").

In the OCAP, the student records problems that are unrelated to the HPI but that nonetheless are active; these do relate to the patient's present health. Each of these areas requires a five-part approach similar to that found in the HPI, although it is usually less extensive. Each typically has its own cardinal symptoms and its own physical and personal components.

Although the HPI is recorded in narrative form, the remainder of the write-up can be recorded in narrative form, outline form, or both; the last is shown with Ms. Jones' write-up in Appendix D.

Health Issues

All health issues (HI) are recorded, as Table 8.2 notes; these include ethical–social–spiritual issues, functional status, health-promoting and health-maintenance activities, and health hazards. When these are relevant, some already will have been recorded in the HPI or OCAP. For example, cigarette-smoking habits are recorded in the HPI for most patients with shortness of breath and possible emphysema. Pertinent details, as Chapter 5 outlines, are provided for all areas (e.g., dates, relevant people, the last occasion that a patient had a Pap smear, the number of cigarettes she or he smokes daily and any efforts to stop).

Past Medical History

The past medical history (PMH) is recorded as Table 8.2 notes, often in the suggested order. Where necessary for providing understanding of the patient's health, it is detailed, but it is abbreviated for past events of little relevance to the patient's current health. For example, with a patient admitted for a hernia repair, the interviewer would obtain extensive data about the patient's coronary artery bypass grafting one year earlier, similar to what she or he would record in the HPI if the patient presented with chest pain. Although pertinent details (e.g., symptoms, secondary data, dates, treatments, doses of medications, types and outcome of adverse reactions to medications, and details of any complicated obstetric problem) are usually recorded in outline form, their inclusion is essential for all major problems.

Social History

The social history (SH) details the information in Table 8.2, usually in narrative rather than in tabular form. Only background and routine data are recorded in the SH. When details pertinent to current psychosocial issues were elicited during the SH part of the interview, they are recorded in the HPI portion of the written record. Similarly, some SH data may be recorded, where relevant, as part of the OCAP or Identifying Data. Again, following the guidelines found in Chapter 5 allows the student to record all relevant data accurately.

Family History

The family history (FH) records information in Table 8.2 and includes a genogram diagram, similar to that shown for Mrs. Jones in Appendix D. The most important knowledge that the interviewer needs is to find out who is available to the patient in a support role; who has had anything like what the patient is experiencing; and what fears she or he might have. As noted, some elements of these data may be included in the HPI/OCAP at times.

System Review Items Not Already Considered: Review of Systems

The review of systems (ROS) simply records the System Review symptoms not already considered during the HPI/OCAP or PMH. The beginning clinical level student often initially spends a lot of time here getting answers in still-unaddressed systems and grouping the positives and negatives together in each system. This detail is necessary for learning purposes. **More advanced students and graduates record only positive items and eventually note only those that are significant.**

Physical Examination

Physical examination findings, which are outside the province of this text, include notations of routine vital signs (temperature, pulse rate, respiratory rate, blood pressure, height, weight) and the details of examination of each system (heart murmur heard on auscultation of the chest, an enlarged uterus on pelvic examination, or wax found on examining the ears).

Initial Diagnostic Formulations and Treatment Interventions

Initial interventions by the interviewer or others, which occur largely in acute situations, are recorded here, although this is also outside the scope of this text. These could include a blood count in someone who is bleeding, an electrocardiogram in someone with chest pain, administration of adrenalin to a patient with an acute allergic reaction, or an x-ray of the abdomen in a patient injured in a traffic accident. These data should not be confused with secondary data that were obtained before the patient came under the interviewer's care and that should already be recorded in the HPI or PMH.

Assessment: The Biopsychosocial Description (The Patient's Story)

At this point, the interviewer gives the complete RPD description and discusses how data were interpreted to arrive at this diagnostic summary (this is also outside the scope of this book, except for the illustration of the RPD designation). Sometimes, however, additional observation and/or diagnostic investigation is required before a full biopsychosocial description can be made. When descriptions are definitive enough to allow identification of a disease, the disease itself is recorded in the disease category. **When descriptions are not sufficient to permit a disease diagnosis, a succinct and pertinent description of the problem is recorded and is called a "problem" to differentiate it from a diagnosis.** Four to six problems or diagnoses are average in ambulatory practices (13).

At whatever level of resolution, the biopsychosocial description is recorded using the RPD components as the following example illustrates.

• Relationship Story

—*Interviewer's response:* liked patient; difficult to talk about possible appendectomy for fear of making patient feel worse about job and home situation. [Note how this links all three RPD components.]

—*Patient's personality:* a few dependent features, within the range of normal.

—*Interaction*: cordial, cooperative; "same wave length."

- Personal Story: worried about losing job because of illness and about increased demand on sick spouse. Is in a new job and does not want to become unemployed again.

- Disease Story (Diagnoses or Problems)

    —*Biomedical*: (a) Abdominal pain of 48-hours duration with recent localization to right lower quadrant, accompanied by absent bowel sounds, involuntary guarding, and rebound tenderness. [This is a "problem" description because a diagnosis is not yet possible. A full discussion of how one arrives at her or his interpretation often is included here with a list of possible disease explanations (differential diagnoses).] (b) Degenerative arthritis of knees and hands [a diagnosis]. (c) Type II (adult-onset) diabetes mellitus [a diagnosis].

    —*Psychiatric*: past history of depression.

Treatment and Investigative Plan

This section is also outside the province of this text, but it does contain the treatment and investigative plans, which follow logically from the preceding assessment. These could include, for example, a blood count, an x-ray of the abdomen, and exploratory surgery for likely appendicitis. Alternatively, a computed tomography (CT) scan of the abdomen could be performed.

Presenting the Patient's Story

Students, graduates, and clinicians frequently tell patients' stories to other professionals. These verbal presentations are valuable for learning and teaching, and they are the medium for communication among professionals. Although these presentations may be difficult at the outset, beginning clinical level students quickly master them. They demonstrate the interviewer's ability to elicit and to synthesize large amounts of data, her or his skills in communicating with others, and the way she or he sees the patient as a person.

Some general guidelines for a presentation follow (Table 8.3). (a) Know beforehand what your goals will be (what the listener expects) and how long you will have. (b) Know the patient thoroughly. (c) Begin preparation for the

TABLE 8.3. GUIDELINES FOR MAKING A PRESENTATION

A. Set goals (what the listener expects) and give the time available.
B. Know the patient.
C. Focus on the problem list and diagnoses.
D. Present only relevant data.
E. Use a standard format: chief complaint and history of present illness, physical examination, and diagnostic investigations.
F. Summarize and invite questions.
G. Be engaging and interesting.
H. Use note cards only for reminders of factual data.
I. Practice and get feedback from colleagues.
J. Observe other good presentations and seek to emulate those.
K. Avoid logistic and other problems.
L. Avoid personalizing and recounting specific conversations.

presentation with the problem list or diagnoses that were identified; clarify uncertainties; know what the differential diagnostic issues are; and know what needs to be done to clarify diagnoses in the future. The entire presentation will be geared to provide evidence, both pro and con, for this definition of the problem (although sometimes presentations may focus on difficult treatment issues for a known diagnosis). (d) Present only relevant data, usually focused on the problem list. The presenter states this much in the fashion of a lawyer presenting a case to a judge. She or he is trying to convince the listener of her or his problem list items or diagnoses by providing all relevant information on both sides of any controversial or unclear issue. In other words, she or he will be presenting the patient's story. (e) Stick to the standard format: start with the CC/HPI; interweave only relevant data from other parts of the interview, and then proceed to the physical exam and, finally, to any diagnostic investigations that were performed. If the patient has prior examinations and laboratory data (from before this illness episode), these are included in the HPI; use only data from the present event when presenting physical examination or laboratory findings. (f) Summarize the presentation and invite questions. (g) Engage and interest the listeners by the way the information is presented. (h) Use note cards only for reminders of factual data; avoid reading a presentation. (i) Practice and get feedback from colleagues. (j) Observe other good presentations and emulate those. (k) Avoid logistic and other problems that may have occupied a lot of interview time but that are irrelevant to the diagnosis or problem list (e.g., Radiology was out of contrast media for a certain study and this caused a delay in obtaining it; or it took several hours to find a relative to obtain permission for a spinal tap). (l) Avoid personalizing and recounting specific conversations that occurred.

Three types of presentations, as follows, are common: very brief, standard, and long. *Very brief presentations* last no more than 1 minute or so and orient a surrogate to key problems in nonurgent situations (e.g., "I'll be in the clinic all afternoon. Mr. Johnson in Room 345 has pneumonia but is doing ok on penicillin. Check his blood cultures when they're out at 4:00 P.M. His wife should be in about then too; let her know all is ok and I'll be back to talk with her around supper time. Thanks.").

The *standard, 3- to 10-minute presentation* conveys full, pertinent information to a listener who is unfamiliar with the patient. Such presentations are useful teaching exercises, as well as a reliable method for transmitting critical information to other caretakers. Students and residents make these presentations to preceptors or senior residents at morning reports, on rounds, and in the clinic. The new clinical student synthesizes personal, primary, and secondary data into a logical diagnosis and then presents it cogently and interestingly. Presentations follow the same format as the write-up, including the logic of clinical reasoning, but they are much more condensed and contain only the most essential data.

The following is an example of a standard presentation using Mrs. Jones, as before, as our subject. (This is a transcript of the junior student's presentation of Mrs. Jones' initial evaluation to her preceptor in the clinic. Although some preceptors may want more detail, most prefer a succinct, pertinent presentation. The student should always ask her or his preceptors to be certain.)

Identifying Data, Source and Reliability of Data, Chief Complaint, and Other Major Agenda Items

The student gives these in one or two sentences, conveying the broad strokes of the situation.

"Joanne Jones is a 38-year-old married white woman who is a lawyer. She is a reliable historian. She self-referred because of headaches of 3 months duration and to get established with a primary care doctor. She also is concerned about stress at work, a past history of ulcerative colitis, and a recent cold."

History of the Present Illness

If we as presenters can organize the history of the present illness (HPI) chronologically, the listener will better understand the subsequent diagnosis or problem identification to which we came. This does not mean that a preceptor will agree with the analysis, but it allows her or him to judge the data and rationale that the presenter used. The presenter should avoid bias and should emphasize pros and cons of diagnostic data. Mrs. Jones' presentation continues with the following.

"Throbbing, nonradiating right temporal headaches associated with nausea and photophobia began suddenly 3 months ago. These have progressively worsened, especially in the last month, so that they now occur two to three times weekly and last as little as 2 and as long as 12 hours, during which time they progressively increase in severity. They are quite severe (worse than having a baby) and make her miss work. An ice bag and dark room seem to help some.

She has been well between headaches and there are no other symptoms, particularly scintillating scotomata or those suggesting neurological disease, meningitis, or head injury. I get no history of arthritis or anything suggesting a collagen disease.

An aunt likely had migraine, and the patient has used birth control pills for 6 years. She had to go to the Emergency Department once a week ago and received a narcotic injection. Only a blood and urine study were done, and we don't have those results yet.

Headaches clearly relate to anger at her boss, who criticizes and disdains her often, and they don't occur when he's not around. She is gradually replacing him as the lead attorney in GHI Corporation here, and he is resisting this more than her Board had said he would. She's mad at them too. She also had headaches as a child when her mother criticized her unfairly and repeatedly. Talking about these problems brought on the headache during our interview. Although her support system is fairly good, she's getting worse; and, if there's no help with this, she may quit her job. She's not depressed and has had no similar problems getting along in the past."

Notice that the student has covered the five components of the HPI we discussed as part of the write-up. The student next reports only pertinent OCAP, HI, PMH, SH, FH, and ROS data.

"Except for chronic stress on the job and being 'workaholic,' she takes good care of herself from a health-maintenance standpoint: seat belts, good aerobics almost daily, low-fat and low-salt diet, no addicting substances, and no risky habits. She has been followed regularly, including Pap smears.

Her past history is significant for what was diagnosed as mild ulcerative colitis in 1982 when she was hospitalized at the University Hospital in her hometown. She'd had bloody diarrhea off and on for 3 months then and re-

sponded to 3 months of prednisone and about a year of sulfasalazine after her work-up was completed. It sounds like both sigmoidoscopy and barium enema were done, as well as several other tests, and I'm sending for the records. She was followed regularly by a Dr. Jergens and was asymptomatic until November 1991 when nonbloody diarrhea occurred and sigmoidoscopy and barium enema showed minimal changes in what she calls the "distal sigmoid colon." No surgery has ever been advised, and she continues without symptoms, having responded almost immediately to another course of sulfasalazine, which she took for 6 months. A sigmoidoscopy 6 months ago was said to be normal.

Except for two uncomplicated obstetric confinements, a mild but now cleared respiratory infection recently, and her only urinary tract infection 8 months ago, she has been in good health.

Aspirin, six to eight daily, is the only other medication. There are no drug sensitivities or allergies.

The SH is significant only in that this job was a big step forward professionally. The FH is not further contributory. ROS reveals nothing more."

Physical Examination

Only the pertinent data are given, both normal and abnormal; they focus from the outset on a vivid general description of the patient and relevant vital signs. (Because the physical examination is outside the province of this text, only a brief report of the exam is presented; some preceptors would prefer that it be more complete and specific.)

"Physical examination shows a normotensive, friendly, and healthy-appearing woman. Head and neck are normal and without bruises or tenderness. Detailed neurological evaluation shows no abnormalities of cranial nerves, reflexes, cerebellar function, extrapyramidal function, or motor/sensory function. She does have a midsystolic click along the left sternal border, but there is no murmur or other abnormality."

Initial Diagnostic and Treatment Interventions

As in the write-up, these actions, which are usually emergency, have been obtained under the student's and her or his team's direction.

"No diagnostic or treatment interventions have been made, and we do not yet have the lab data from a week ago."

Assessment: Biopsychosocial Description (The Patient's Story)

The assessment should be equally cogent, as Mrs. Jones' story shows.

(a) "We got along well, and she indicated liking my approach. I liked her, but I think I cut the conversation short when she was talking about some sexual problems she had. I didn't know what to say. (b) Mrs. Jones is under severe stress from the conflict with her boss on a new job. (c) In turn, this has precipitated migraine headaches, with a typical clinical picture of intermittent throbbing and photophobia and a family history. The birth control pills could be a factor as well. Less likely is a stress tension headache—I wouldn't expect this to be so intermittent, severe, or throbbing. Meningitis, subdural hematoma, and a vasculitis all are extremely unlikely. She has ulcerative colitis, the recent cold, a urinary tract infection last summer, and probably mitral valve prolapse that is not symptomatic."

Treatment and Investigative Plan

This is equally brief and to the point, as Mrs. Jones' case that follows demonstrates. In complicated cases, this and the assessment are much more extensive.

"For the headaches, I'd suggest we start her on either sumatriptan tablets or ergotamine tartrate with caffeine tablets for the acute headaches. Prophylactic treatment, with a beta-blocker or calcium channel blocker, may be necessary; but I'd like to see first what our other measures do. Likewise, if she doesn't do better, we may need to stop the birth control pills. We've already discussed strategies for working with her boss, and I'd like to follow-up in about a week to see how this is progressing and perhaps to develop some new ones. I think she'd also benefit from knowing a relaxation procedure that I can show her. I don't think any laboratory investigation is needed now; but, should she not respond, we might want to reconsider. We'll get records from the Emergency Department and from Dr. Jergens, and I think she needs a referral to gastroenterology for evaluation and a colonoscopy; I've read that cancer can be a risk in patients with ulcerative colitis. A return appointment for 1 week is okay with her."

As noted, the student included the five components of the written HPI: chronological overview of the story, the dimensions of each symptom, pertinent positives and negatives, the course of the problem and relevant secondary data, and the personal contextual aspects. All RPD components are included in the assessment so that the listener obtains the full, integrated biopsychosocial description.

Long presentations more closely resemble the written report. These usually are used for presenting an interesting patient problem for teaching purposes (10 to 15 minutes) or for evaluating students' grasp of their patients (30 to 45 minutes). The time available determines how much information is included. The student allows relatively more time for the assessment and its discussion, either to pose the problem for discussion or to show her or his understanding of the patient.

Not only does the student investigate and formulate the problem beforehand but, once the presentation is outlined, she or he can also practice doing the presentation; audiotaping and feedback from other students can be especially helpful. Presentations work best when notes are kept to a minimum; brief presentations use no notes. Longer presentations usually require notes, which are not read but which are referred to for organizational purposes. Concluding summaries are helpful as they demonstrate the student's ability to synthesize the problem.

SUMMARY

This chapter addresses a very practical need of most students: summarizing the patient's story and transmitting it to others both in a written record and as a verbal presentation.

LEARNING EXERCISES

1. What are the reasons for using a multidimensional diagnostic approach like the RPD designation?*
2. What is the content for each of the five paragraphs in the write-up of the patient's HPI?
3. List several guidelines for an effective case presentation.*
4. Define the types of presentations.

*Good test questions.

PRACTICE EXERCISES

1. Perform a complete new-patient history on a colleague, simulated patient, or real patient and then write up your findings. Make a diagnosis according to the RPD format.
2. Present the same case in 30 minutes, in 5 to 7 minutes, and in 1 to 2 minutes. In each instance, make a diagnosis in the RPD dimensions that is appropriate to the amount of time available.

References

1. Barrows HS, Pickell GC. *Developing clinical problem-solving skills. A guide to more effective diagnosis and treatment.* New York: WW Norton Medical Books, 1991.
2. Tresolini CP, Pew-Fetzer Task Force. *Health professions education and relationship-centered care.* San Francisco: Pew Health Professions Commission, 1994.
3. Inui TS. What are the sciences of relationship-centered primary care? *J Fam Pract* 1996;42:171–177.
4. American Psychiatric Association. *Diagnostic and statistical manual of mental disorders,* 4th ed. Washington, D.C.: American Psychiatric Association, 1994.
5. Smith RC, Hoppe RB. The patient's story: integrating the patient- and physician-centered approaches to interviewing. *Ann Intern Med* 1991;115:470–477.
6. Kravitz RL, Callahan EJ. Patients' perceptions of omitted examinations and tests—a qualitative analysis. *J Gen Int Med* 2000;15:38–45.
7. Marple RL, Kroenke K, Lucey CR, et al. Concerns and expectations in patients presenting with physical complaints—frequency, physician perceptions and actions, and 2-week outcome. *Arch Intern Med* 1997;157:1482–1488.
8. Regier D, Goldberg I, Taube C. The de facto mental health services system. *Arch Gen Psychiatry* 1978;35:685–693.
9. Mitchell WJT, ed. *On narrative.* Chicago: University of Chicago Press, 1981.
10. Kerby AP. *Narrative and the self.* Bloomington, IN: Indiana University Press, 1991.
11. Bohm D. *Wholeness and the implicate order.* London: Routledge and Kegan Paul, 1980.
12. Anderson H, Goolishian HA. Human systems as linguistic systems: preliminary and evolving ideas about the implications for clinical theory. *Fam Proc* 1988;27:371–393.
13. Williams BC, Philbrick JT, Becker DM, et al. A patient-based system for describing ambulatory medicine practices using diagnosis clusters. *J Gen Int Med* 1991;6:57–63.

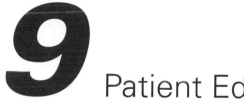

Patient Education

Patient education often is overlooked in medical communication textbooks. Educating patients means giving them information and, if necessary, motivating them to act on it. To this point, I have addressed only gathering information from the patient and establishing a relationship. However, as soon as this database permits, educating the patient becomes equally important. Only a small percentage of interactions lead to mechanical, doctor-given treatments, such as an injection or a manipulation. Most treatment occurs as instructions to patients who then carry out the treatment themselves. They take their pills, go for x-rays and tests, and keep their appointments. We as clinicians cannot do it for them. Therefore, educating the patient is a key element in therapeutics (1–4).

Although patient education occurs throughout the entire encounter, we usually emphasize that function toward the end of an interaction or at subsequent visits. Consider the following patients that were seen during a single clinic morning. The *first,* new to our care and similar to Mrs. Jones, requires information about the interviewer's present findings, answers to her questions, and diagnostic and treatment plans for the future. The *second* patient is here on a follow-up visit; he wants to resume an exercise program after he recovers from a badly sprained ankle. He makes this request while the interviewer is using the patient-centered process. The interviewer devotes a large part of the interaction, following the doctor-centered process and physical examination, to explaining an exercise program. The *third* patient asks for no information, but the interviewer wants to discuss a topic that she has not asked about. He first listens to her needs using the patient-centered process and then attends to the necessary details using the doctor-centered process. He also wants to discuss the need for the patient to stop smoking cigarettes, which he learned about during a previous visit. Education thus involves items that stem from either patient-centered or physician-centered concerns.

Education occurs in two categories. (a) Sometimes the interviewer needs to provide information—either good or bad news—but she or he is not challenged by the additional task of motivating the patient to act on it. (For example, in the above paragraph, the second patient is taught about his improving ankle and the exercise program that he requested.) (b) Often we as interviewers have to give information and then motivate our patients to act on it. (For example, the third patient may not be ready to agree to a cigarette cessation program.) We must then enlist the patient as an active decision maker and partner in therapy (2,5–7). Such negotiation may be implicit and easily agreed upon. Often, though, the interviewer must explicitly negotiate with the patient about both the patient's and doctor's behaviors and roles, as in the case of the cigarette smoker.

The interviewer needs patient-centered skills that have not yet been addressed to educate patients effectively. As the reader might expect, understanding the personal context of the educational issue and developing a healthy relationship remain essential (8).

Providing Information

Giving Routine Data

Much of our informing seems simple—prescribing treatment and diagnostic tests, giving results of tests, and explaining causes of problems. But many patients do not understand information that is provided in either spoken or written form, and, still worse, they forget 40% of it (9). Equally problematic, most doctors underestimate their patients' desire for information, especially that of shy or inarticulate patients, and thus spend a minimal amount of time informing patients (10,11).

The following eight steps, outlined in Table 9.1, greatly enhance patient understanding and memory (12,13). (a) Determine the patient's present understanding. For example, interviewers often should ask, "Before I start explaining things, let me check first and see what you already know about heart tests." (b) Give the most important instructions and advice before the other information and stress their top priority (e.g., "I'm going to start with what is most important for your health, so this is what you most need to remember."). This enhances the likelihood of recall and compliance with what is most important. (c) Categorize data where possible (e.g., "First, let's talk about your heart medicines and then . . ."). (d) Make a clear, short statement

---

TABLE 9.1. PROVIDING INFORMATION

A. Check baseline understanding.
B. Give the most important instructions first.
C. Categorize information.
D. Make clear, simple, and short statements about one major bit of information at a time.
E. Advise concerning specific patient behaviors.
F. Encourage questions.
G. Check understanding.
H. Repeat the message. Write it down if necessary.

---

about just one bit of data at a time and use simple words. (e) Recommend specific behaviors for the patient to perform (e.g., "In the mornings, walk around the block for 15 minutes, sit and rest for 15 minutes, and then repeat this once more. Do the same in the evenings."). (f) Encourage patients to ask questions. (g) Ask questions to check the patient's understanding of the major points. Do not provide more data until the initial material is clarified and assimilated. (h) Repeat the most important messages; be prepared to write the information down if necessary. Also be sure that the patient can read the writing and can understand the words.

Giving Bad News

Sometimes, as clinicians, we have to deliver bad news to our patients, a task where research shows we often falter badly, particularly by not being patient-centered (14). We can expect that they will find such news difficult to hear (e.g., diagnosis of cancer or AIDS). In addition to maintaining a patient-centered attitude and supportive approach, the following guidelines, which are summarized in Table 9.2, are useful (15).

Plan Ahead

The student or clinician must ensure that data are complete and accurate, that she or he fully understands them, and that she or he knows how to proceed. Patients will almost certainly ask questions about diagnosis, prognosis, and subsequent treatment. The interviewer must also consider her or his own feelings of grief and loss. Failure to attend to one's personal responses often leads to their unplanned, deleterious intrusion into the patient's situation; for ex-

TABLE 9.2. GIVING BAD NEWS*

A. Plan ahead.
  1. Be sure information is complete and well understood.
  2. Attend to one's own reactions.
  3. Have others who are necessary present.
  4. Rehearse, especially in light of patient's personality and other unique features.
B. Arrange the meeting personally, be sure enough time is available, and avoid use of intermediaries or a telephone.
C. Ensure a safe, comfortable setting.
D. Determine patient's readiness to hear the information and his or her level of understanding of the situation.
E. Give the bad news clearly and succinctly.
  1. Give only one bit at a time.
  2. Encourage questions and answer directly.
  3. Encourage emotional expression.
  4. Always convey hope, but do not falsely reassure.
  5. Be comfortable with silence, and do not rush the patient.
  6. Accept that the interviewer may be able to do nothing but be there with the patient.
  7. Encourage follow-up questions and check patient's understanding.
  8. Provide necessary additional information.
  9. Explore impact on patient's life and her or his beliefs about the implications of the bad news.
  10. Determine if the patient is suicidal; make necessary immediate arrangements if so.
F. Develop a plan.
  1. Ensure a support system.
  2. Inform others.
  3. Schedule follow-up visits or telephone calls explicitly; give home telephone number.
  4. Initiate follow-up if patient does not.
  5. Use appropriate diagnostic and treatment considerations.

*Emotion-seeking and emotion-handling skills are used throughout.

ample, a doctor might provide a patient with a falsely reassuring picture because of her or his own unrecognized feeling of loss in learning that a well-liked patient has widespread metastatic cancer.

The clinician or student must also determine whether anyone else needs to be informed and if this person should be at the initial meeting. A responsible person must be present when the patient is young or is of limited competence. Similarly, a psychologically fragile patient or one who is in denial needs a responsible and supportive person. If such a supportive person is available, many of us as humans, whether strong or weak, benefit from that person's presence. On the other hand, the patient may not want anyone else present; the student or clinician should accept this initially. When bad news can be anticipated, she or he should arrange a follow-up meeting and should negotiate in advance who will be present.

In rare instances, giving bad news might be medically or psychologically dangerous; for example, a student or clinician might have additional bad news for a patient who is having an acute heart attack or a patient who is suicidal. Even here, I advise against long delays in notifying the patient. Sometimes, families ask that information be withheld from the patient, often to "protect" her or him. The interviewer may accommodate this briefly—for example, to bring a close relative home—but a delay should not be prolonged. Patients have the right to have information about themselves.

The student or clinician should note the important points that she or he plans to make prior to the difficult discussion. She or he can even rehearse the key statements aloud. Sometimes, doing so can make for a more coherent message and a more sensitive interaction. Incorporating information about the patient's personality style, spiritual life, beliefs, and support system into the preparation also helps.

Personally Arrange a Meeting with the Patient

If the student or clinician has not made advance arrangements, she or he should personally make them but should avoid giving the bad news on the phone. She or he might call the patient and say, "Some of your lab tests are back. They're too complicated to talk about on the phone, so I'd like you and your wife to come in later today so we can discuss them." Although this "message framing" sounds innocuous, it will probably worry the patient, so one should arrange the meeting for as soon as possible and should provide a sufficient amount of time for it.

Ensure a Safe and Comfortable Setting

A private office or room will suffice. Avoid conducting discussions in hallways, coffee shops, or any other place where privacy and comfort are unlikely. The student or clinician should establish an atmosphere of warmth and safety by the use of nonverbal means (e.g., shake hands) and by giving undivided and unhurried attention, ensuring the patient's physical comfort, and arranging the situation so that no interruptions occur.

Determine the Patient's Readiness to Listen and Her or His Understanding of the Situation

As clinicians, we try to learn how ready and able the patient is to hear the bad news. We need to learn about what other things might be going on in her or his life at this time that might be more important and more stressful (8). If the patient is not ready at the beginning of the meeting, the clinician or student can help the patient by allowing her or him to control the pace and flow of information. This can include allowing her or him to address issues that she or he perceives as needing management (e.g., answering a business call) or as more pressing (e.g., being certain that the baby sitter knows where the patient is); she or he then gently asks if the patient is ready to proceed with addressing a serious health matter. At this point, she or he would look for emotional content; in doing so, the interviewer may discover fear of anticipated bad news or exaggerated anxiety about its implications. Rarely, the patient may resist hearing the news by seeming not to understand it. The interviewer must consider this situation; in such cases, she or he tries to inform other responsible parties.

The interviewer next determines the patient's understanding of the problem. This includes her or his knowledge about the diagnosis and her or his beliefs about its implication for prognosis and treatment. The student or clinician establishes these data with focused, open-ended questions such as, "Tell me first about your understanding of the situation and what concerns you have."

Give the Bad News

The clinician or student should preface the bad news by indicating that a problem exists (e.g., "I'm afraid I have some difficult news to give you."). This lessens the shock of the news and allows the patient to brace herself or himself for what is to come. She or he then gives a clear, direct, and brief message. Only one bit of the most important information is given at a time (e.g., "Your mammogram is very indicative of cancer."). The interviewer cannot assume a common understanding of terms, such as cancer; she or he should be ready to give clarification.

The student or clinician follows the patient's lead in deciding how far and fast to proceed by accepting questions and listening for emotions. She or he gives clear answers and explanations and clarifies any misperceptions or overreactions (e.g., "Yes, surgery will be needed but they usually don't remove the entire breast any more."). If the patient's emotions are not forthcoming, the interviewer uses emotion-seeking skills and emotion-handling skills. The interaction will evolve as the patient expresses emotion and a desire for more information. However, the student or clinician in this situation must tread a fine line. She or he does not want the patient to feel pushed or overwhelmed. Nor does the interviewer want to leave the patient isolated with her or his fear, anger, or grief. Gentle emotion-seeking and emotion-handling usually work best.

The interviewer must avoid false reassurance but should still convey hope. For example, she or he might say to a newly diagnosed AIDS patient, "I know it looks bad but treatment is working better all the time, and there's a lot of research now indicating that we should consider it a chronic rather than a fatal disease." Sometimes, though, the interviewer herself or himself provides the only immediate hope. Therefore, she or he must make her or his presence and support explicit and must convey the appropriate nonverbal support (arm around shoulder, holding hand), which is often the first link in eventually restoring meaning and hope. The student or clinician must reassure the patient that she or he will not abandon the patient, which is a common and weighty fear. Silence and a quiet presence are powerful (16). The interviewer's own genuine emotions are appropriate and are often consoling (17). The alleviation of suffering can be most successful when the student or clinician abandons her or his efforts at reassurance and recognizes that she or he may be able to do nothing but to be available and to provide support. This is most effective if the interviewer can establish and develop this relationship over many encounters, as might occur in a primary care setting (17). The first visit is just the beginning.

After the initial shock passes, the interviewer should encourage the patient to ask questions and should check her or his understanding. Many people do not assimilate information well in tension-laden situations, and they can develop an erroneous understanding, one that is often worse than the reality. For example, when patients are informed of cancer or AIDS, many expect to die within a few months. Tape recording the interaction and then giving the tape to the patient can help to offset this (17,18).

As additional information is exchanged, the patient may display further feelings; the interviewer again addresses these using emotion-seeking skills and the naming, understanding, respecting, and supporting (NURS) tetrad. As the interaction evolves, the interviewer must reinforce the patient's other supports, her or his strengths, and her or his prior abilities in dealing with adversity. The clinician or student needs to learn the impact of the bad news on her or his life and on the lives of family and friends. The interviewer must also gauge how well the patient is handling the information and should try not to overwhelm her or him. Additional meetings are often necessary to allow the sufficient assimilation of all information. She or he also must determine if the patient is suicidal. This can be done only by direct inquiry (e.g., "This is a lot to throw at you and I know you're quite down. Do you have thoughts of hurting yourself, you know, taking your life?"). Although students will learn about the suicidal patient in psychiatry rotations, if they detect suicidal intent, they need to hear more about it and to ask for immediate outside help.

Develop a Plan

The student or clinician must ensure satisfactory support. This can include medical and psychological professionals, as well as family, friends, church, support groups, and others. The interviewer may need to assist in obtaining support for some patients, either because she or he has too little of it or she or he is too defeated to seek it out.

If the interviewer plans to inform significant others, she or he should negotiate specific plans with the patient beforehand. Usually this presents no problem—the patient wants certain others informed, or she or he will inform them personally. On occasions, though, the student or clinician must discuss any plans to exclude concerned others with the patient. These others, such as partners of a patient who has been newly diagnoised with AIDS, may need to be informed for medical, legal, and humanistic reasons.

The interviewer should schedule a follow-up visit in the very near future; she or he may make a follow-up telephone call later the same day. She or he may also give the patient her or his home phone and should initiate follow-up actions if the patient fails to make a scheduled visit or call.

The student or clinician should initiate any psychological or medical interventions. A sedative or a brief course of a tranquilizing agent can be beneficial. Prescribing specific tasks can help the overwhelmed patient (e.g., discussing who and how to tell the news, writing down questions, and talking to others with similar problems). Also, she or he should arrange additional diagnostic and therapeutic interventions (e.g., referral to a surgeon).

Providing Information and Motivating Patients to Act on It

Simply informing patients, as I have covered to this point, is only part of the task with the group of patients that I now consider. This section demonstrates how the interviewer also attempts to persuade the patient to accept a course that she or he has not previously chosen. Focusing on the clinician's agenda to correct an adverse health habit, such as smoking cigarettes or losing weight, can lead to a conflicted interview and can jeopardize the doctor–

patient relationship. Although the interviewer encourages her or his agenda, doing so requires skillful negotiation to establish the patient as responsible and in charge.

Prochaska and his colleagues clarified this process of behavioral change (19,20). Their research shows that five stages of change are seen: (a) precontemplation (not considering change in the next 6 months), (b) contemplation (intending to change in the next 6 months), (c) preparation for change (intending to take action in the next month), (d) action (have made overt modifications of lifestyle in last 6 months), and (e) maintenance of change (6 months to 5 years of behavioral change). Patients do not progress through these stages linearly, however; but rather, they cycle back and forth among stages.

In general, among recruits for change programs, 40% are precontemplators, 40% are contemplators, and 20% are preparing; a few may already be in action. Prochaska and his colleagues' research shows that success is a function of matching different treatments to different stages; that is, as clinicians we cannot treat all patients the same (19,20). We can focus on raising the issue to full awareness in the 80% of patients who are in *early stages* (precontemplation, contemplation) and on encouraging insight, outlining key decisions with their pros and cons, conducting environmental reevaluation and self-reevaluation, and encouraging readiness for change. However, patients in the *preparation and action stages* no longer need knowledge or help with decision making but instead require specific procedures, such as stimulus control, deconditioning from unhealthy behaviors, reinforcement of good behaviors, commitment, contingency assessment, environmental control, and social support. Thus, for early change, we try to instill insight, whereas we encourage commitment and provide specific behavioral techniques for later change. Or, stated differently, in early stages we emphasize the positive results of changing, whereas in later stages we focus on the difficult aspects of actually changing. A reasonable clinical goal is to progress one stage at a time. Wadland and Stoffelmayr (21,22) have outlined in detail how we can use these principles for cigarette cessation and also have shown how to maintain abstinence effectively via counseling by nurses at office visits or by telephone.

The role of the doctor–patient relationship continues to be prominent, perhaps even more so than usual. The research of Williams and colleagues (23,24) shows the importance of enhancing patient autonomy as a key dimension of patient-centered behavioral change in these patients. They need to have a sense of being guided by their own values, which greatly enhances the relationship and the likelihood of success. Also of great interest with regard to the relationship is the research of Ockene and her colleagues (25–27) who have shown that physicians can learn to deliver smoking cessation programs effectively when they use patient-centered counseling approaches that emphasize open-ended inquiry and exploration of emotion rather than simply giving information.

My own research (28) (Appendix A) shows that physicians can learn a specific patient-centered model for informing and motivating, which is presented next and is summarized in Table 9.3. This evidence-based method was developed by Stoffelmayr and his coworkers (1) and encompasses both the five stages of change and the doctor–patient relationship. It is presented here with the caveat that patients often will not go through all steps linearly. The method is most effective when we as clinicians target patients in the early stages to establish an information base and to motivate the patient, whereas we target patients in later stages to evoke a commitment and to negotiate a specific plan. The relationship is essential throughout these stages.

TABLE 9.3. INFORMING AND MOTIVATING*

A. Establish an information base and motivate the patient.
    1. Determine knowledge base, the patient's specific situation, and readiness for change.
    2. Give clear information about adverse potential of health habit that needs change.
    3. Make brief, explicit recommendation for change.
    4. Motivate patient.
        a. Inform of health and other benefits from change.
        b. Use knowledge of personality.
        c. Highlight patient's capacity for change.
        d. Emphasize that help is available.
        e. Indicate that past failures do not bode poorly.
    5. Check understanding and desire for change.
B. Obtain a commitment.
    1. Reinforce commitment.
    2. Set expectations for success.
    3. Reaffirm commitment.
    4. (Manage a decision against advice.)
C. Negotiate a specific plan.
    1. Start with detailed understanding of the role in the patient's life of the habit to be changed.
    2. Involve patient actively in plan, including when to begin and the specific details of its implementation.
    3. Include medical interventions where applicable.
    4. Check understanding and reaffirm plan.
    5. Set follow-up.

---

*Emotion-seeking and emotion-handling skills are used throughout.

I now consider the three following steps of my own evidence-based method for educating a patient to change behaviors: informing and motivating, obtaining a commitment, and negotiating a specific plan (1,28). When no commitment is obtained with the precontemplators and contemplators, the interviewer works to maintain the relationship and to keep the door open for other problems, as well as for later educational activities.

We can assume that, when dealing with these matters, we are working with emotionally charged material. Therefore, the student or clinician uses emotion-seeking and emotion-handling skills throughout, particularly at points of resistance. She or he needs a sound clinical base to educate the patient effectively. Here I present only a general guide because the specific approach to each adverse health habit is unique and varied. As students learn clinical medicine, they easily learn to fit specific clinical information into the template outlined in Table 9.3 (1).

Establish an Information Base and Motivate the Patient

As always, the interviewer begins by determining the patient's knowledge base and readiness to change (e.g., "What do you know about the health impact of cigarette smoking? Where are you in thinking about quitting?"). Following this, she or he informs the patient, as necessary, about the adverse potential of her or his present actions (e.g., smoking cigarettes, alcohol or drug use, lack of exercise, overweight, stressful life, not using condoms). For example, she or he might inform a patient who was not aware of an adverse impact that smoking cigarettes is associated with a 10% risk of developing lung cancer, a greater chance of developing bronchitis and emphysema, even more risk for developing cardiovascular disease (heart attack, stroke), and a general reduction of 6 to 7 years in life expectancy.

Next, the student or clinician should make a brief, explicit recommendation (e.g., "For health purposes, you need to quit smoking completely."). She or he follows with a statement that details what improved health and other benefits (cost, odor) will follow (e.g., "By quitting cigarettes your health improves immediately; after being off them a year, the risk for heart attacks and strokes is almost as though you'd never smoked. The risk for emphysema and cancer decreases also.").

To maximize the impact of the information and to enhance the relationship, the interviewer also incorporates awareness of the patient's personality style into the interview to increase the patient's motivation. For example, specific discussion of the medical literature would enhance acceptance with an obsessive-compulsive patient; indicating the potential adverse effect on appearance would appeal to a histrionic person; and appealing to a patient with a self-defeating style on the grounds that smoking could prevent her or his continued care of a spouse would be compelling for him or her.

The interviewer also persuades by emphasizing with which of the patient's interests the habit interferes (e.g., see grandchildren grow up), as well as her or his capabilities for change (e.g., "You've really done a lot at the church and are known as a doer. You could add this to your list of achievements, set a good example for many, and gain the benefit of saving a lot of money."). Gauging from both the patient's style and response to suggested interventions, the interviewer's roles may vary and can include acting as a cheerleader, politician, diplomat, confidant, and/or disciplinarian. She or he must communicate in the way that the patient understands best. On the other hand, the more that we as clinicians pressure the patient to change her or his behavior, the more likely she or he is to resist. The patient must lead. When we find out what she or he wants to do, then only can we offer the appropriate help.

The interviewer can remind the patient that help is available and effective (e.g., "I'll be working with you weekly on this if you decide to go ahead. There are smokers' groups and medications that are helpful as well. We've had some great results."). This offsets the pessimistic view that nothing can be done. To further encourage the patient, she or he can say that having failed before at changing a bad habit bodes well for future efforts because most successful patients have had many unsuccessful previous attempts.

The clinician or student should repeatedly intersperse emotion-seeking ("How're you doing with this? It's a lot to ask of you.") and emotion-handling skills ("It has been difficult for you to quit. I know and I understand what it's like. I'm impressed that you're considering that we might work together on it."). These skills are more effective with recalcitrant patients than are repeated education or encouragement efforts. As interviewers, we need to try to understand the patient more and to convey this to her or him. Usually, she or he already understands us. Still, we must check the patient's understanding, particularly of the recommendation that is being made (e.g., "We've talked about a lot of stuff and I want to be sure I haven't confused the issue. What do you hear me telling you?").

Obtain a Commitment

Trying to obtain a commitment may be the most awkward part of the interaction, and tension can lead the interviewer to be vague and indirect or to provide a loophole for escape. To someone in the preparation stage, the interviewer might say, "We need to decide now if you want to make a commitment to work on this." The student or clinician must permit the existence of the silence and awkwardness that often follows such a statement. The patient is indeed on the spot and needs to wrestle with the issue. She or he may have little experience in making such decisions, but she or he must make this one.

If the patient does commit to a change, the student or clinician should support the plan and should reaffirm her or his availability and that of other help. In addition, she or he should set the expectations of success and should provide reinforcement for the patient making a change ("I'm impressed that you're willing to work on such a big change. I know it will be a stretch but I think you can do it.").

Before moving to the next stage, the interviewer should check once again and should ask the patient to affirm her or his decision. For example, she or he might say, "To be sure we're clear, could you repeat what you want to do?"

Negotiate a Plan

The student or clinician must understand the details of the behavior to be changed so that an effective plan can be agreed on. With the example of cigarette smoking, the interviewer wants the details of when the patient smokes, the most important times for smoking (e.g., while drinking coffee), what stresses prompt smoking (e.g., work), who else in her or his environment smokes (e.g., best friend), and what situations might make the patient resume smoking once she or he has stopped (e.g., "having a beer with the boys"). Strategies for change must address these issues yet, at the same time, must be compatible with the patient's daily life.

As usual, the interviewer actively involves the patient in identifying problem areas and solutions. For example, a cigarette smoker might first identify drinking beer with his friends as a difficult time, and the interviewer might then facilitate the patient's decision not to join these friends at the tavern for the first month or so after quitting. The patient also decides to tell them and others that he is quitting smoking. (Some patients do not want to let others know.) He agrees to stop smoking over an upcoming holiday so he will be away from his smoking friends and the stress at work. (Some prefer to quit while they can stay busy.) He also decides to drink herbal tea instead of coffee and to chew gum to replace the cigarettes. Whatever the patient's plan is, a student or clinician who facilitates the patient's active involvement achieves the greatest success. Only the patient can find those solutions unique to her or his life circumstance.

With some habits, the interviewer encourages a "step at a time" approach. For example, although smoking requires complete abstinence, a diet often works best when a few foods at a time are decreased. For instance, in initiating a low-cholesterol diet, the interviewer may negotiate decisions about which foods to reduce (e.g., eggs), the amount of reduction (e.g., one instead of three), and the meal from which they are reduced (e.g., breakfast). Further negotiation will be required only if the cholesterol does not fall; options then would be to stop the remaining egg at breakfast, to omit margarine and butter, and to reduce red meat intake to twice weekly.

When applicable, the student or clinician negotiates medical interventions as well. For example, the medical community seldom uses medications for elevated cholesterol until dietary measures have been shown to be ineffective. On the other hand, we sometimes use nicotine replacement regimens (gums, patches, inhalers, nasal sprays) and other medications initially if the patient wants this help to stop smoking. Similarly, some patients might want to participate in a group for support from the ongoing efforts of others. Some patients, however, want no medications, no group work, or no other medical interventions and prefer to "do it on my own." Here, more closely spaced follow-up visits can be helpful but, often, only if they are framed as something other than support.

After negotiating a plan, the interviewer asks the patient to repeat the specific plan that will be implemented. This reinforces it and allows any misunderstanding to be clarified. Agreement on the timetable is especially important. She or he must also reinforce and support the patient's commitment and should set follow-up plans before ending the interaction. Sometimes, writing this out for the patient to take home is necessary. Typically, we provide close follow-up for patients who are undergoing major changes, such as quitting cigarettes or adopting a low-fat diet. They not only benefit from the support but also may need help with additional problem solving.

When a Commitment Is Not Obtained

A negotiated approach allows for and accommodates the option that the patient (precontemplators and contemplators) may discard the interviewer's advice to change right now. She or he should nonjudgmentally inquire about refusal, taking care that the patient does not feel pressured, and should clarify any misunderstanding. Because these patients represent 80% of the population needing change, as clinicians, we must maintain effective contact and must recall that simply changing the patient from one stage to another bodes well for subsequent success (e.g., getting a precontemplator to the contemplator stage).

When the patient rejects a recommendation, the interviewer can ask, "What would it take to make you change your mind?" (29). The cigarette smoker, for example, might answer with, "Well, a heart attack or cancer, I guess." The answer itself sometimes helps the patient realize how really dangerous the habit is and encourages stage change.

The interviewer must make her or his acceptance of the patient's decision explicit. She or he should defuse differences or tension that might interfere with subsequent care. She or he should reassure the patient that she or he will not pressure or abandon him or her but that she or he will continue to explore gently the patient's readiness to change. One empathic technique is to express understanding of the patient's dilemma (e.g., "I can see you are caught in a bind. On the one hand, you're tired of these chest colds and want to stop smoking. On the other hand, you enjoy smoking and find it releases stress at work. So you both want to quit and want not to. That's a real squeeze!").

SUMMARY

Treating and educating the patient involve both patient-centered and doctor-centered processes. The interviewer checks the patient's readiness for the information, establishes a baseline of the patient's understanding and desires, informs her or him to the extent necessary, determines her or his commitment to action where needed, and negotiates specific plans. Sometimes, especially with adverse health habits, interviewers also must try to motivate the patient to act on the information provided, carefully identifying the patient's specific stage of change and working hard to enhance the relationship in a difficult circumstance. The student or clinician frequently checks the patient's comprehension and always reaffirms plans. The more difficult the situation is, the more the she or he must use emotion-seeking and emotion-handling skills.

LEARNING EXERCISES

1. At what point in the interaction does patient education usually occur? At which visit?
2. List several circumstances where you might provide routine data; where you might need to give bad news; where you may want not only to inform the patient but also to motivate her or him to action.
3. List and define the various stages of change.
4. What skills are required for patients in early stages of change; in later stages of change?*
5. In which patient education category is an extra focus on the doctor–patient relationship most important? In addition to using NURS, what other factor(s) enhance the relationship for motivating the patient to change?*

*Good test questions.

PRACTICE EXERCISES

1. In role-play, inform the patient of the necessary details of her or his treatment program that includes several medications to be taken at different times of day (e.g., an antibiotic, decongestant, vaporizer, and oxygen for a patient with mild ["walking"] pneumonia).
2. In role-play, give a patient bad news (e.g., that she or he has AIDS, an abnormal mammogram, abnormal amniocentesis, elevated blood sugar, or a cancerous-appearing lump in a chest x-ray).
3. In role-play, inform and motivate a patient to stop or change a deleterious habit (e.g., to stop smoking cigarettes, to change to a low-fat diet, or to begin a program of progressively increasing exercise).
4. When facile in role-play, conduct all exercises with real or simulated patients.

References

1. Stoffelmayr B, Hoppe RB, Weber N. Facilitating patient participation: the doc-tor–patient encounter. *Primary Care* 1989;16:265–278.
2. Grueninger UJ, Duffy FD, Goldstein MG. Patient education in the medical en-counter: how to facilitate learning, behavior change, and coping. In: Lipkin M,

Putnam SM, Lazare A, eds. *The medical interview*. New York: Springer-Verlag, 1995:122–133.

3. Grueninger UJ, Goldstein MG, Duffy DF. Patient education in hypertension: five essential steps. *Hypertension* 1989;7(suppl 3):s93–s98.

4. Prochaska JO, DiClemente CC. Towards a comprehensive model of change. In: Miller WR, Heather N, eds. *Treating addictive behaviors: processes of change*. New York: Plenum Press, 1986:3–27.

5. Lazare A, Eisenthal S, Frank A, et al. Studies on a negotiated approach to patienthood. In: Stoeckle JD, ed. *Encounters between patients and doctors*. Cambridge, MA: The MIT Press, 1987:413–432.

6. Lazare A, Eisenthal S, Wasserman L. The customer approach to patienthood: attending to patient requests in a walk-in clinic. *Arch Gen Psychiatry* 1975;32: 552–558.

7. Quill TE. Partnerships in patient care: a contractual approach. *Ann Intern Med* 1983;98:228–234.

8. Waitzkin H, Britt T. Processing narratives of self-destructive behavior in routine medical encounters: health promotion, disease prevention, and the discourse of health care. *Soc Sci Med* 1993;36:1121–1136.

9. Ley P. Doctor-patient communication: some quantitative estimates of the role of cognitive factors in non-compliance. *J Hypertens* 1985;3:51–55.

10. Waitzkin H. Doctor-patient communication: clinical implications of social scientific research. *JAMA* 1984;252:2441–2446.

11. Waitzkin H. Information giving in medical care. *J Health Soc Behav* 1985;26: 81–101.

12. Ley P. Memory for medical information. *Br J Soc Clin Psychol* 1979;18: 245–255.

13. Ley P, Whitworth MA, Skilbeck CE, et al. Improving doctor–patient communication in general practice. *J Roy Coll Gen Pract* 1976;26:720–724.

14. Eggly S, Alfonso N, Rojas G, et al. An assessment of residents' competence in the delivery of bad news to patients. *Acad Med* 1997;72:397–399.

15. Quill TE, Townsend P. Bad news: delivery, dialogue, and dilemmas. *Arch Intern Med* 1991;151:463–468.

16. Frank AW. Just listening: narrative and deep illness. *Fam Systems Health* 1998; 16:197–212.

17. Fallowfield LJ, Lipkin M. Delivering sad or bad news. In: Lipkin M, Putnam SM, Lazare A, eds. *The medical interview*. New York: Springer-Verlag, 1995: 316–323.

18. Smith RC. Review: providing recordings or summaries of consultations may help patients with cancer. *ACP J Club* 2000;133:28.

19. Prochaska JO, DiClemente CC, Norcross JC. In search of how people change—applications to addictive behaviors. *Am Psychol* 1992;47:1102–1114.

20. Prochaska JO, Velicer WF. The transtheoretical model of health behavior change. *Am J Health Promotion* 1997;12:38–48.

21. Wadland WC, Stoffelmayr B. Cigarette smoking. In: Weiss BD, ed. *20 Common problems in primary care*. New York: McGraw-Hill, 1999:3–26.

22. Wadland WC, Stoffelmayr B, Berger E, et al. Enhancing smoking cessation rates in primary care. *J Fam Pract* 1999;48:711–718.

23. Williams GC, Freedman FR, Deci EL. Supporting autonomy to motivate patients with diabetes for glucose control. *Diabetes Care* 1998;21:1644–1651.

24. Williams GC, Cox EM, Hedberg VA, et al. Extrinsic life goals and health-risk behaviors in adolescents. *J Appl Soc Psychol* 2000;30:1756–1771.

25. Ockene JK, Kristeller J, Goldberg R, et al. Increasing the efficacy of physician-delivered smoking interventions. *J Gen Intern Med* 1991;6:1–8.

26. Ockene JK, Kristeller J, Pbert L, et al. The physician-delivered smoking intervention project: can short-term interventions produce long-term effects for a general outpatient population? *Health Psychol* 1994;13:278–281.

27. Ockene JK, Quirk ME, Goldberg JR, et al. A residents' training program for the development of smoking intervention skills. *Arch Intern Med* 1988;148: 1039–1045.

28. Smith RC, Lyles JS, Mettler J, et al. The effectiveness of intensive training for residents in interviewing. A randomized, controlled study. *Ann Intern Med* 1998; 128:118–126.

29. Williams GC, Quill TE, Deci EL, et al. "The facts concerning the recent carnival of smoking in Connecticut" and elsewhere. *Ann Intern Med* 1991;115:59–63.

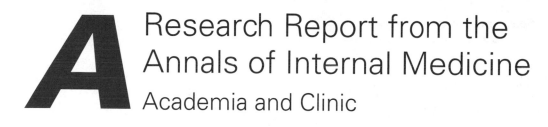

Research Report from the Annals of Internal Medicine
Academia and Clinic

Robert C. Smith, M.D.; Judith S. Lyles, PH.D.; Jennifer Methler, M.A.;
Bertram E. Stoffelmayr, PH.D.; Lawrence F. Van Egeren, PH.D.;
Alicia A. Marshall, PH.D.; Joseph C. Gardner, PH.D.;
Karen M. Maduschke, M.A.; Jennifer A. Stanley, M.A.;
Gerald G. Osborn, D.O.; Valerie Shebroe, PH.D.;
Ruth B. Greenbaum, M.N.

The Effectiveness of Intensive Training for Residents in Interviewing: A Randomized, Controlled Study

Background

Interviewing and the physician–patient relationship are crucial elements of medical care, but residencies provide little formal instruction in these areas.

Objective

To determine the effects of a training program in interviewing on (a) residents' attitudes toward and skills in interviewing and on (b) patients' physical and psychosocial well being and satisfaction with care.

Design

Randomized, controlled study.

Setting

Two university-based primary care residencies.

Participants

Sixty-three primary care residents in postgraduate year 1.

Intervention

A 1-month, full-time rotation in interviewing and related psychosocial topics.

Measurements

Residents and their patients were assessed before and after the 1-month rotation. Questionnaires were used to assess residents' commitment to interviewing and psychosocial medicine, their estimate of the importance of such care, and their confidence in their ability to provide such care. Knowledge of interviewing and psychosocial medicine was assessed with a multiple-choice test. Audiotaped interviews with real patients and videotaped interviews with simulated patients were rated for specific interviewing behaviors. Patients' anxiety, depression, and social dysfunction; role limitations; somatic symptom status; and levels of satisfaction with medical visits were assessed by questionnaires and telephone interviews.

Results

Trained residents were superior to untrained residents in knowledge (difference in adjusted post-test mean scores, 15.7% [95% CI, 11% to 20%]); attitudes, such as confidence in psychological sensitivity (difference, 0.61 points on a 7-point scale [CI, 0.32 to 0.91 points]); somatization management (difference, 0.99 points [CI, 0.64 to 1.35 points]); interviewing real patients (difference, 1.39 points on an 11-point scale [CI, 0.32 to 2.45 points]); and interviewing (data gathering) simulated patients (difference, 2.67 points [CI, 1.77 to 3.56 points]). Mean differences between the study groups were consistently in the appropriate direction for patient satisfaction and patient well being, but effect sizes were too small to be considered meaningful.

Conclusion

An intensive 1-month training rotation in interviewing improved residents' knowledge about, attitudes toward, and skills in interviewing.

Reference

Smith RC, Lyles JS, Mettler J, et al. Research report. *Ann Intern Med* 1998;128:118–126. This paper is also available at *http://www.acponline.org*

Medical interviewing justifiably reigns as the premier skill in medicine (1–4), and it is the vehicle for physician–patient interaction and exchange of information in almost all circumstances (3,4). The interview alone produces the data required for diagnosis more than three-fourths of the time, and it establishes more diagnoses than physical examination and laboratory data combined (5–8). Interviewing generates most of the data required for treatment and prevention and serves as the primary means for transmitting information from physician to patient (4,9). It also defines the physician–patient relationship, and the quality of the physician–patient relationship influences the quality of the data exchanged (4,10,11). Against this background and with the knowledge that most physicians perform more than 200,000 interviews during their careers (3), the fact that interview often gets short shrift is a matter of national concern in the United States (3).

Most medical schools teach at least some interviewing skills (12), but instruction in interviewing receives scant attention in residencies (9,13—16), despite strong, research-based recommendations in favor of such training (13,17–20). Surveys of internal medicine program directors (14,21) showed that formal training in interviewing averaged only 5 to 13 hours per year during residencies. This is far less than the 1 month of full-time training that is often recommended (13,17—20,22,23), but educators have few empirical data to guide them with respect to what and how to teach residents in intensive interview training programs. A recent literature review produced only 12 studies of intensive training programs, and six of the 12 had nonexperimental designs (13). Of the six with quasiexperimental designs, four (17—20) specifically addressed interviewing, interpersonal skills, or the physician–patient relationship and showed positive results, thus supporting a "patient-centered" approach. The other two studies (24,25) did not inform the question (13).

We developed an intensive training program for primary care residents in interviewing and related psychosocial topics in medicine. Using a randomized, controlled study design, we tested two hypotheses: (a) that trained residents, compared with controls, could gain more knowledge, confidence, and skill in gathering data, building relationships with patients, managing somatizing patients, and educating patients and (b) that the patients of trained residents would have greater satisfaction, fewer somatic symptoms, less social dysfunction, less depression and anxiety, and reduced functional disability.

Methods

Participants

We trained 65 medical and family practice residents in postgraduate year 1 and asked them to participate in a study to evaluate the interviewing training program. Thirty-six men and 27 women accepted; two residents who were trained refused to participate in the evaluation. Each participant was paid $100 to participate in the evaluation.

Training Program

As we have described elsewhere (26,27), the training was experiential and was skills-oriented, and it was guided by competency-based (28) objectives that were both learner-centered and teacher-centered (29,30). We used the four interviewing models described in the following to enhance learning of complex new material. Each model described the step-by-step behaviors needed to conduct a complex interaction with a patient efficiently, placed these behaviors in sequence, and prioritized them.

Basic Patient-Centered Interviewing and Physician–Patient Relationship Model One of the authors formulated a basic model of the entire interview to serve as an infrastructure that learners could use as a guide (4). The model incorporated a rich body of literature that is reviewed elsewhere (4). (A textbook from the American Academy on Physician and Patient is a particularly useful guide for teachers [31].) We restricted our focus to the often unfamiliar patient-centered interviewing process, which places the patient's needs and the physician–patient relationship first (4), because residents were already relatively skilled with the physician-centered interviewing process that is aimed at diagnosing disease. The patient-centered process, which was usually used at the start of the interview, was easily learned and was structured so that, with experience, it usually took no more than 3 to 10 minutes.

Other Patient-Centered Interviewing Models Other interviewing models used the basic patient-centered model and integrated it with the following additional patient-centered skill areas: (a) interacting with patients who had chronic somatization by using cognitive-behavioral principles developed by one of the authors (32,33); (b) informing the patient and motivating the patient to take a new course of action (such as losing weight) by using a model developed by one of the authors (34) and others (4,35–39,39a); and (c) giving patients bad news by using published approaches (4,40).

Noninterviewing Training Objectives This learning experience encompassed several important objectives apart from interviewing skills. It was intended to help residents develop self-awareness of potentially harmful personal reactions (41–43); to enable them to make accurate neuropsychiatric diagnoses for conditions common in primary care settings (44–48); to improve their skill with practical psychopharmacology in a medical setting (44); and to increase their skill in treating anxiety, depression, and chronic somatization in primary care settings (32,33,44,45,47,49).

Training took place during a required, full-time, 4-week block rotation, in which three or four residents matriculated at a time. The rotation had a core seminar component and a core supervisory component. Core seminar sessions of 3 hours each took place three times weekly in a private conference room. A brief discussion of the interviewing model (or other objective) was followed by demonstration of and repeated practice with the model through role-playing (50). The training allowed residents to achieve significant mastery of new, complex, and often counterintuitive interviewing skills before they tried them with actual patients, and it was designed to foster confidence (30,51,52,52a). Supervisory sessions lasting 3 hours each took place daily and involved inpatient and outpatient interviews that were observed directly by investigators or were watched from prerecorded audiotapes. The focus of the seminar and supervisory teaching sessions was efficient data gathering, emotion-handling, patient education, and management of psychosocial and psychiatric problems common in primary care settings. Integrated throughout was a strong emphasis on the development of residents' self-awareness, as detailed elsewhere (4,41–43). We gave residents a syllabus of required readings and other materials. (Copies of these documents are available from the authors.)

Experimental Procedure

Residents were randomly assigned to receive training either during the first 6 months of postgraduate year 1 (training group) or later in postgraduate year 1 after they served as controls (control group). An effort to assign equal numbers of men and women to the training and control groups was limited by scheduling constraints. Fifteen women and 16 men (16 graduates of international schools and 15 graduates of U.S. schools) served as trainees, and 12 women and 20 men (15 international graduates and 17 U.S. graduates) served as controls. No international graduates were U.S. citizens.

Residents' interviewing skills were assessed through evaluations of audiotaped recordings of outpatient clinic visits (for all residents during all 4 years of the study) and videotaped recordings of simulated patient visits (for the final 49 residents evaluated during the last 3 years of the study). Outpatient interviews were used to assess residents' skills in information gathering only.

Adult patients were approached before clinic visits and were asked to participate in the study after being informed that the visit would be recorded and after being told about other data-gathering aspects of the study; 11% of internal patients refused to participate. Interviews and measurements, described in the following, were obtained between approximately 4 weeks before and after a resident's training rotation (or a similar period for controls). A resident interviewed different patients before and after the training or control period.

Six women and 10 men, ranging in age from the early twenties to the early seventies, served as paid trained simulated patients. Twenty-eight simulated patient scenarios were constructed to assess the three major interviewing models addressed in the training program: gathering data and establishing a relationship, managing somatization, and informing and motivating patients. Each scenario described the patient's presenting story, social and occupational background, personality, and medical history. Somatization scenarios described patients with physical symptoms for which no organic basis could be found despite thorough and repeated clinical investigations. Informing and motivating scenarios described patients who needed help in reducing a health risk, such as smoking.

Residents were instructed to interview a simulated patient as they would an actual patient; before, they were given the patient's name, age, chief problem, and pertinent history and (in the case of somatizing patients) the results of previous clinical evaluations. They received specific instructions about their interviewing task, depending on the type of patient involved. Residents were to gather information as needed with all patients, to explain symptoms, and to initiate realistic management plans when a patient presented as a somatizer. For a patient who needed to change a harmful health habit, residents were instructed to help the patient make behavioral changes.

Measurements

Attitudes We developed a 38-item questionnaire to assess the attitudes toward psychosocial skills used in medical care (26). Each questionnaire item was written in three forms to assess confidence in using the skill (self-efficacy), the perceived importance of the skill to the success of patient care (outcome expectation), and the personal commitment to using the skill (commitment). Five scales were developed for each of the three forms by using factor analysis of the self-efficacy questionnaire; the five scales addressed emotional sensitivity to patients, psychological sensitivity to patients, directive facilitation of the interview, nondirective facilitation of the interview, and recognition and management of somatizing patients. The reliability of measurement scales was estimated by computing Cronbach a coefficients of internal consistency. Coefficient values of 0.70 or more are generally considered satisfactory (53); the values obtained ranged from 0.71 to 0.91.

Knowledge We developed a 35-item multiple-choice test to assess basic knowledge of core topics in psychosocial medicine (26).

IInterviewing Skills The first 15 minutes of 238 interviews with actual patients were evaluated because we were interested in the data-gathering skills that should have been used during that time. The total interview was evaluated for simulated patient interviews (N = 349), which were limited to 15 minutes. Fifteen 11-point rating scales were developed to assess key interviewing behaviors specifically addressed in the training program. Ten items represented behaviors that were considered characteristic of effective interviewers, regardless of type of interview: encouraging patient responses; allowing the patient to talk; responding to emotions; not completely pursuing biomedical data initially; including psychosocial data initially; not dominating the interview; building rapport; tracking the patient by pursuing topics that the patient has initiated, whether psychosocial or disease-oriented; effectively managing the interview; and being patient-centered. These ten items were applied to all interviews, actual and simulated. During interviews with simulated patients, four additional rating scales were used to assess each resident's ability to provide information, to motivate behavioral change, to support patients in the achievement of health-related goals, and to manage somatizing patients (when applicable). The fifteenth scale was a rating of the overall quality of the interview. Rating scales were anchored at the upper and lower ends with examples of criterial behaviors. For example, the upper end of "encouraging patient responses" had examples such as "uses exploratory questions," "uses echoing," or "uses paraphrasing." Criteria for the lower end of this scale included such examples as "uses directive questions" and "dismisses patient's responses."

Six graduate students in communications or psychology who were experienced in research were trained to serve as raters. Rater-training materials (available from the authors) consisted of a glossary of key terms; a training manual giving examples of behaviors at four different levels of each scale, and a set of 25 scored training tapes of interviews. Two members of the research faculty rated the 25 training tapes independently. Discrepancies between scores were discussed until an agreement was reached and gold standard scores were established.

The six graduate student raters were trained in a sequence of steps: recognition of key interview behaviors, assignment of ratings to interview behaviors, review of rating assignments, correction of errors, and re-rating of interviews until agreement with gold standard ratings was reached. Training tapes were used to establish the accuracy and reliability of each rater.

After training, graduate student raters were assigned taped interviews stratified according to study group (training or control), data collection point (before or after the intervention), and interview type (actual or simulated). The purpose of stratification was to remove systematic rater biases from the study results. Raters were blinded to group assignments and data collection points.

Two graduate students independently rated each interview tape. Rater accuracy and inter-rater agreement were assessed periodically by assigning additional training tapes and comparing a rater's scores with the gold standard scores. In some instances, two raters' scores for the same tape were compared. Large deviations from comparison scores (2 points) were discussed, and rating criteria were clarified until consensus was reached in order to bring ratings within a 2-point range.

Patient Satisfaction and Well Being A patient satisfaction questionnaire developed locally (27), the General Health Questionnaire (GHQ) (54), and the Functional Health Survey (FHS) (55) were administered to the patient participants before and after a resident's rotation. Information on patient satisfaction was collected over all 4 years of the study, whereas GHQ and FHS measures were collected over the last 3 years of study; this resulted in 394 patients who contributed information on satisfaction and 203 who contributed information on health status. At each data collection point, patients completed the GHQ and FHS immediately before a medical visit and (in a telephone interview) 3 months after the visit. They completed the satisfaction questionnaire immediately after a visit. The instruments were administered to one set of patients before a resident's rotation and to a different set of patients after the rotation.

The patient satisfaction measure (27) was a 29-item questionnaire with four clearly interpretable, independent factors of satisfaction with medical interviews, as indicated by factor analysis: (a) opportunity to disclose concerns, (b) physician's empathy, (c) confidence in physician's abilities, and (d) the visit overall. Cronbach-coefficient reliability estimates for factor scale scores ranged from 0.71 to 0.89.

The GHQ (54) provided estimates of the patient's anxiety, insomnia, social dysfunction, depression, and somatic symptoms. The FHS (55) provided estimates of role limitations and physical limitations. Cronbach-coefficient reliability estimates ranged from 0.86 to 0.94 for the GHQ scales and from 0.77 and 0.79 for the two FHS scales.

Statistical Analysis

Residents had one to four interviews tape-recorded at each data collection point for each type of interview (one actual patient and three types of simulated patients). The number of patient satisfaction questionnaires that were completed for each resident varied from one to six (average, three). The number of patients completing sets of GHQ and FHS questionnaires for each resident varied from one to five (average of two) at each data collection point. Changes in the patient's health status were estimated by subtracting baseline scores from later scores. Measures obtained from patients to assess a resident were averaged at each data collection point for that resident. The scores obtained by the two raters who assessed each patient interview were also averaged. When a measure was incomplete for a resident, that measure for that resident was omitted and the data were analyzed with fewer participants.

The influence of the training program was assessed by analyses of covariance; a pretraining measure served as a covariate. Preliminary tests of models that included sex and medical education (a U.S. or international medical school) as factors showed that the effects of these influences on training were too small to be of interest. All analyses were performed with SAS software, version 6.12 (56).

Results

Knowledge and Attitudes

Knowledge of interviewing and psychosocial medicine was greater among trained than untrained residents at the end of the training period (difference in adjusted post-test mean scores, 15.7% [95% CI, 11% to 20%]).

Adjusted post-test means and differences for attitude measures are shown in Table A.1. At the end of the training period, trained residents expressed more favorable attitudes toward interviewing and psychosocial medicine than did untrained residents. The training group effect was especially clear for feelings of self-confidence (self-efficacy) with respect to performance of interviewing skills. Trained residents expressed greater confidence in their abilities to be sensitive to patients' psychological (difference, 0.61 points on a 7-point scale [CI, 0.32 to 0.91 points]) and emotional concerns (difference, 0.61 points [CI, 0.28 to 0.94 points]), to directively (difference, 0.67 points [CI, 0.33 to 1.0 points]) and nondirectively (difference, 0.55 points [CI, 0.20 to 0.91 points]) facilitate communication, and to manage somatization problems (difference, 0.99 points [CI, 0.64 to 1.35 points]).

TABLE A.1. ANALYSIS OF ATTITUDE QUESTIONNAIRES COMPLETED BY RESIDENTS

Variable	Post-Test Means*		Difference (95% CI)	P Value
	Untrained Residents (N = 26)	Trained Residents (N = 31)		
Self-efficacy				
Psychological sensitivity	4.9	5.5	0.61 (0.32 to 0.91)	<0.001
Emotional sensitivity	5.3	5.9	0.61 (0.28 to 0.94)	<0.001
Directive facilitation	5.1	5.7	0.67 (0.33 to 1.00)	<0.001
Nondirective facilitation	5.1	5.6	0.55 (0.20 to 0.91)	0.003
Somatization management	4.6	5.6	0.99 (0.64 to 1.35)	<0.001
Outcome expectation				
Psychological sensitivity	6.0	6.1	0.14 (−0.13 to 0.41)	>0.2
Emotional sensitivity	5.5	5.9	0.34 (−0.04 to 0.72)	0.075
Directive facilitation	5.7	5.8	0.18 (−0.19 to 0.54)	>0.2
Nondirective facilitation	5.3	5.7	0.42 (−0.01 to 0.84)	0.055
Somatization management	5.8	6.2	0.40 (0.06 to 0.75)	0.024
Commitment				
Psychological sensitivity	5.9	6.1	0.22 (−0.12 to 0.57)	0.195
Emotional sensitivity	5.5	5.9	0.44 (0.07 to 0.81)	0.022
Directive facilitation	5.7	5.9	0.18 (−0.17 to 0.53)	>0.2
Nondirective facilitation	5.5	5.9	0.46 (0.01 to 0.91)	0.045
Somatization management	5.6	6.2	0.57 (0.16 to 0.99)	0.008

*On a 7-point scale adjusted for pretest scores. Because of missing data, means for outcome expectation and commitment are based on a sample size of 56.

Interviewing Patients

Interview rater accuracy was evaluated by comparing ratings of training tapes with gold standard ratings, and interview rater consistency was evaluated by comparing ratings of training tapes to ratings of other raters. The mean accuracy value (absolute deviation from standard) ranged from 0.87 to 1.37

points on an 11-point scale, depending on the interview behavior. The mean inter-rater consistency value (absolute deviation between paired raters' ratings), computed in the same way, ranged from 0.70 to 0.98 points when inter-rater discrepancies were corrected and from 0.73 to 1.83 points when inter-rater discrepancies were not corrected. The results indicate acceptable levels of rater accuracy and consistency.

Means and 95% CIs for interview behaviors are shown in Tables A.2 and A.3. At the end of the training period, trained residents interviewed simulated patients and actual patients more skillfully than untrained residents did. For example, trained residents more often responded effectively with actual patients to patients' expressions of emotions (difference, 2.33 points on an 11-point scale [CI, 1.01 to 3.64 points]), with simulated patients who enacted data-gathering scenarios (difference, 3.35 points [CI, 2.31 to 4.38 points]), and with simulated patients who enacted somatization management scenarios (difference, 2.42 points [CI, 1.53 to 3.31 points]). In addition, with both actual and simulated patients, trained residents pursued psychosocial information more often, and they were more patient-centered (Tables A.2 and A.3). Differences between trained and untrained residents were clearer and more consistent in interviews with simulated patients than in interviews with

TABLE A.2. RATINGS OF RESIDENTS' DATA-GATHERING SKILLS IN INTERVIEWS WITH ACTUAL PATIENTS

Variable	Post-Test Means*		Difference (95% CI)	P Value
	Untrained Residents (N = 27)	Trained Residents (N = 28)		
Encourages responses	5.5	5.9	0.42 (−0.44 to 1.28)	<0.2
Allows talking	6.5	7.2	0.68 (−0.08 to 1.43)	0.078
Responds to emotions[†]	4.0	6.3	2.33 (1.01 to 3.64)	0.001
Pursues biomedical data	7.8	7.1	−0.73 (−1.58 to 0.11)	0.086
Pursues psychosocial data	2.6	4.6	1.94 (0.54 to 3.34)	0.008
Dominates interview	5.1	4.6	−0.44 (−0.94 to 0.05)	0.078
Builds rapport	6.2	6.7	0.51 (−0.08 to 1.10)	0.090
Tracks patient	6.2	6.8	0.61 (−0.10 to 1.31)	0.090
Manages interview	5.5	6.2	0.67 (−0.14 to 1.49)	0.104
Uses patient-centered approach	5.0	6.1	1.16 (0.30 to 2.03)	0.009
Overall rating	4.2	5.6	1.39 (0.32 to 2.45)	0.011

*On an 11-point scale adjusted for pretest scores.
[†]This item was rated only when patients mentioned an emotion that should have elicited a response. 40 participants were rated on this item.

TABLE A.3. RATINGS OF THREE TYPES OF

Variable	Untrained Residents* (N = 19)	Trained Residents* (N = 22)	Difference (95% CI)	P Value
	Data-Gathering Skills			
Encourages responses	6.0	8.5	2.54 (1.92 to 3.17)	<0.001
Allows talking	6.6	8.3	1.72 (0.94 to 2.50)	<0.001
Responds to emotions†	4.5	7.9	3.35 (2.31 to 4.38)	<0.001
Pursues biomedical data	8.3	8.5	0.16 (−0.43 to 0.76)	>0.2
Pursues psychosocial data	4.5	7.8	3.37 (1.97 to 4.76)	<0.001
Dominates interview	5.3	4.5	−0.88 (−1.33 to −0.42)	<0.001
Builds rapport	6.2	7.4	1.17 (0.63 to 1.71)	<0.001
Tracks patient	6.3	8.2	1.93 (1.07 to 2.79)	<0.001
Manages interview	6.4	7.9	1.47 (0.71 to 2.22)	<0.001
Uses patient-centered approach	5.6	8.2	2.60 (1.75 to 3.45)	<0.001
Overall rating	5.2	7.8	2.67 (1.77 to 3.56)	<0.001
Informs patient**	—	—	—	—
Motivates patient**	—	—	—	—
Willing to help**	—	—	—	—
Manages somatization	—	—	—	—

*Values given are post-test means on an 11-point scale adjusted for pretest scores.
†This item was rated only when patients mentioned an emotion: thus, 39 residents were rated for this item on data-gathering skills: 17 were rated for this item on informing and motivating skills; and 32 were rated for this item on managing somatization skills.
**Only 26 residents were rated for this item because of missing data.

actual patients. Ratings of overall interview quality were higher for trained residents with actual patients (difference, 1.39 points on an 11-point scale [CI, 0.32 to 2.45 points]), in data gathering with simulated patients (difference, 2. 67 points [CI, 1.77 to 3.56 points]), in informing and motivating patients (difference, 1.73 points [CI, 0.63 to 2.83 points]), and in managing somatization (difference, 2.75 points [CI, 1.65 to 3.86 points]). Trained residents were not expected to pursue biomedical data more often than untrained residents, and no statistically significant difference was seen for this variable.

Patient Satisfaction and Well Being

Patients seen by trained residents after the training period expressed slightly greater satisfaction with medical visits than did the patients seen by untrained residents, and they had greater measured physical and psychological well being. However, the differences were too small to be statistically or practically

INTERVIEWING SKILLS WITH SIMULATED PATIENTS

Informing and Motivating Skills				Managing Somatization Skills			
Untrained Residents* (N = 14)	Trained Residents* (N = 13)	Difference (95% CI)	P Value	Untrained Residents* (N = 18)	Trained Residents* (N = 15)	Difference (95% CI)	P Value
5.7	6.7	1.00 (0.03 to 1.98)	0.045	6.2	7.5	1.29 (0.38 to 2.20)	0.007
6.4	6.8	0.38 (−0.45 to 1.22)	>0.2	6.3	7.4	1.13 (0.40 to 1.86)	0.004
5.3	5.9	0.61 (−0.64 to 1.86)	>0.2	5.2	7.6	2.42 (1.53 to 3.31)	<0.001
6.6	6.4	−0.20 (−2.31 to 1.89)	>0.2	7.0	6.0	−0.97 (−2.21 to 0.27)	0.12
4.5	3.9	−0.59 (−2.97 to 1.78)	>0.2	6.4	6.9	0.51 (−0.88 to 1.91)	>0.2
5.9	5.2	−0.68 (−0.04 to −1.32)	0.039	5.3	5.2	−0.08 (−0.72 to 0.56)	>0.2
6.4	7.1	0.73 (0.06 to 1.39)	0.034	6.3	7.5	1.22 (0.47 to 1.98)	0.002
6.6	7.6	0.95 (0.12 to 1.78)	0.027	6.2	7.9	1.65 (0.79 to 2.51)	0.001
6.1	7.3	1.24 (−0.09 to 2.57)	0.066	6.0	7.5	1.59 (0.53 to 2.54)	0.005
5.7	6.7	1.03 (−0.19 to 2.24)	0.094	6.1	7.8	1.69 (0.64 to 2.74)	0.003
5.6	7.3	1.73 (0.63 to 2.83)	0.004	5.0	7.7	2.75 (1.65 to 3.86)	<0.001
5.9	7.5	1.56 (0.30 to 2.82)	0.018	—	—	—	—
5.0	7.7	2.65 (1.17 to 4.13)	0.001	—	—	—	—
5.1	7.4	2.35 (0.94 to 3.76)	0.002	—	—	—	—
—	—	—	—	2.2	6.0	3.80(1.80 to 5.81)	0.001

significant. For example, on the patient satisfaction scale, patients of trained residents were only slightly different from those of untrained residents with respect to confidence in the physician (difference, 0.13 points on a 5-point scale [CI, 0.05 to 0.30 points]) or general satisfaction (difference, 0.13 points [CI, 0.07 to 0.33 points]). Similarly, on the GHQ, the greatest difference seen between trained and untrained residents (possible range, +3 to -3) occurred with somatic symptoms and was miniscule (difference, 0.16 points on a 7-point scale [CI, 0.06 to 0.386 points]) (P = 0.14).

Discussion

Use of a randomized, controlled study design enabled us to distinguish the effects specific to training, from the more general effects of residency training (57). Trained residents, whom we believe were representative of a primary-care resident population, improved in knowledge about, in positive attitudes toward, in self-confidence in, and in skills in interviewing patients; in dealing with physician–patient relationships; in managing somatization; and in educating patients. Data on our secondary hypotheses about the effects of residents' training on patient outcomes, although consistently in the predicted direction, were not statistically significant.

Four findings suggest that the data on gains in interviewing skills have considerable generalizability. First, gains occurred in both male and female residents. Second, gains were unrelated to whether the resident was a graduate of a U.S. or international medical school. Third, gains were seen in interviews of both actual and simulated patients. Fourth, gains occurred in three different kinds of interviews with simulated patients: data gathering and establishing a relationship, informing and motivating patients, and managing somatization.

Not surprisingly, the mean scores with actual patients were lower than the mean scores with simulated patients. Not only was a performance factor (desire to do well in a situation specifically designed for testing) likely to be operational with the simulated patients, but also more control was possible. Simulated patients were specifically trained to present residents with an opportunity to perform all aspects of the interviewing models and to test the residents' maximal skill levels. Actual patient interviews provided a sense of what was used in addition to how well it was used. Because actual patients were usually residents' own patients, more variation was present in the amount of information already known by the resident and in the reasons for the medical visit. The fact that responding to emotions, eliciting psychosocial data, and being patient-centered were the strongest effects with actual patients suggests that importance was attached to these skills and that they were valued and used. This is especially gratifying because these skills are central to establishing relationships with patients.

Unfortunately, considerations of cost and imposition on residents' time precluded our ability to obtain quantitative follow-up data on skill use. However, an extensive qualitative evaluation of the long-range effect of our training, conducted by one of the authors, showed that the value of interviewing skills to residents and the use of these skills by residents increased during the 3 to 5 years after training (58).

One limitation of our study was its low power to detect the effects of residents' training on their patients. Scatterplots indicated that residents' patients were not very emotionally distressed or physically limited; this may have contributed to the failure to show much effect on patient outcomes. A second factor that weakened the evaluation of training effects on patients was the tendency of patients to rate their satisfaction with nearly all physicians as very high; this may have resulted from self-selection. Another limitation was that our satisfaction measures concerned only physician–patient factors; therefore, they may have missed other determinants of satisfaction, such as the convenience of appointments, waiting times, and parking (a "halo effect"). The generalizability of the study was additionally limited because measures of residents' learning were obtained in situations in which the residents knew that they were being studied and that their patients were being assessed, which could have enhanced their performance. In addition, data collection was incomplete for some measures for several reasons, none of which could be expected to bias the results. For some measures, data collection began some time after the start of study. In other instances, patients could not be recruited at both data-collection points for a particular resident, patients or residents failed to fill out questionnaires, scorable events did not appear in a particular resident's simulated patient interview, or scheduling a simulated patient interview for a resident was impossible. Finally, some "contamination" of controls by trained residents undoubtedly occurred and could have reduced the observed effects of training.

Reports of others' experience with this model of interview training are needed. Evaluation of other forms of intensive training, such as training for an equal number of hours distributed over an entire year rather than 1 month, also merits consideration. We believe that the interviewing models and other material can be easily adapted to longer training periods. We also propose that the basic patient-centered (and physician–patient relationship-centered) interviewing model was the major factor producing our positive results. As the most important and proximate skill, it received, by far, the most attention and was also integrated into the other models. For programs with less time available for teaching interviewing, the data support a focus restricted to the basic patient-centered interviewing model. Because, in many respects, the expertise expected of residents is similar to that of other learners in patient-centered interviewing, the study provides a basic data-based patient-centered interviewing model for students, faculty, and persons in continuing medical education. Study of each group, however, is needed to confirm this. In addition, we discourage an isolated focus on models other than the basic model unless learners have previously demonstrated mastery of basic patient-centered interviewing.

McWhinney, Engel, Feinstein, and others (59–68) have argued that if medicine is to advance as a unique science, clinicians must take the lead and must redefine the science of medicine around the personhood of the individual patient. To accomplish this, we are challenged to develop better methods and better models. Inui and Carter (57) make the following assertion explicit: to be successful, these methods and models must have a solid empirical base.

Our study, building on recent advances (59,60,69–74), shows that patient-centered methods of interviewing (described by the models) can be made behaviorally specific, systematic, user-friendly, and efficient. As we disseminate more refined and consistent patient-centered clinical methods, we can encourage the personhood of the individual patient to reemerge in clinical medicine. We will thus increase the applicability and the utility of working concepts, such as the biopsychosocial model (61,75), that integrate determinants of health and disease extending from molecular to physiological to psychological to societal. We can better operationalize these concepts by addressing more explicitly the processes by which they are identified and through which they operate. In so doing, we face formidable challenges. This study, by providing data-based interviewing models, is one attempt to shift the paradigm of medicine in the desired direction (61,75,76).

Acknowledgments

The authors thank the Fetzer Institute in Kalamazoo, Michigan; the biopsychosocial programs at the University of Rochester; and the American Academy on Physician and Patient. They also thank the medical school deans; department chairs in medicine, psychiatry, and family practice; program directors in medicine and family practice; general internal medicine division chiefs; and residents at Michigan State University. This work was supported by a grant from the Fetzer Institute, Kalamazoo, Michigan.

References

1. Lipkin M Jr. The medical interview as core clinical skill: the problem and the opportunity. *Gen Intern Med* 1987;2:363–365.
2. Stoeckle JD, Billings JA. A history of history-taking: the medical interview. *J Gen Intern Med* 1987;2:119–127.
3. Davidoff F. Medical interviewing: the crucial skill that gets short shrift. In: Davidoff F. *Who has seen a blood sugar? Reflections on medical education.* Philadelphia: American College of Physicians, 1996:76–80.
4. Smith RC. *The patient's story: integrated patient-doctor interviewing.* Boston: Little, Brown and Company, 1996.

5. Peterson MC, Holbrook JH, Von Hales D, et al. Contributions of the history, physical examination, and laboratory investigation in making medical diagnoses. *West J Med* 1992;156:163–165.

6. Schmitt BP, Kushner MS, Wiener SL. The diagnostic usefulness of the history of the patient with dyspnea. *J Gen Intern Med* 1986;1:386–393.

7. Hampton JR, Harrison MJ, Mitchell JR, et al. Relative contributions of history-taking, physical examination, and laboratory investigation to diagnosis and management of medical outpatients. *Br Med J* 1975;2:486–489.

8. Linfors EW, Neelon FA. Interrogation and interview: strategies for obtaining clinical data. *J Roy Coll Gen Pract* 1981;31:426–428.

9. Smith RC, Hoppe RB. The patient's story integrating the patient- and physician-centered approaches to interviewing. *Ann Intern Med* 1991;115:470–477.

10. Watzlawick P, Beavin JH, Jackson DD. *Pragmatics of human communication: a study of interactional patterns, pathologies, and paradoxes.* New York: WW Norton, 1967.

11. Foss L, Rothenberg K. *The second medical revolution: from biomedicine to infomedicine.* Boston: New Science Library, 1987.

12. Novack DH, Volk G, Drossman DA, et al. Medical interviewing and interpersonal skills teaching in US medical schools. Progress, problems, and promise. *JAMA* 1993;269:2101–2105.

13. Smith RC, Marshall AA, Cohen Cole SA. The efficacy of intensive biopsychosocial teaching programs for residents: a review of the literature and guidelines for teaching. *J Gen Intern Med* 1994;9:390–396.

14. Merkel WT, Margolis RB, Smith RC. Teaching humanistic and psychosocial aspects of care: current practices and attitudes. *J Gen Intern Med* 1990;5:34–41.

15. Burns BJ, Scott JE, Burke JD Jr, et al. Mental health training of primary care residents: a review of recent literature (1974–1981). *Gen Hosp Psychiatry* 1983;5:157–169.

16. Strain JJ, George LK, Pincus HA, et al. Models of mental health training for primary care physicians. *Psychosom Med* 1985;47:95–110.

17. Merkel WT, Nierenberg BP. Behavioral science training in family practice residency education: a first evaluation. *Soc Sci Med* 1983;17:213–217.

18. Breunlin DC, Richman JS, Lattimer A. An evaluation strategy for behavioral pediatrics training. *Fam Syst Med* 1990;8:48–56.

19. Roter DL, Cole KA, Kern DE, et al. An evaluation of residency training in interviewing skills and the psychosocial domain of medical practice. *J Gen Intern Med* 1990;5:347–354.

20. Smith RC, Osborn G, Hoppe RB, et al. Efficacy of a one month training block in psychosocial medicine for residents: a controlled study. *J Gen Intern Med* 1991;6:535–543.

21. Strain JJ, Pincus HA, Gise LH, et al. Mental health education in three primary care specialties. *J Med Educ* 1986;61:958–966.

22. Williamson PR, Smith RC, Kern DE, et al. The medical interview and psychosocial aspects of medicine: block curricula for residents. *J Gen Intern Med* 1992;7:235–242.

23. Novack OH, Goldberg RJ, Rowland Morin P, et al. Toward a comprehensive psychiatry/behavioral science curriculum for primary care residents. *Psychosomatics* 1989;30:213–223.

24. Thompson TL 2nd, Stoudemire A, Mitchell WD. Effects of a psychiatric liaison program on internists' ability to assist psychosocial problems. *Int J Psychiatry Med* 1982—1983;12:153–160.

25. Schubert DS, Billowitz A, Gabinet L, et al. Effect of liaison psychiatry, rate of consultation, and psychosocial documentation. *Gen Hosp Psychiatry* 1989; 11:77–87.

26. Smith RC, Metter JA, Stoffelmayr BE, et al. Improving residents' confidence in using psychosocial skills. *J Gen Intern Med* 1995;10:315–320.

27. Smith RC, Lyles JS, Mettler JA, et al. A strategy for improving patient satisfaction by the intensive training of residents in psychosocial medicine: a controlled, randomized study. *Acad Med* 1995;70:729–732.

28. Houpt JL, Weinstein HM, Russell ML. The application of competency-based education to consultation-liaison psychiatry. *Int J Psychiatry Med* 1976;7:295–328.

29. Knowles MS. *The modern practice of adult education: from pedagogy to andragogy*. New York: The Adult Education Company, 1980.

30. McKeachie WJ, Pintrich PR, Lin Y, et al. *Teaching and learning in the college classroom*, 2nd ed. Ann Arbor, MI: Regents of the University of Michigan, 1990.

31. Lipkin M, Putnam SM, Lazare A, eds. *The medical interview: clinical care, education, and research*. New York: Springer-Verlag, 1995.

32. Smith RC. A clinical approach to the somatizing patient. *J Fam Pract* 1985;21:294–301.

33. Smith RC. Somatization disorder: defining its role in clinical medicine. *J Gen Intern Med* 1991;6:168–175.

34. Stoffelmayr B, Hoppe RB, Weber N. Facilitating patient participation: the doctor-patient encounter. *Primary Care* 1989;16:265–278.

35. Grueninger UJ, Duffy FD, Goldstein MG. Patient education in the medical encounter: how to facilitate learning, behavior change, and coping. In: Lipkin M, Putnam SM, Lazare A, eds. *The medical interview: clinical care, education, and research*. New York: Springer-Verlag, 1995:122–133.

36. Williams GC, Quill TE, Deci EL, et al. "The facts concerning the recent carnival of smoking in Connecticut" and elsewhere. *Ann Intern Med* 1991;115:59–63.

37. Waitzkin H. Information giving in medical care. *J Health Soc Behav* 1985;26:81–101.

38. Waitzkin H. Doctor–patient communication. Clinical implications of social scientific research. *JAMA* 1984;252:2441–2446.

39. Prochaska JO, Di Clemente CC. Towards a comprehensive model of change. In: Miller WR, Heather N, eds. *Treating addictive behaviors: processes of change*. New York: Plenum, 1986:3–27.

39a.Vispoel WP, Chen P. Measuring self-efficacy: the state of the art. Paper presented at annual meeting of the American Educational Research Association. Boston. 1990.

40. Quill TE, Townsend P. Bad news: delivery, dialogue, and dilemmas. *Arch Intern Med* 1991;151:463–468.

41. Smith RC. Use and management of physicians' feelings during the interview. In Lipkin M, Putnam SM, Lazare A, eds. *The medical interview: clinical care, education, and research.* New York: Springer-Verlag, 1995:104–109.

42. Smith RC. *Teaching supplement for the patient's story: integrated patient-doctor interviewing.* East Lansing, MI: Michigan State University, 1996.

43. Marshall AA, Smith RC. Physicians' emotional reactions to patients: recognizing and managing countertransference. *Am J Gastroenterol* 1995;90:4–8.

44. Andreason NC, Black DW. *Introductory textbook of psychiatry.* Washington, D.C.: American Psychiatric Press, 1991.

45. American Psychiatric Association. *Diagnostic and statistical manual of mental disorders: DSM-III-R,* 3rd ed. Washington, D.C.: American Psychiatric Association, 1987.

46. Depression Guideline Panel. *Depression in primary care.* Vol. 1. *Detection and diagnosis.* Rockville, MD: U.S. Dept of Health and Human Services, 1993. AHCPR publication no. 93-0550.

47. National Institute of Mental Health. *Panic disorder in the medical setting.* Rockville, MD: U.S. Dept of Health and Human Services. Public Health Service. Alcohol, Drug Abuse, and Mental Health Administration, National Institute of Mental Health, 1989. DHHS publication no. (ADM) 89-1629.

48. Folstein MF, Folstein PR. "Mini-mental state." A practical method for grading the cognitive state of patients for the clinician. *J Psychiatr Res* 1975;12:189–198.

49. Depression Guideline Panel. *Depression in primary care.* Vol. 2. *Treatment of major depression.* Rockville, MD: U.S. Dept of Health and Human Services, Public Health Service, Agency for Health Care Policy and Research, 1993.

50. Simpson MA. How to use role-play in medical teaching. *Med Teach* 1985;7:75–82.

51. Bandura A. Self-efficacy: toward a unifying theory of behavioral change. *Psychol Rev* 1977;84:191–215.

52. Schunk DH. Self-efficacy and classroom learning. *Psychol Schools* 1985; 22:208–223.

52a.Tresolini CP, Stritter FT. Medical students' development of self-efficacy in conducting patient education for health promotion: an analysis of learning experiences. Paper presented at the annual meeting of the American Educational Research Association. San Francisco. 1992.

53. Nunnally JC. *Psychometric theory.* New York: McGraw-Hill, 1978.

54. Goldberg DP, Hillier VF. A scaled version of the General Health Questionnaire. *Psychol Med* 1979;9:139–145.

55. Greenfield S, Kaplan S, Ware JE Jr. Expanding patient involvement in care. Effects on patient outcomes. *Ann Intern Med* 1985;102:520–528.

56. *SAS/STAT users guide,* 4th ed, version 6. Cary, NC: SAS Institute, 1989.

57. Inui TS, Carter WB. Problems and prospects for health services research on provider-patient communication. *Med Care* 1985;23:521–538.

58. Lyles J. *An examination of the long-term effects of psychosocial teaching on the practice of medicine.* [thesis] East Lansing, MI: Michigan State University, 1996.

59. McWhinney I. The need for a transformed clinical method. In: Stewart M, Roter D, eds. *Communicating with medical patients.* London: Sage, 1989:25–42.

60. McWhinney I. *An introduction to family medicine.* New York: Oxford University Press, 1981.

61. Engel GL. The need for a new medical model: a challenge for biomedicine. *Science* 1977;196:129–136.

62. Engel GL. The care of the patient: art or science? *Johns Hopkins Med J* 1977;140:222–232.

63. Engel GL. Physician-scientists and scientific physicians. Resolving the humanism-science dichotomy. *Am J Med* 1987;82:107–111.

64. Feinstein AR. The intellectual crisis in clinical science: medaled models and muddle mettle. *Perspect Biol Med* 1987;30:215–230.

65. Feinstein AR. An additional basic science for clinical medicine. I. The constraining fundamental paradigms. *Ann Intern Med* 1983;99:393–397.

66. Feinstein AR. An additional basic science for clinical medicine. II. The limitations of randomized trials. *Ann Intern Med* 1983;99:544–550.

67. Feinstein AR. An additional basic science for clinical medicine. III. The challenges of comparison and measurement. *Ann Intern Med* 1983;99:705–712.

68. Feinstein AR. An additional basic science for clinical medicine. IV. The development of clinimetrics. *Ann Intern Med* 1983;99:843–848.

69. Lazare A, Eisenthal S, Wasserman L. The customer approach to patienthood. Attending to patient requests in a walk-in clinic. *Arch Gen Psychiatry* 1975;32:552–558.

70. Levenstein JH, McCracken EC, McWhinney IR, et al. The patient-centered clinical method. 1. A model for the doctor-patient interaction in family medicine. *Fam Pract* 1986;3:24–30.

71. Levenstein JH, Brown JB, Weston WW, et al., eds. *Communicating with medical patients.* London: Sage, 1989.

72. Rogers CR. *Client-centered therapy: its current practice, implications, and theory.* Boston: Houghton Mifflin, 1951.

73. Lipp MR. *Respectful treatment the human side of medical care.* Hagerstown, MD: Harper & Row, 1977.

74. Lipkin M Jr, Quill TE, Napodano RJ. The medical interview: a core curriculum for residencies in internal medicine. *Ann Intern Med* 1984;100:277–284.

75. Engel GL. The clinical application of the biopsychosocial model. *Am J Psychiatry* 1980;137:535–544.

76. Kuhn TS. *The structure of scientific revolutions,* 2nd ed. Chicago: University of Chicago Press, 1962.

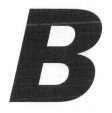 Foreword to the First Edition

Being Scientific in the Human Domain: From Biomedical to Biopsychosocial

> We include as biology not only the data obtained by observing other individuals and things but also those that we reach through [our own inner experiences of living].
> The biologist is himself of the same material of which are composed the living things that he studies.
>
> H.S. Jennings, 1933

Biologist Herbert Spencer Jennings' early insistence that "inner experiences" are proper data for biology was my first encounter with the idea that the use of subjective data need not violate the conventional requirement for scientific respectability. Quite by chance, in 1937 as a college student, I had stumbled on Jennings' *Behavior of the Lower Organisms* (1). As a biologist, Jennings deemed his inner experience as a living organism no less integral for understanding living systems than his outward observations that were customarily relied on for information about the physical (nonliving) universe. However, some 20 years would pass before the complementarity of outer observation and inner experiencing fully took hold for me as a physician and helped me define the requirements for being scientific in the human domain (2–9).

As a profession and an institution, medicine owes its origin to three distinctively human attributes. First, we humans are aware of death and its inevitability and we realize that feeling and/or looking bad ("sick") may be its portent. Second, we suffer when our interpersonal bonds are sundered and we feel solace when they are reestablished. Third, we are capable of examining our own inner life and experience and of communicating them to others via a spoken and written language. Critical for all three and for the work of the physician is the distinctively human capability of using words to communicate both what is being observed in the outer world, as well as what is being experienced within the inner world. For each of us the distinction between sick and well is preeminently manifest as inner experience, which must be communicated verbally in characteristic ways to become known. *Surely, as scientists dedicated to organizing our experiences and formulating observations, we should be careful to define science in such a way as to be able to include verbal reporting as legitimate data.*

From *biomedical* to *biopsychosocial* refers to an historical transition in scientific thinking that has been taking place over the past century and a half (6). Particularly pertinent for medicine is its explicit attention to *humanness*. That alone identifies biopsychosocial as a more complete and inclusive conceptual framework for guiding clinicians in their everyday work with patients. Physicians have always depended on what patients have been able to tell them about the experiences that led them to seek medical attention. This is testimony that the importance of verbal exchange between patient and physician is the primary source of the data required for the clinician's task. Scientists studying sick, diseased, or even dying animals or plants do not have a comparable resource; they are limited to what can be observed, as are all scientists dealing with physical or infrahuman systems.

That we humans are able to participate actively in our own study by looking inward and by contributing information that is otherwise not available should be a great scientific advantage. Yet, paradoxically, biomedical thinking, a 20th-century derivative of 17th-century natural science, categorically excludes from science what patients have to tell us on the grounds that it is nonmaterial in form and not measurable or subjective and not objective. On those grounds alone even posing such a question is axiomatically disallowed. Instead, the human domain as a whole is seen as the art of medicine, subject neither to systematic inquiry nor to the possibility of teaching.

However, the history of medicine as far back as the papyri of Egypt of 5 millennia ago documents that information provided by patients was deemed sufficiently valuable to justify writing ways that doctors might improve their skills in eliciting such (10). Paradoxically, its exclusion from medicine by medicine's science notwithstanding, few clinicians would seriously argue that what patients tell us can therefore simply be disregarded. Rather, the issue hinges on what has become a cultural imperative of western society, namely, that the canons of science as defined in the 17th century continue to apply. The possibility that the premise itself is a fallacy is simply ignored. This is what we now examine.

> *What we observe is not nature itself but nature exposed to our method of questioning.*
>
> *W. Heisenberg (11)*

Physicist Heisenberg's dictum exemplifies a fundamental distinction between 17th- and 20th-century scientific thinking, the latter of which is derived from such conceptual developments as evolution, relativity, quantum mechanics, general systems theory, far-from-equilibrium thermodynamics, and, more recently, chaos and complexity theory. Loosely speaking, we are applying biomedical and biopsychosocial as labels to contrast the two positions (8).

Actually, what Heisenberg enunciates is what clinicians have known from time immemorial—namely, that the answers you get from a patient depend on the questions you pose and how you do so. More broadly, it exposes the fallacy of the 17th-century natural science position that what scientists discover exists entirely external to and independent of themselves. In fact, rather than simply examining or observing something "out there," scientists devise mental constructs of their experiences with the observed as a means of characterizing their understanding of its properties and behavior. This change in perspective began in physics with relativity theory, which required acknowledgment that the location of the observer cannot be ignored relative to what is being observed. The rediscovery of the obvious occurred in that transformation—namely, that science itself is a human activity. The lesson is that humanness and human phenomena cannot be excluded from science. Medicine's long history of successful utilization of what patients have to say about their experience of illness itself surely suffices to justify reviving earlier efforts at developing more systematic (i.e., scientific) approaches to so doing.

It is important to ask questions of patients because with the help of these questions one will know more exactly some of the things that concern disease and one will treat the disease better.

Rufus of Ephesus, 1,000 A.D. (12)

The first formal document solely about the value of the information patients can provide is credited to Rufus of Ephesus. Surely, his words "will know more exactly" eloquently reveal his advocacy of an approach more scientific than those solely dependent on chance, fate, magic, or mysticism that were so commonplace in those days and that are still evident today in some instances of so-called alternative medicine. Rufus thereby revealed his intuitive awareness that the very universality of sickness and death as human experiences rendered the patient a logical source of primary data.

The sick person's appeals for help and the helping responses evoked thereby already reflect a biologic social interdependency with a long evolutionary history, which, in humans, was evident early in the response to the crying of an infant. In that biologic constellation are already suggested the origins not just of sick role behavior but also of the profession's and institution's responses thereto. What originated in infancy as nonspecific cries of distress are eventually differentiated to include personal and social awareness of being sick as a distinctive category of distress. Similarly, what may have begun merely as helping responses comes to oblige the helper to differentiate sickness from other types of distress. The mother's inquiry of her child as "What's wrong?" or "Are you feeling all right?" can hardly result from anything other than learning by living and experiencing; she has already gone through the same steps in growing up, as have most of us.

Intuitively, doctors tend to take such lay opinions seriously if for no other reason than that they often do prove to be correct. But such judgments by physicians are still mainly extensions of natural reactions with which we all have grown up. They are not yet scientifically based. Biopsychosocial thinking aims to provide a conceptual framework suitable for developing a scientific approach to what patients have to tell us about their illness experiences. But to accommodate the human domain, *science* and *being scientific* must be redefined.

> *The object of science is to render as reliable as possible whatever claims to knowledge we make... [and is achieved] by reasoned efforts that ultimately depend on evidence that can be consensually validated.*
>
> *Charles E. Odegaard, 1986 (13)*

Historian Odegaard's succinct statement may be viewed as an effort to provide a more generic definition of science and being scientific, one that is independent of domain or method. With respect to the patient's verbal report of an illness experience and the doctor's version thereof, both constitute claims to knowledge about what each believes he or she knows about what has happened and about what the patient's experiences were like. These constitute the data on which the doctor depends for further study and decision making. Doing so scientifically requires the discipline to enhance the reliability of the very process of data acquisition itself.

To explore scientific acquisition of verbal data, we can exploit the fact that every reader has surely experienced falling ill. I propose that readers pause and mentally reconstruct a recent occurrence of not feeling well, no matter how trivial, just as one might in anticipation of seeing her or his physician. I will do the same; but please do not look at my account until you are satisfied that what you have put together really represents what you think you would want to share with your own doctor. Our respective offerings may then be examined to see how useful Odegaard's generic definition may be for the scientific handling of what patients tell us about feeling ill. You might find it worthwhile to put your thoughts in writing as I do now.

I had another of those unpleasant episodes last night. I awakened early, about 5 A.M., feeling vaguely uncomfortable. Then gradually I became aware of a steady, annoying sensation in my throat, a familiar recurring experience awakening me from sleep. The sensation is hard to describe—it is clearly located at the level of the suprasternal notch, I can indicate it with my fingers, as a "full" feeling, as though somehow being stretched; slightly achy, steady; a little lump, a little sore in the throat.

I wanted very much to sleep longer and hence tried to ignore it, but it was in vain. Then I realized I had slipped down from the semiupright position and was lying flat, my head raised but slightly against a pillow. From past episodes I had learned the mitigating effects of sleeping semiupright. I immediately sat up, swung around and, leaning forward slightly, lowered my legs to the floor. In a minute or so, I belched with prompt relief. I lay back against the pillows, propped up at about a 70-degree angle, hoping I might now be able to sleep. But the unpleasant sensation soon returned. Determined to get more sleep, I did the next thing that usually helps; I got up and, while standing and moving about, drank a few swallows of hot water. Soon came the first of three belches and again prompt relief.

Confident that I would enjoy another couple of hours of sleep, I returned to bed, again propped up. I awakened symptom-free, but feeling a little sad, remembering how in the past when my wife had noticed I had slid down, she would try to help me get repositioned before symptoms developed. She has been in a nursing home for more than a year.

From this representative sample of human (patient-derived) data, however idiosyncratic, how may its acquisition and processing be rendered as scientific as possible?

[The scientist] devises mental constructs of his experiences with [nature] as a means of characterizing his understanding of its properties and behavior. . . [They, in turn,] are predominantly communicated by language, it being difficult

> *to communicate them in any other way than by speaking about them.*
>
> M. Delbruck, 1986 (14)

> *The whole of science is nothing more than a refinement of everyday thinking.*
>
> A. Einstein, 1950 (15)

The raw data patients proffer are in the form of speech, gesture, and posture and not much else; that is, they are bits of distinctively human behavior, verbal and nonverbal. Physicists Delbruck and Einstein remind us of two things: that 20th-century conceptual transformations render self-evident the dependence of *science* and *being scientific* on a spoken and written language and that the efforts of the person feeling sick to figure out what is happening call on the same mental operations humans ordinarily employ whenever confronted with threats to their sense of well-being. But in contrast to the distress evoked by threatening external events or circumstances, feeling sick and falling ill more often begin as private experiences that are not necessarily apparent to anyone else. Hence, the truly scientific physician not only must access that private world but also must be reasonably assured that the information (data) can be relied on. Critical is the recognition that the patient is both an initiator and a collaborator in the process, not merely an object of study. The physician in turn is a participant–observer who in the process of attending to the patient's reporting of inner-world data taps into his or her own personal inner-viewing system for comparison and clarification. The medium is dialog, which at various levels includes communing (sharing experiences), as well as communicating (exchanging information). Hence, *observation* (outer viewing), *introspection* (inner viewing), and *dialog* (interviewing) are the basic methodologic triad for clinical study and for rendering patient data scientific (9).

My written account of illness provides an opportunity to examine a patient's inner viewing that has not yet been influenced either by the physical presence of or by dialog with the doctor. It derives both from what I literally strove to remember and to reconstruct from what I had experienced a couple of hours earlier, as well as from much else that came into my mind in the course of so doing. The actual written material available to the reader, however, is already limited by the fact that I am obliged to convey that information not only in words but also in writing and in a textbook to boot. Moreover, you have no means to ascertain on what basis my final words were selected from the myriad of associations with which I was bombarded in the process of writing it. Clearly, this process is very different from what would have gone on in my head were I seated in the doctor's waiting room rehearsing what I would want to tell her or him.

Such a state of affairs at once identifies long-known barriers to being scientific in the handling of human (patient-derived) clinical data. Painfully evident is the fact that what can be communicated of such data to others is limited both by the frailty of human memory and by the constraints imposed by the requirement to convey in words actual experiences for which suitable words may not exist. Gaps are inevitable between what patients experience and what they can effectively communicate to the doctor; between the words of the patient and what the doctor remembers and may select as relevant; and ultimately between the preceding and what the doctor reports orally or writes in the record, which is the public data available for clinical reasoning.

Yet, the fact remains that, notwithstanding such formidable obstacles, experienced clinicians using observation, introspection, and dialog can be remarkably successful in documenting the existence of explicit pathologic bodily processes and of associated nondisease issues as first inferred simply from what the patient had to say. Thus, a clinician knowledgeable about physiology surely would quickly consider problems with the esophagus as one plausible explanation for the attacks I described and would accordingly pursue appropriate inquiries to test such an hypothesis (16). Moreover, the experienced clinician would recognize the interrelationship of my disease process and my personal life. Consider, for example, how my sadness about my wife's incapacity might affect my esophageal symptoms; for example, they might be worse since she went to the nursing home.

Biomedical education has an *a priori* assumption that such patient-derived data and the means of their acquisition are neither teachable nor subject to systematic study, which needs to be examined. To do so let us consider two dimensions of such data by again using my case protocol.

> [The] relationship between doctor and patient partakes of a peculiar intimacy presuppos[ing] on the part of the physician, not only knowledge of his fellow man, but sympathy... [D]esignated as the art [of medicine] . . . [intimacy], should most properly be called [its] essence.
>
> W.T. Longcope, 1932 (17)

> [The] widened, vicarious experience [provided by] narrative is memorable precisely because it is necessarily enmeshed with past and future, cause and consequence.
>
> [Patients'] life stories cultivate . . . interest in their oddities and their ordinariness and a tolerance of both.
>
> The narrative in each case belongs to a human being who is an object of scientific study and to that person's world of lived experience and belief. . . . [It] remains central to knowledge in medicine [precisely] because the patient is the focus.
>
> K.M. Hunter, 1991 (18)

Odegaard proposed defining *science* as independent of domain (13). But a universal requirement for being scientific is that we understand and respect the natural state of whatever domain we are concerned with. Thus, just as marine biologists must master functioning underwater to study marine life scientifically, so too must clinicians accommodate to what is distinctive about the human condition and the environment of patients. And what is more distinctive about being human than how we communicate and interact?

In effect, Longcope's "intimacy" refers to a unique quality of the doctor's relationship with the patient, one that he felt was so indispensable that medicine "would cease to be" medicine without it. Where in my protocol, if anywhere, does *intimacy* reveal itself? I, in my anticipation of meeting with my doctor, deliberately included one item that, on the face of it, would seem to contribute little or nothing to his understanding of the symptom complex that I was struggling to make clear to him. (Actually, it did contribute something, as I already mentioned.) It was my reference to my wife's residence in a nursing home. His response to that intensely personal and poignant item would, I anticipated, give a clue as to where we stood with each other, whether my confidence in our *intimacy* was shared by him.

By the same token, while imagining myself telling my doctor what I had just gone through, my recollections quite naturally took on a narrative form, as my story. That is, after all, how we humans ordinarily communicate our experiences to others, especially to those to whom we would turn for help. As Hunter reminds us, narrative style facilitates vicarious participation of the listener in whatever the patient was or is experiencing. That, in itself, implies an element of intimacy between the two participants and helps direct attention to what is distinctive about the individual whose story is unfolding.

Readers need only review their own experiences with doctors taking their histories to appreciate the difference between encouraging narration and requiring reporting. The latter approach is deliberately interrogative with the doctor assuming the initiative and agenda and the patient as an object of study rather than an active participant in his own study. Eighteen seconds has been reported as the mean length of time that elapses before doctors interrupt the patient's first response (19). Small wonder that patients complain that doctors do not listen. Interrogation generates defensiveness; narration encourages intimacy.

Do the words intimacy and narration refer to phenomena about which consensual agreement with regard to criteria can be achieved? The answer to that question is key to whether the concepts that the words express fall within the scope of science. The history of science is a record of repeatedly rendering the tacit manifest, the difficult easy, and the impossible possible. We all agree the answer to our question is difficult for many reasons that have already been cited. Others insist that the very consideration of such questions in medical matters is impossible. But surprise is also characteristic of science—the unexpected, sudden discovery or technologic development in one field that fosters a corresponding progress in another.

> ...[R]ejoice in the discovery of a great and final instrument of drama [one], which all the other arts have had since time immemorial, which the oldest art, the theatre, lacked until today; . . . [an] instrument that gives it precision and scientific serenity.
>
> R. Boleslavsky, 1933 (20)

What discovery could be so important to a noted stage director and teacher of acting to inspire him to announce it as finally providing the theater "precision and scientific serenity?" Astonishingly, Boleslavsky awarded that high honor to the newly introduced "talkie" motion pictures, which at that very moment were being ridiculed by traditional theatre as an outrageous degradation of the stage and its art for purely commercial purposes. For Boleslavsky films finally made possible the preservation of the art of the actor and of the theatre. "Do you realize," he passionately exclaimed, "that with the invention of spontaneous recording of the image, movement, and voice, and consequently of the personality and soul of an actor, the theatre is no more a passing affair but an eternal record?"

Written more than 60 years ago, Boleslavsky reveals an impressive grasp of one of the essentials of being scientific—namely, to have publicly available and lasting records of natural phenomena that are otherwise evanescent or not accessible to direct human perception. The introduction of talkies, an early stage of audiovisual (AV) technology, marked the first time in history that humans could observe the behavior not only of another but also of one's self and could do so repeatedly and in public! Although I have made use of AV technology for teaching and research for almost 50 years, appreciation of that momentous change for humankind came to me only on reading Boleslavsky's *Acting. The First Six Lessons.*[1]

---

[1] When I first came upon Boleslavsky's little "dialog" with the fictional "Creature" as an inexperienced, stage-struck young ingenue in 1992, it seemed to me that both he and I had been struggling with the same problem: his concern—how to teach actors—mine and my colleagues—how to teach medical students—was the common domain of *human phenomena not subject to reexamination. G.L. Engel, 1995 (21)*

The conclusion seems inescapable. However powerful the cultural imperative was that was engendered by the 17th-century scientific revolution, medicine's resistance or, more accurately, blindness to the need to address the issue of being scientific with human data stems not just from the inherent difficulty of so doing but also from a lack of any dependable means to do so, an altogether common occurrence in the history of science. For the human domain, AV technology fills that gap just as did telescopy for astronomy and microscopy for biology.

A successful dialogue between patient and physician is at the heart of working scientifically with patients.

G.L. Engel, 1995 (21)

Those words epitomized my final tribute to John Romano (1908–1994); they also epitomize this book. What they recall is the impact of my seeing Romano in 1941 sit down with a patient on medical rounds and engage with him as though in the privacy of his office. That single experience was to inaugurate an association between us that culminated in Romano's concept of human biology (22) and in my move *beyond* the biomedical to the biopsychosocial and finding synthesis and subsistence in the Rochester medical curriculum as an integrating, driving reality. Bob Smith's book represents an effort to extend that reality by examining its operation at the very heart of the doctor–patient encounter in the process of the interview.

The Patient's Story: Integrated Patient-Doctor Interviewing makes progress in key areas, although such a claim becomes possible only after we see how the book works in students' and other learners' hands. In the final analysis, research on how effectively learners pick up this approach will be important (23), as will the impact that its patient-centeredness has on the patient (24). For example, can it be shown that patients feel better or do better when the interviewer uses this approach (24)?

Identifying a basic infrastructure of the interview carries much potential for medicine as a science. The benefit, of course, is that a basic interviewing approach allows us to obtain human data in a more systematic way by one interviewer on multiple occasions or across many interviewers. To the extent that it is successful, this addresses Odegaard's concern that, as a means of acquisition of data, the interview process should be demonstrated to be as reliable as possible. Smith's emphasis on how idiosyncratic and confusing the approaches to teaching interviewing to students have been in the past is well taken. The lack of a basic methodology to medical interviewing may itself have encouraged students to acquire patient data erratically and unsystematically. Although this method provides sufficient structure and necessarily detailed instructions for the beginner, the overall approach is still flexible enough to offer promise that the personhood of the patient and humanity of the interviewer will both be enhanced.

As Smith cautions, this interviewing approach must not be seen as a final destination for the interviewer but rather as a point of departure. This prospect is facilitated by the text's incorporation of teaching directed specifically at enhancing the doctor–patient relationship, especially by fostering the effectiveness of the intimacy between doctor and patient; by considering in trospection at the level of better understanding oneself and the importance of opening such self-awareness to the patient; and by actively incorporating the relational dimension of interviewing instruction and placing it on equal footing with the informational aspects of interviewing.

An important distinction this book makes, often overlooked or misunderstood, is that although the biopsychosocial model provides a basis for the description of the patient and the patient's problems, the ability to interview effectively is indispensable for operationalizing the model, hence my earlier reference to the significance of a "successful dialog."

George L. Engel

References

1. Jennings HS. *Behavior of the lower organisms.* New York: Columbia University Press, 1923.
2. Engel GL. Homeostasis, behavioral adjustment, and the concept of health and disease. In: Grinker R. *Mid-century psychiatry.* Springfield, IL: Charles C Thomas, 1953:33—59.
3. Engel GL. Selection of clinical material in psychosomatic medicine: the need for a new physiology (special article). *Psychosom Med* 1954;16:368–373.
4. Engel GL. A unified concept of health and disease. *Perspect Biol Med* 1960;3:459–485.
5. Engel GL. *Psychological development in health and disease.* Philadelphia: WB Saunders, 1962.

6. Engel GL. The need for a new medical model: a challenge for biomedicine. *Science* 1977;196:129–136.

7. Engel GL. The clinical application of the biopsychosocial model. *Am J Psychiat* 1980;137:535–544.

8. Engel GL. How much longer must medicine's science be bound by a seventeenth century world view? In: White KL, ed. *The task of medicine: dialogue at Wickenburg.* Menlo Park, CA: Henry J. Kaiser Family Foundation, 1988:113–136.

9. Engel GL. On looking inward and being scientific. A tribute to Arthur H. Schmale, M.D. *Psychother Psychosom* 1990;54:63–69.

10. Sigerist HE. *A history of medicine.* Vol I. *Primitive and archaic medicine.* New York: Oxford University Press, 1951.

11. Heisenberg W. *Physics and philosophy. The revolution in modern science.* New York: Harper, 1958.

12. Sigerist HE. *A history of medicine,* vol I. *Primitive and archaic medicine.* New York: Oxford University Press, 1951.

13. Odegaard CE. *Dear doctor. A personal letter to a physician.* Menlo Park, CA: The Henry J. Kaiser Family Foundation, 1986.

14. Delbruck M. *Mind from matter? An essay on evolutionary epistemology.* Palo Alto, CA: Blackwell, 1986.

15. Einstein A. *Out of my later years.* New York: Philosophical Library, 1950.

16. Gignoux C, Bost R, Hostein J, et al. Role of upper esophageal reflex and belch reflex dysfunctions in noncardiac chest pain. *Dig Dis Sci* 1993;38:1909–1914.

17. Longcope WI. Methods and medicine. *Bull Johns Hopkins Hosp* 1932;50:420.

18. Hunter KM. *Doctors' stories, the narrative structure of medical knowledge.* Princeton, NJ: Princeton University Press, 1991.

19. Beckman HB, Frankel RM. The effect of physician behavior on the collection of data. *Ann Int Med* 1984;101:692–696.

20. Boleslavsky R. *Acting. The first six lessons.* New York: Theatre Arts Books, 1962.

21. Engel GL. For whom the bells toll a second time. John Romano, physician and psychiatrist (1908–1994). *Rochester medicine.* University of Rochester: 1995;1012:36.

22. Romano J. Basic orientation and education of the medical student. *J Am Med Assoc* 1950;143:409–412.

23. Smith RC, Mettler JA, Stoffelmayr BE, et al. Improving residents' confidence in using psychosocial skills. *J Gen Intern Med* 1995;10:315–320.

24. Smith RC, Lyles JS, Mettler JA, et al. A strategy for improving patient satisfaction by the intensive training of residents in psychosocial medicine: a controlled, randomized study. *Acad Med* 1995;70:729–732.

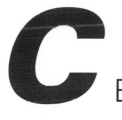

Examples of Emotions

Abandoned	Blamed	Confused	Dissatisfied
Afraid	Blissful	Consumed	Distracted
Aggravated	Blocked	Contented	Distraught
Agitated	Blue	Contrite	Distressed
Alienated	Bored	Controlled	Distrustful
Alive	Bothered	Creative	Disturbed
Alone	Bugged	Crummy	Dominated
Amazed	Bummed-out	Crushed	Doubtful
Ambiguous	Burdened	Curious	Down
Ambivalent			Downtrodden
Amused	Calm	Deceitful	Drained
Angry	Capable	Deceived	Driven
Annoyed	Captivated	Defeated	Dumb
Anxious	Cautious	Defiant	
Appalled	Challenged	Degraded	Eager
Apprehensive	Charmed	Dejected	Ecstatic
Ashamed	Cheated	Delighted	Edgy
Astonished	Cheerful	Depressed	Elated
Astounded	Childish	Despair	Embarrassed
At ease	Clever	Destructive	Empty
Awed	Combative	Determined	Encouraged
Awkward	Comfortable	Devastated	Energetic
	Committed	Different	Engrossed
Bad	Compassionate	Dirty	Engulfed
Bashful	Concerned	Disappointed	Enlightened
Betrayed	Condemned	Discouraged	Enraged
Bitchy	Confident	Disgusted	Enthusiastic
Bitter	Conflicted	Disoriented	Envious

Euphoric
Evil
Exasperated
Excited
Exhausted

Fearful
Flustered
Foolish
Forgotten
Forlorn
Fragmented
Frantic
Frenzied
Fretful
Friendly
Frightened
Frustrated
Funny
Furious

Gloomy
Glum
Good
Grateful
Gratified
Great
Grief
Groovy
Grouchy
Guilty
Gullible

Happy
Hassled
Hateful
Helpful
Helpless
Hesitant

High
Hopeful
Hopeless
Horrible
Horrified
Hostile
Hurt

Ignorant
Ignored
Impatient
Important
Impulsive
Inadequate
Incompetent
Independent
Indifferent
Inferior
Infuriated
Insecure
Insensitive
Inspired
Interested
Intimidated
Involved
Irritated
Isolated

Jealous
Jittery
Joyful
Jubilant
Jumpy

Lazy
Left out
Let down
Lethargic
Light hearted

Listless
Lonely
Longing
Loved
Loving
Low

Mad
Manipulated
Marvelous
Maudlin
Mean
Meek
Melancholy
Mellow
Miserable
Misunderstood
Mixed up
Modest
Morose
Mystified

Needed
Negative
Neglected
Nervous
Numb
Nutty

Obnoxious
Obsessed
Odd
Oppressed
Outraged
Overwhelmed

Pained
Panicked
Patient

Peaceful
Perplexed
Persecuted
Perturbed
Petrified
Phony
Picked on
Pity
Pleasant
Pleased
Positive
Preoccupied
Pressured
Proud
Pushed
Put down
Put upon
Puzzled

Quarrelsome
Quiet

Rage
Refreshed
Regretful
Rejected
Rejuvenated
Relaxed
Relieved
Remorseful
Renewed
Resentful
Resigned
Restless
Rewarded
Righteous
Rotten

Sad
Safe

Satisfied	Stuck	Tormented	Upset
Scared	Stunned	Torn	Uptight
Scattered	Stupefied	Tranquil	Useful
Screwed up	Stupid	Trapped	Useless
Secure	Successful	Tremendous	
Selfish	Suffering	Troubled	Violent
Sensitive	Superfluous	Turned off	Vital
Sensuous	Superior	Turned on	Vivacious
Serious	Surprised		Vulnerable
Shattered	Suspicious	Ugly	
Shocked	Sympathetic	Uncertain	Warm
Shy		Uncomfortable	Wary
Smothered	Tense	Uneasy	Weak
Solemn	Tentative	Unfortunate	Weepy
Sophisticated	Terrible	Unhappy	Whimsical
Sorrowful	Terrific	Unimportant	Whole
Sorry	Terrified	Uninvolved	Wicked
Spiteful	Testy	Unlucky	Wonderful
Strange	Threatened	Unpleasant	Worried
Strong	Thwarted	Unsettled	Worthless
Stubborn	Tired	Unwanted	Worthwhile

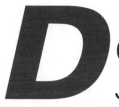

Complete Write-Up Of Mrs. Jones' Initial Evaluation

Joanne Elizabeth Jones

Clinical Center #12 34 56

February 29, 1994

Identifying Data

This is the first visit to the Clinical Center for this 38-year-old married white woman who is a local attorney with GHI Corporation. J. White, a third-year medical student, conducted the interview.

Source and Reliability of Information

The patient was cooperative and reliable. No other informants or data sources were available.

Chief Complaint or Agenda

The chief complaint is (a) headaches in the context of the problem, (b) difficulties with her boss. Other agenda items are (c) cough, (d) "colitis," and (e) she wants to know if medications for colitis need to be added.

History of the Present Illness

The patient's headache began rather suddenly at work 3 months ago. The headaches have been accompanied by nausea during the last month, and she vomited once last week during the most severe headache ever, which prompted this appointment.

The headaches are located diffusely over the right temporal region and do not radiate elsewhere. They feel like they are deep within the head, are not associated with tenderness or increased sensitivity of the scalp, and are described as pounding and throbbing. They begin suddenly and then increase in intensity and are described as "worse than having a baby" when severe. Mrs. Jones has had to miss work a few days because of the intense pain. The headaches occur two to three times per week and can last as long as 12 hours at a time, although initially they occurred no more often than once weekly and lasted only a couple of hours. The headaches are getting worse but seem to clear on the weekends when she is not at work. Nevertheless, the headaches have progressively worsened and are interfering with her life. Bright lights make the headache worse (photophobia). Lying in a dark room and placing an ice bag on her head seem to help. Drinking wine may also have been a precipitant once or twice. Nausea accompanies all headaches, and she vomited a small amount of nonbloody material with one severe headache a week ago. The patient feels entirely well between her spells of headache and nausea.

Except for being carsick a couple of times as a youngster, no other associated symptoms in neurologic, gastrointestinal, or other body systems have occurred. In particular, no loss of consciousness, change in vision, paralysis, stiff neck, rash, fever, chills, change in memory, or history of seizures have occurred. She feels well otherwise, has a good appetite, and enjoys outside activities. No history of joint pain or swelling is found.

An injection in the emergency room 1 week ago provided relief, but we do not yet know the exact medication; only blood and urine tests were obtained, the results of which are not yet available. Except for no more than six to eight aspirin daily and this one injection, she takes nothing for the headaches and has seen no other caretakers. Regarding possible causative factors, she has been taking birth control pills for 6 years and an aunt has a possible history of migraine. She has no history of head or neck injury. As noted in the following, the headaches seem clearly to be precipitated by the stress she is having on the job.

Mrs. Jones' headaches occur at times of conflict with her boss. She is the corporation's new lead attorney; she was brought in to replace the man who is now her boss and was promised there would be no problem during a year of transition prior to his retirement. He has been pushing and criticizing her, which makes her angry, and this leads to the headaches. She is also angry with the Board for promising that this problem would not occur. The relationship of anger and headache is similar to what she experienced as a child when her mother would unfairly criticize her. She believes her boss is the problem because, when she can avoid him, she has no headaches. She wants help with the headaches and coping with the stress because she is afraid they will adversely affect her and her family's personal lives. She is considering leaving her job. She has friends who provide support at work and her husband is supportive, but he doesn't say much because he encouraged her to take the job.

Health Issues

Ethical–Social–Spiritual Issues

1. Mrs. Jones has never considered advance directives. She and her husband have arranged for power of attorney, but she does not think it includes directions for health issues.

2. She wants to resume church activities, which have faltered during the last few years as life got busier; but, she says, "I don't want all that guilt stuff." Mrs. Jones indicates that her children have brought her more meaning in life than anything else and that she and her husband are often able to "get out of ourselves" through them.

Functional Status

Mrs. Jones has no functional limitations.

Health-Promoting and Health-Maintenance Activities

1. The patient adheres carefully to a low-fat, low-salt diet and exercises actively in an aerobics class four to five times weekly for 45 minutes

or so; this is vigorous enough to bring her pulse rate to 150 beats per minute and to prompt a drenching sweat. Her weight is stable in the 120-pound range. She always uses her seat belt, but she does not have airbags or antilock brakes. She does not ride bicycles or motorcycles; no weapons exist in the home; all medications are out of reach of the children; and the furnace is checked yearly for carbon monoxide emissions. She would like to take time for relaxation, but she does not do so now. She enjoys painting but worries that she is getting so busy that it will fall into the background. She describes herself as a "workaholic" and says that this prevents her from doing more interesting things like her painting but that it does not keep her away from her children. She would like to curtail her work activities but sees no way to do this now in a busy new job. She and her husband also "socialize" a lot. It is part of both their businesses and she sees no alternative, although neither seems to enjoy it much.

2. She has had regular physical examinations with Dr. Jergens, who has also been her primary care physician, including a Pap smear 1 year ago; she does not know what blood tests he performed, but some were done. She thinks her cholesterol was normal when she was hospitalized in 1982. She has not seen a dentist since a cavity was filled 4 years ago, although she has no symptoms. She examines her breasts regularly about a week after each menstrual period.

3. She has had all of the usual "baby shots" but does not know exactly what they were. A tetanus shot was given 2 years ago following a puncture wound to the hand. She does not think flu shots work and does not want any more because she got sick after the last one 3 years ago.

Health Hazards

1. Except for a rare cup of coffee and glass of wine, the patient has not used addicting substances.

2. The patient and her husband are monogamous and heterosexual. She had two other sexual partners prior to marriage. She has no history of sexually transmitted diseases or sexual abuse. Mrs. Jones had been satisfied with her sexual life until the last 3 months when her interest

decreased and her husband had problems with inconstant impotence. Sexual intercourse now occurs about once weekly but was three to four times weekly before starting this job. She is not worried about this; she thinks that it relates to her work problems and was not interested in discussing it further.

3. She has no history of physical or sexual abuse directed toward her, nor has she ever been abusive.

Past Medical History

Hospitalizations

1. **1982.** She was hospitalized for 3 days, and a diagnosis of mild ulcerative colitis was made. She presented with a 3-month history of periodic loose stools with occasional blood and mild abdominal cramping. Tests for "parasites and other germs" were negative at the University Hospital in the city where she was attending law school. She was cared for by a Dr. Jergens. Sigmoidoscopy and barium enema led to the diagnosis of ulcerative colitis, and she was told she didn't need surgery but did need to follow-up closely, which she did at about 6-month intervals. She took prednisone for the first 3 months following discharge, starting at 40 mg daily and slowly reducing the dosage. She also took sulfasalazine, starting at eight tablets daily (presumably 500-mg tablets but not yet verified). After 3 months, when the prednisone was stopped, the dose of sulfasalazine was gradually reduced to four tablets daily over the ensuing 3 months. This was stopped altogether a year later. She was asymptomatic until November 1991 when some diarrhea without blood developed. Sigmoidoscopy by Dr. Jergens showed a mild flare-up, and a barium enema showed only minor changes in the "distal sigmoid colon." Again, no surgery was advised, and she was treated with sulfasalazine (she brought this pharmacy label), 1.0 gm qid, for about 2 months. It was then gradually reduced to 0.5 gm qid for 6 months, and then it was stopped. No recurrence of symptoms has occurred. At her most recent sigmoidoscopy with Dr. Jergens 6 months ago, she was told her colon looked essentially normal and that nothing further was necessary, except for close follow-up.

2. Two uncomplicated obstetric confinements at 6 and 8 years ago produced healthy children. She was hospitalized less than 72 hours each time.

3. Tonsillectomy and adenoidectomy were performed as a child.

Other Medical, Surgical, or Psychological Problems

1. As was noted above, she followed regularly with Dr. Jergens for her ulcerative colitis; he also acted as her primary physician until she moved here 5 months ago, since which time she has seen no one except for one emergency room visit. Dr. Jergens urged her to get a primary care physician when she moved here.

2. She had a cough and stuffy nose 3 weeks ago, with a slight persisting cough. There was no sore throat, earache, or fever; and the cough is nearly gone. She took an over-the-counter cough medication for a week at the beginning, but she doesn't recall the name.

3. Her first and only episode of urinary tract infection occurred in July 1993 with symptoms of increased frequency and dysuria. She felt well otherwise, and there was no hematuria, fever, chills, or back pain. She received a 7-day course of trimethoprim/sulfamethoxazole tablets (twice daily) from an emergency room in Colorado, where they were vacationing, and was symptom-free within 2 days.

4. She had a fracture of the left ulna 21 years ago as the result of a fall. It was casted for several weeks, and there has been no problem since.

5. She knows she had measles and chickenpox as a child, and she thinks she had a mild case of the mumps.

Screen for Major Diseases

1. She has no history of rheumatic fever, scarlet fever, diabetes mellitus, cancer, tuberculosis, heart disease, venereal disease, or stroke.

2. She has never received blood transfusions, insulin, digitalis, blood thinners, heart medications, or blood pressure medications.

Medications and Other Treatments

1. Aspirin, six to eight 5-grain tablets daily with her headaches during the last four to six weeks and with smaller amounts during the preceding 6 weeks. No adverse effect.

2. "Birth control pill" of uncertain type. She will call in the dosage and type.

3. No use of laxatives, vitamins, other hormones, nerve pills, tonics, or over-the-counter medications.

4. Except for Dr. Jergens, she has seen no one else; she has not sought care from alternative healers, nor does she use any nontraditional healing remedies.

Allergies and Drug Reactions

1. No history of allergies to drugs or other drug reactions.

2. No known allergic disease and no history of asthma, hives, or hay fever.

3. No known food or environmental substances to which she is sensitive.

Menstrual and Obstetric History

1. Menses began at age 12; and they are attended by only slight discomfort for a day or so. They last 5 days, require five pads daily, and occur regularly every month since she has been on the birth control pill.

2. She is gravida (pregnancies) 2, para (deliveries) 2, abortus (spontaneous and induced abortions) 0, with two healthy living children.

There have been no complications of her pregnancies, both of which were vaginal deliveries.

Social History

Current Personal Situation

The patient is 38 years old, and she just moved here with her husband and two children 5 months ago. She left a job as a corporate attorney in the city where she had trained as a lawyer to come here with GHI Corporation as the lead attorney. See the history of present illness (HPI).

She views her new job here as a big step upward professionally in corporate law. It provides the opportunity for leadership and creativity that didn't exist previously. Her husband also is a lawyer with GHI, but he works in a different area. His job was a big step up for him also, and he has been quite happy here and is getting along well. Both were happy in their previous jobs but felt the need to progress professionally.

She has no financial problems, and she is well-covered by health insurance.

Other Personal Factors

The patient was born in a small farming community in Kansas on 8-12-55. She had one younger sibling, a brother born 3-14-58. Her parents were her primary caretakers, although her father's mother lived in the area and frequently assisted in raising the two children. Her father owned the local hardware store, and the family had no financial problems but was not wealthy—she described them as "pretty much middle class." Her father was a loving, caring man but was "always at work." She had a good relationship with him, and she frequently helped him out in the store. She could run the store in his absence by the time she was in her teens. Her mother was "more critical", and she was always pushing her to do more things. She was insistent that the patient do well in school, that she not date boys with no future, and that she go to college. Her mother frequently lamented not having gone to college; the patient described her as "very bright, but clever and biting in things she said."

The patient never felt as close to her mother as she did to her father, but nonetheless she got along well with her, always understood what she wanted, and "knew that she loved me." She loved her younger brother greatly, and they always had a special relationship, which continues to this day. She scarcely knew her mother's parents but grew up close to her paternal grandparents, developing a very close relationship with her grandmother, who was "very loving and accepting."

Her kindergarten through twelfth grade schooling occurred in the same small town; there were about 100 students in her graduating class. She did well in school, she was well-liked, and she had many extracurricular activities. She dated frequently, but she never had a steady boyfriend or close relationship. The patient and her family attended church, but they "weren't very religious."

It was difficult to leave many friends and family when she went off to college very far from home on scholarship. She recalls "moping around" for several weeks but then getting over it as she got into the flow of school and began to meet other new students. She did well in school and graduated 4 years later. During college, she had two serious relationships, which included sexual activity; but in both cases she decided against marriage because of her desire to go to law school and to forego a family.

She attended law school at the same university and did extremely well. She also periodically resumed one of the close relationships from college during this time, but she didn't want to marry as her boyfriend did. She preferred to date casually and to attend to her studies.

She began working with a large, prestigious law firm in the same city following graduation in 1980. She slowly worked her way up to a mid-level position in their hierarchy and was happy until the last year or so when she realized that she would never have the chance for independence and creativity that she wanted.

She met her husband at work in 1981, and they were married in 1982 after her colitis cleared. He had similar professional values and ideas about children, and she describes their relationship as very compatible, until the current problems with their sexual lives. Their oldest son was born in 1985, and the second son was born in 1987. She describes her children as "the best thing I ever did" and as having produced real meaning in her life. She was "quite happy and satisfied" with life "until I got here." She has several friends at work and locally.

Family History

General and Specific Inquiry

The patient is aware of no known diseases that seem to run in the family; and, in particular, she is aware of no familial problems with the following: tuberculosis, cancer, heart disease, bleeding problems, kidney failure, dialysis, alcoholism, tobacco use, weight problems, asthma, or mental illness. Her paternal grandmother has diabetes mellitus.

Genogram

Figure D.1 is an example of Mrs. Jones' genogram.

Review of Systems (System Review)

General: nothing additional.

Integument: had rash while traveling that seemed to be caused by harsh soaps; no recurrence since moving here.

Hematopoietic: excessive bruising years ago when taking prednisone but none since.

Endocrine: nothing additional.

Musculoskeletal: nothing additional.

Eyes, Ears, Nose, Throat: uses reading glasses when doing much reading.

Head and Neck: nothing additional.

Breasts: breasts are generally "lumpy" around her periods but never has felt any masses. Did not nurse her children.

Cardiovascular and Pulmonary: nothing additional.

Gastrointestinal: nothing additional except moderately painful hemorrhoids in the later stages of each pregnancy.

Urinary: nothing additional except for brief period of enuresis around age 5.

Genital: nothing additional.

Neuropsychiatric: nothing additional.

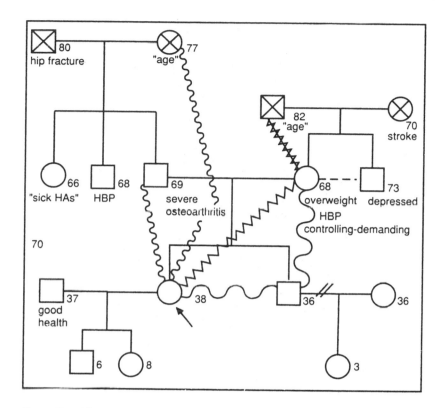

Figure D.1. Mrs. Jones' genogram. Age of family members appears to the right of each. Under some figures is listed the cause of death (deceased persons) or the current status of living persons. Key: □, male; ○, female; ⊠, deceased; —⫽—, divorced; ∿, close (good) relationship; ⋀⋀⋀⋀, conflicted relationship; ⋁⋁⋁⋁, close and conflicted relationship; ...., distant relationship; ——, the patient.

Abbreviations: HA, headaches; HBP, high blood pressure.

Adapted with permission from Mullins HC, Christie-Seely J. Collection and recording family data: the genogram. In: Christie-Seely J, ed. Working with the family in primary care: a systems approach to health and illness. New York: Praeger; 1984:179—191.

Physical Examination[1]

[I summarize only pertinent findings because this text does not address the physical examination.]

---

[1] Included for completeness but not addressed in this book.

Mrs. Jones had a blood pressure of 110/70, a pulse rate of 66, and 12 respirations per minute. She had no evidence of neurological or gastrointestinal abnormality; these are the areas most likely to have explanatory value for her symptoms if abnormalities were found. Except for a midsystolic click along the left sternal border heard on auscultation of the heart (suggests mitral valve prolapse), no other abnormalities existed on physical examination either.

Initial Diagnostic and Treatment Interventions[2]

None.

Assessment: Biopsychosocial Description (The Patient's Story)[3]

Relationship Story

Student's Responses

1. Liked her and felt good about her compliments.

2. Uncomfortable when she spoke of her sexual problems and might have cut the conversation short.

3. Uneasy not knowing more about diseases that cause headaches.

Mrs. Jones' Personality Style

Minor obsessive features within the range of normal.

Interaction

1. Warm and respectful. The patient made good eye contact and indicated several times that she valued the work.

---

[2] Included for completeness but not addressed in this book.
[3] Included for completeness but not addressed in this book, except to note how assessments are made using the Relationship story, Personal story, and Disease story/diagnoses (RPD) way of recording. Many supervisors request that the Assessment or Problem List contain an extensive discussion of the student's reasoning, as well as a comprehensive review of the literature about the problem.

2. The patient developed a headache while discussing problems involving her boss and her mother.

[Note how subsequent personal and disease dimensions interact with the relational.]

Personal Story

1. Severe stress from a critical boss, resulting in anger (closely associated with headaches) at him and the Board that recruited her.

2. Similar relationship of headaches and anger since childhood, when they occurred in response to a critical mother.

Disease Story

Biomedical

1. Intermittent right temporal headaches, throbbing; associated with nausea and photophobia; increasing in frequency and severity over 3 months; on birth control pills; associated with severe stress; and without historical or physical exam evidence of neurological dysfunction. The following are the diagnostic possibilities, in order of likelihood:
   a. migraine headache.
   b. stress-tension headache.
   c. chronic meningitis—very unlikely.
   d. vasculitis (e.g., systemic lupus erythematosus)—very unlikely.
   e. chronic subdural hematoma—very unlikely.

2. Nausea with one episode of vomiting. Most likely part of the preceding picture.

3. Recent respiratory tract infection ("cold"), cleared.

4. Idiopathic ulcerative colitis, quiescent and mild by her report, but these patients can have a higher incidence of cancer of the colon.

5. Past history of one lower urinary tract infection 8 months ago.

6. Probable mitral valve prolapse, asymptomatic and likely of no clinical importance.

Psychiatric

None.

Treatment and Investigative Plan[4]

Headaches

1. Obtain records from recent emergency room visit.

2. Start treatment of migraine headaches with ergotamine tartrate and caffeine or sumatriptan tablets.

3. Will consider later addition of prophylactic treatment with a beta-blocker or calcium channel blocker if #2 is not effective.

4. Also, will need to consider discontinuing the birth control pill and finding an alternative means of contraception if #2 and #3 are not effective.

5. Defer any investigation of the headaches until observing the impact of treatment on what appears to be typical migraine.

6. Further discuss specific strategies for dealing with her boss at the next visit in 1 week.

7. Instruct her in a relaxation procedure.

Ulcerative Colitis

1. Obtain outside records from Dr. Jergens.

2. Referral to gastroenterology for evaluation and colonoscopy.

[4] Included for completeness but not addressed in this book.

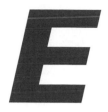

Mental Status Evaluation

Complete Mental Status Evaluation

Appearance

The interviewer observes the gestalt or overall appearance of the patient: whether she or he appears older or younger than her or his age, the presence of unique physical attributes (prosthetic leg), grooming and neatness, depressed or anxious appearance, and apparent state of health (ill appearing).

Attitude

The interviewer observes the patient's attitudes, both exhibited and expressed, during the interview and particularly looks for cooperativeness. Other attitudes include anger, guarded, suspicious, attentive, seductive, playful, and obsequious.

Activity

The student or clinician notes the patient's motor activity: increased (hyperactive, agitated), decreased, catatonic, and abnormal movements (tics, tremors). She or he also asks the patient to draw a simple figure, such as a clock set at a specific time or a square inside a circle, to assess visual-motor integrity.

Mood

The interviewer determines, primarily by inquiry, the patient's sustained, day-in and day-out emotional feelings (e.g., sad, happy, anxious, angry, depressed, detached, irritable).

Affect

Primarily by observation, the interviewer notes how the patient expresses her or his immediate emotional state. Is the patient fully and appropriately responsive to stimuli and circumstances? Or are her or his responses flat or blunted (dulled emotional responsivity), inappropriate (laughing when most would be serious), anhedonic (no enjoyment of anything), or labile? To combine mood and affect, she or he might say, "The patient's mood was depressed and the affect blunted."

Speech

Students or clinicians should observe for the following speech characteristics: normal, slowed, reduced, increased, pressured, mute, dysarthric, punning, or rhyming.

Language

Interviewers can observe the patient's use of language for the following characteristics: bizarre, distracting, colorful, word salad (incoherent mix of words and phrases seen in psychotic states), circumstantial, tangential, loosening of associations (connections that are difficult to follow), and neologistic (coining new words).

Thought Content

The student or clinician determines the presence or absence of the following features of the patient's thought content via the patient's speech and language: logical, incoherent, derailed, content-poor, obsessive, delusional, paranoid. She or he also notes the content of thought, describing any delusions in detail.

Perceptions

The interviewer asks about abnormal perceptions, typically hallucinations, which may be visual, auditory, olfactory, or tactile. Hallucinations are abnormal sensory perceptions in the absence of a stimulus (voices coming from a picture on the wall), whereas illusions are misinterpretations of stimuli (belief that the doorbell ringing is someone speaking). Depersonalization is the patient's perception that her or his own body is strange and unreal, as though it is apart from the patient. Derealization is a similar perception of unreality and estrangement of objects in the environment.

Judgment and Insight

The clinician or student determines if the patient is realistic or unrealistic about the problem and other issues. An apparent obliviousness to a serious problem is called *la belle* indifference.

Neuropsychiatric Evaluation

(a) The student or clinician observes the patient's level of consciousness (e.g., comatose, stuporous, drowsy, alert, hyperalert). (b) She or he carefully investigates the patient's attention and concentration by asking the patient to repeat a series of from three to eight digits (e.g., repeat the following: 8-1-6-3-9); having her or him subtract from 100 by 7 and continuing to do so with each answer, so-called "serial 7s" (e.g., $100 - 7 = 93$; $93 - 7 = 86$; and so on); spelling a word ("world") backward; and inquiring about immediate occurrences in the environment (e.g., repeating the interviewer's name after she or he clearly states it). (c) The interviewer also assesses the patient's language function for fluency, comprehension, naming, repetition, reading, and writing. In addition to observing and listening to the patient, the clinician or student asks the patient to read and to explain a simple text and to write a sentence or two on her or his own (without giving the sentence). Such exercises should be appropriate to the patient's level of education. (d) Recent memory is tested by determining the patient's orientation to time, place, and person (e.g., the patient is asked to describe the day, date, year, time, place, and her or his name and identity). Recent memory also is tested by asking the patient to recall three objects immediately after the interviewer mentions them (e.g., comb, dog, the color yellow), then warning the patient that she or he will be asked to recall the three objects in 3 to 5 minutes and, finally, testing the patient's recall at that time. Remote memory is evaluated by inquiring about events of several days earlier, as well as about events from months and years earlier (e.g., "What day did you come into the hospital?" or "Who is the President?" or "What are your daughters' names?"). (e) Other higher functions include how well the patient thinks abstractly. Interpreting proverbs (e.g., "People who live in glass houses shouldn't throw stones.") can vary from bizarre to very concrete to quite abstract and interpretive. Similarly, the student or clinician can determine the capacity for abstract thinking by inquiring how an apple and orange are alike and how they are different. Calculations and testing general intelligence also can be helpful at times.

Subject Index

Page numbers followed by a *t* indicate tables; those followed by an *f* indicate figures.